D0464021

*Sensory Processes
at the Neuronal
and
Behavioral Levels*

CONTRIBUTORS

J. A. Altman

A. V. Baru

A. V. Bertulis

J. Bureš

O. Burešova´

G. V. Gersuni

V. D. Glezer

L. H. Hicks

V. A. Ivanov

Richard Jung

T. A. Karaseva

Yasuji Katsuki

I. N. Kondratjeva

N. B. Kostelyanets

L. I. Leushina

A. M. Maruseva

N. F. Podvigin

A. V. Popov

E. A. Radionova

G. I. Ratnikova

I. A. Shevelev

I. M. Tonkonogii

G. A. Vardapetian

I. A. Vartanian

SENSORY PROCESSES AT THE NEURONAL AND BEHAVIORAL LEVELS

Edited by **G. V. GERSUNI**

Pavlov Institute of Physiology
The Academy of Sciences of the U.S.S.R.
Leningrad, U.S.S.R.

Translated by **JERZY ROSE**

Laboratory of Neurophysiology
University of Wisconsin
Madison, Wisconsin

1971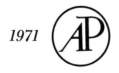

Academic Press • *New York* • *London*

ACADEMIC PRESS, INC.
111 Fifth Avenue, New York, New York 10003

United Kingdom Edition published by
ACADEMIC PRESS, INC. (LONDON) LTD.
Berkeley Square House, London W1X 6BA

LIBRARY OF CONGRESS CATALOG CARD NUMBER: 78 - 127682

PRINTED IN THE UNITED STATES OF AMERICA

CONTENTS

LIST OF CONTRIBUTORS

Numbers in parentheses indicate the pages on which the authors' contributions begin.

J. A. ALTMAN *(157, 221), Pavlov Institute of Physiology, The Academy of Sciences of the U.S.S.R., Leningrad, U.S.S.R.*

A. V. BARU *(265, 287), Pavlov Institute of Physiology, Academy of Sciences of the U.S.S.R., Leningrad, U.S.S.R.*

A. V. BERTULIS *(19), Pavlov Institute of Physiology, The Academy of Sciences of the U.S.S.R., Leningrad, U.S.S.R.*

J. BUREŠ *(127), Institute of Physiology, Czechoslovak Academy of Sciences, Budejovicks, Praha, Czechoslovakia*

O. BUREŠOVÁ *(127), Institute of Physiology, Czechoslovak Academy of Sciences, Prague, Czechoslovakia*

G. V. GERSUNI *(85, 157, 287), Pavlov Institute of Physiology, The Academy of Sciences of the U.S.S.R., Leningrad, U.S.S.R.*

V. D. GLEZER *(19), Pavlov Institute of Physiology, The Academy of Sciences of the U.S.S.R., Leningrad, U.S.S.R.*

L. H. HICKS *(57), Department of Psychology, Howard University, Washington, D. C.*

V. A. IVANOV *(19), Pavlov Institute of Physiology, The Academy of Sciences of the U.S.S.R., Leningrad, U.S.S.R.*

RICHARD JUNG *(1), Neurologische Universitätsklinik mit Abteilung für Neurophysiologie, Freiburg, West Germany*

T. A. KARASEVA *(287), Institute of Physiology, Academy of Sciences of the U.S.S.R., Leningrad, U.S.S.R.*

YASUJI KATSUKI *(115), Department of Physiology, Tokyo Medical and Dental University, Yushima Bunkyoku, Tokyo, Japan*

I. N. KONDRATJEVA *(47), Institute of Higher Nervous Activity and Neurophysiology, Academy of Sciences of the U.S.S.R., Moscow, U.S.S.R.*

N. B. KOSTELYANETS *(19), Pavlov Institute of Physiology, The Academy of Sciences of the U.S.S.R., Leningrad, U.S.S.R.*

L. I. LEUSHINA *(69), Laboratory of Physiology of Vision, Pavlov Institute of Physiology, Academy of Sciences of the U.S.S.R. Leningrad, U.S.S.R.*

A. M. MARUSEVA *(157, 181), Pavlov Institute of Physiology, The Academy of Sciences of the U.S.S.R., Leningrad, U.S.S.R.*

N. F. PODVIGIN *(19), Pavlov Institute of Physiology, The Academy of Sciences of the U.S.S.R., Leningrad, U.S.S.R.*

A. V. POPOV *(301), Sechenov Institute of Evolutionary Physiology and Biochemistry, Pavlov Institute of Physiology, Academy of Sciences of the U.S.S.R., Leningrad, U.S.S.R.*

E. A. RADIONOVA *(135, 157), Pavlov Institute of Physiology, The Academy of Sciences of the U.S.S.R., Leningrad, U.S.S.R.*

G. I. RATNIKOVA *(157), Pavlov Institute of Physiology, The Academy of Sciences of the U.S.S.R., Leningrad, U.S.S.R.*

I. A. SHEVELEV *(57), Institute of Higher Nervous Activity and Neurophysiology, U.S.S.R. Academy of Sciences, Moscow, U.S.S.R.*

I. M. TONKONOGII *(287), Pavlov Institute of Physiology, Academy of Sciences of the U.S.S.R., Leningrad, U.S.S.R.*

G. A. VARDAPETIAN *(245), Pavlov Institute of Physiology, Academy of Sciences of the U.S.S.R., Leningrad, U.S.S.R.*

I. A. VARTANIAN *(157, 201), Pavlov Institute of Physiology, Academy of Sciences of the U.S.S.R., Leningrad, U.S.S.R.*

PREFACE

The papers presented in this volume are devoted to problems of functional organization of the visual and auditory systems. The various articles deal with single unit data or with the results of behavioral and psychophysical studies of visual and auditory functions. All investigators agree that an integration of data obtained from different experimental approaches (psychophysical, behavioral, and electrophysiological) is urgently needed for the promotion of our understanding of perception and sensation. Such an integration, however, is not achieved by a mere comparison of data obtained by different methods. A new synthesis, rather, is required which will hopefully lead to new insight regarding the problems of sensory mechanisms. Attempts to provide such new viewpoints in sensory studies have grown considerably in the last decade, but they are only initial attempts in a very difficult task.

In this volume some conclusions concerning visual mechanisms are drawn based on behavioral, psychophysical, and single unit work. With respect to audition an attempt is made to contrast and compare the most obvious discrepancies and similarities between electrophysiological and behavioral studies.

Most of the authors were participants in the symposium "Sensory Processes at the Neuronal and Behavioral Levels" which was held at the XVIII International Congress of Psychology (Moscow, August 1966).

I am greatly indebted to the Planning Committee of the XVIII International Congress of Psychology and its chairman Professor A. R. Luria for the opportunity to publish this volume and to Professor J. Rose for his invaluable help in editing the English version of the Russian papers.

ix

*Sensory Processes
at the Neuronal
and
Behavioral Levels*

I. Vision

1
Neuronal Mechanisms of Pattern Vision and Motion Detection

Richard Jung

Neuronal responses to motion and pattern stimulation in the cat's cortex in conjunction with some of their human psychophysiological correlates are examined in this chapter. The study is restricted to luminance differences; spectral responses and the effects of eye movements are not included.

Two Basic Neuronal Pathways (B and D) for Brightness and Darkness Information

To understand neuronal transformations in the cortex previous studies on sensory coding in the retinogeniculate system should be considered briefly. Sensory coding was first elucidated in the retina by Kuffler's analysis of receptive fields [27]. Two parallel neuronal channels with antagonistic functions carry all visual impulses from the retina to the cortex. These channels constitute two reciprocal subsystems: the B system (on-center neurons) signals "brighter"; the D system (off-center neurons) signals "darker" [20, 21]. Contrast coding by these two neuronal subsystems begins in the retina with antagonistic organization of their receptive fields: B neurons have on-centers with lateral inhibition; D neurons have off-centers with lateral activation by illumination of the surrounding field [2, 6]. B Neurons inhibit D Neurons having the same field location and vice versa [21].

The two reciprocal subsystems, B and D, provide specific information to the brain, transmitted by activation or inhibition of each neuronal system.

The invariant of the coding process in these dual systems is the transmission of spatial and temporal differences of luminance rather than its level. The required stimulus is the contrast of spatial or temporal changes of illumination, regardless of whether the response is elicited by turning a light on or off [2].

Thus, a B neuron that usually responds to diffuse light with on-activation and off-inhibition will reverse to on-inhibition and off-activation when its receptive field projects to a black area. Therefore, we prefer not to refer to the B and D systems as "on-neurons" or "off-neurons." At light-on, the information transmitted to the brain corresponds to the luminance difference in the patterns projected on the receptive fields (simultaneous contrast); at light-off, it corresponds rather to successive contrast and its afterimages [21]. At the neurons' receptive field center, increased B discharges invariably signal "brighter," either brighter than surroundings (in simultaneous contrast), or brighter than preceding stimulation (in successive contrast). Conversely, increased D discharges always signal "darker" in these contrast conditions. This was made clear by Baumgartner's contrast experiments [2, 7] with bright and dark stripes projected on different parts of the receptive field of the recorded neurons at light-on and -off. These contrast stimulations demonstrated a progressive contour enhancement on three levels—retina, lateral geniculate, and cortex [Fig. 1(d)]. Cortical neurons signal edges and contour patterns selectively with reduction of information regarding bright and dark surfaces. Figure 1(a)-(c) shows a photographic model of contour abstraction. It might be compared to progressive effects of contrast enhancement in retinal, geniculate, and cortical neurons, although Barlow [1] has expressed doubts as to whether lateral inhibition at different levels would be a sufficient explanation.

Many correlations of neuronal phenomena with subjective vision were described in earlier papers [20, 21], mainly for brightness and darkness, flicker, brightness enhancement, afterimages, simultaneous contrast, local adaptation, and attention.

The five types of neuronal responses in the visual cortex, A, B, C, D, and E, which we distinguished earlier with diffuse light stimulation [19] and other classifications [20], were useful only for the first descriptive order and the analysis of neuronal convergence of visual, reticulothalamic, vestibular, and other multisensory afferents. For pattern vision, the conception of dual B and D subsystems [21] provides a better key to cortical neuronal transformations.

In the lower visual system, all neurons of the retina and geniculate body respond to diffuse light or darkness. However, many neurons in the visual and paravisual cortex show less constant response or no response at all to diffuse changes of illumination. These cortical neurons, referred as type A in earlier papers, are not only a stabilizing system precluding mass discharges at sudden changes of illumination [24], but represent the most important nerve cells for higher visual information processing. They respond only to selected optic patterns or movements, and their adequate stimulus has to be sought out carefully

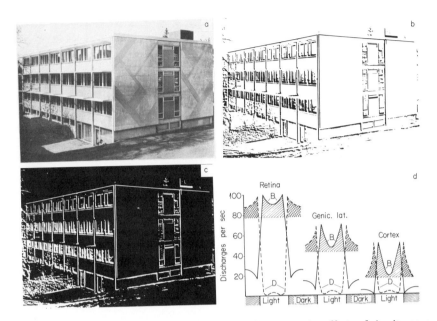

FIG. 1. Contour abstraction in the visual system by progressive effects of simultaneous contrast, modified from Jung and Baumgartner [23]. (a), (b), and (c) Imitation of contour enhancement by Barlow's photographic procedure [1] as a model for the neuronal effects; (b) and (c) are copies of displaced positive and negative transparencies of (a). The results in (b) and (c) are contour versions of the original picture. The effects are similar to contoured line drawing with suppression of flat surfaces. The black lines in (b) correspond to contrast enhancement with lateral activations in off-center neurons. The white lines in (c) are the result of a reverse contrast process by lateral disinhibition of on-center neurons. The pattern information of (b) and (c) nearly equals that of (a). (d) Schematic drawing of neuronal on-responses of the two antagonistic systems, B and D, to contrasting stimuli of large light bar with progressive contour enhancement from retina to cortex. In (d), B indicates on-center neurons (_____), D, off-center neurons (- - - -). The on-responses to various patterned parts of light bars with black contrasting surrounds are compared with uncontrasted stimulation, B discharge in diffuse illumination (. . . . .), and D discharge in darkness. The discharge difference between patterned and uniform stimulation is hatched for B (on-center neurons with lateral inhibition) and cross-hatched for D (off-center neurons with lateral activation).

as it is often difficult to find. Only those neurons of this group which respond both to specifically oriented contours and lines and to moving patterns have been studied extensively for monocular- and binocular-patterned stimuli by Baumgartner, Hubel, and Wiesel. Other specialized neurons require investigation by selective stimulation, e.g., stereoscopic neurons for depth discrimination, which would be activated by contours presented to noncorresponding points of the two retinas.

Transformation of Visual Messages in Cortical Neurons

After some preprocessing in the retina and the lateral geniculate, the visual radiation pathways with their dual B and D channels carry all visual messages to area 17. Although some brightness or darkness information from the two reciprocal subsystems B and D is preserved in the first stages of cortical neuronal integration, the organization of receptive fields is changed in the cortex as shown by Hubel and Wiesel [15-17] and Baumgartner [6, 23]. These field reorganizations occur in several neuronal steps (Figs. 2 and 4). They represent only one aspect of the transformation processes in the higher visual system toward selectivity of neuronal responses to specific stimuli.

Neurons in the visual cortex are distinguished from retinal and geniculate neurons by eight characteristics: (1) stronger and quicker adaptation to stationary visual stimuli with less intense or null responses to diffuse uniform light; (2) greater variety of neuronal response types; (3) slower discharge rates; (4) binocular interaction; (5) altered forms of receptive fields with response specificity to certain axis orientations; (6) columnar arrangement of neurons with similar orientation of their receptive field axes; (7) further specialization of visual neuronal responses to complex optic forms in paravisual and contralateral areas 18 and 19; (8) convergence of specific, nonspecific, and multisensory afferents at many cortical neurons.

These characteristics of visual cortex neurons define basic mechanisms required for transformation of monocular retinogeniculate responses to diffuse and contrasting bright and dark surfaces into specialized cortical responses to oriented visual contours, moving patterns, and binocular stereopsis. Complex integration with other senses by multisensory interaction [25] and attentive selection [24] are other processes in which cortical neurons cooperate with subcortical centers to handle information on environmental events.

The exact synaptic connections of the neuronal chains for higher visual information processing are still unknown. The general tendencies of these neuronal transformations may be defined as differentiation and integration for abstracting visual information. The increase of selected and abstracted information in specialized neurons is related to a reduction of general information in the same neuronal channels. Among these abstractive neuronal processes only those for pattern and motion detection are discussed here.

Neuronal Mechanisms of Pattern Vision
and Contour Selection

In the visual cortex, contrast-enhanced B and D messages from local retinal areas of brightness and darkness are transformed into specialized representations of oriented edges. Thus, information about surface brightness is reduced in favor of selective neuronal responses to contours [23]. The border contrast accentuation of neuronal responses was discovered by Baumgartner in 1959, using black and white stripes for stimulation of cortical neurons [7]. Hubel and Wiesel [15-17] then made precise experiments on the optimal orientation of line stimuli and discovered the axis orientation of cortical cells. The contour enhancement of patterns is elaborated on several neuronal levels of the primary visual cortex (area 17) and the paravisual areas 18 and 19. At every stage of neuron integration, the responses to contours become more selective for certain patterns.

The field organization of cortical neurons differs from that of retinal and geniculate cells by the presence of oblong receptive fields with definite orientations in the coordinates of the visual field (Fig. 2). Hubel and Wiesel explain this specific axis orientation by the convergence of several neighboring concentric fields in certain directions [16]. Higher-order neurons with complex fields respond optimally to similarly oriented line stimuli, but their position in the visual field can vary up to $10°$. The critical stimulus is still a small contrast in luminance at a definite angle to the vertical meridian. Thus, form generalization and abstraction of oriented contours by these neurons is possible [23].

After further transformations in paravisual areas 18 and 19, higher-order neurons signal still more selective patterns—lines of certain lengths, and lines with discontinuities, curves, or angles. Hubel and Wiesel [18] have shown that these cells called "higher-order hypercomplex" detect oriented curvatures or corners. Although these higher-order neurons receive binocular inputs, some monocular dominance is also maintained in the higher levels of area 19.

All of these contour-sensitive neurons, henceforth referred to as K neurons, show maximal responses to contrasting edges or lines of certain critical inclinations and forms. Luminance differences in nearby regions of the visual field remain the effective stimulus, and in simple field K neurons a B or D type with on- or off-field center may be preserved. In other K neurons, edges of white-black contours direction-specific for one side of the axis are optimal stimuli [13]. In most K neurons that receive B afferents from the geniculate, maximal activation is obtained by centering a white line, or the bright contour of a black line, on the respective field center. Conversely, dark-sensitive neurons that receive D afferent from retinogeniculate input are stimulated maximally by centering on a black line or on the black border of a white area. If these neurons signal contours from the border of a patterned form, this contour detection may operate for both bright or dark surfaces of this form.

An abstract accentuation of contours similar to that which Baumgartner, Hubel, and Wiesel have demonstrated in visual cortex neurons is used in line drawings. The selective neuronal K responses to oriented edges of contrasting surfaces which occur in the visual cortex can therefore be compared to the

Retina   Geniculatum   Cortex (area 17)

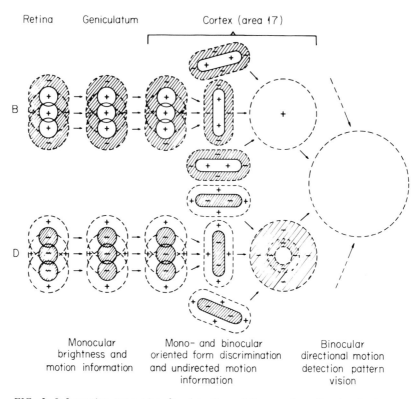

B

D

| Monocular brightness and motion information | Mono- and binocular oriented form discrimination and undirected motion information | Binocular directional motion detection pattern vision |

FIG. 2. Information processing for detection of form and motion in visual neurons with their receptive fields, modified after Jung and Baumgartner [23]. B and D demonstrate the two antagonistic neuronal systems signaling brighter (+, on-field center) and darker −, off-field center). It is assumed that each spot in the visual field is connected with both B and D systems and that correlated B or D signals from the same retinal part are mutually exclusive. In area 17, convergence of several concentric receptive fields results in longitudinal fields possessing oblong axes of different orientation which prepare local contour detection of critical axis orientation. Further convergence results in larger receptive fields which again may resume concentric configurations. Several of these cells converge to direction-specific cells for motion detection, and to complex cells signaling special oriented contours and forms over large retinal regions. Only direction-specific motion or axis inclination of contour, not retinal localization per se, is a selective stimulus for those neurons. In this way, form generalization and motion direction may find their neuronal correlates. + indicates activation; −, inhibition by light-on. Conversely, at light-off + represents neuronal inhibition, − represents activation. For further explanation, refer to Fig. 4.

drawing procedure with de-emphasis of plane surfaces and accentuation of oriented contour [23]. The critical stimuli in both cases are straight and curved contours or lines with certain inclinations to the meridian of the visual field. Oriented contours and lines with curves are a common basis of pattern vision and Gestalt recognition. Thus, one may consider the selective neuronal K responses to contours as basic processes of pattern detection in the visual cortex.

Neuronal Mechanisms of Motion Detection

Experiments with moving visual patterns have disclosed special motion-sensitive neurons in the cat's visual cortex [3, 5]. They can be distinguished from contour detectors by their optimal response to directional movement without signaling slow-moving contrast borders per se. There are transitions to contour-sensitive K neurons which are activated by specific moving patterns drawn slowly over their receptive field in one direction more than in others. Motion-sensitive neurons with clear directional preference may be called M neurons. These M neurons do not show selective responses for certain stationary oriented forms. Higher-order M neurons are direction specific; they signal movements of various patterns in one direction only (Fig. 3). After prolonged stimulation they may signal motion in the opposite directions.

Neurons responding predominantly to patterns moving in certain directions were first described by Hubel 1959 in unrestrained cats [14]. However, they could not be analyzed accurately in the presence of eye and head movement.

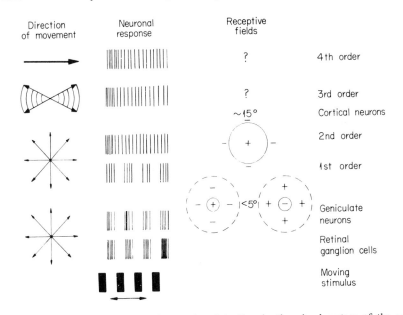

FIG. 3. Neuronal mechanisms for motion detection in the visual system of the cat. From Jung and Baumgartner [23]. From the lower to the upper rows, progressive specialization of neuronal responses is indicated schematically from retinal neurons to higher-order cortical cells. Arrows in the first column show direction of the stimulus which causes neuronal activation. The striped patterns of the moving stimuli are shown in the lowest row of the second column. Above, the neuronal responses in different levels are drawn schematically. The third column signifies the organization of the receptive fields (+ indicates activation; −indicates inhibition by light-on).

Baumgartner and co-workers [3, 5] made more detailed studies on motion-sensitive neurons in the cat's cortex after eliminating eye movement by curare. They found special neurons responding to directed movements of certain velocities in areas 17 and 18. The arrangement of these neurons on different levels is still hypothetical since it is impossible to record different neuronal and synaptic stages in the same experiment.

The progressive specialization to movement detection on successive levels and the reduction of response to contrast borders and spatial patterns is shown by the tendency toward continuous discharges in response to alternate black and white stripes moving in specific directions over their receptive fields. Receptive fields of these motion detectors cover a larger area than those of K neurons and extend widely over the retina [3]. Some M neurons receive input from large retinal regions including the peripheral parts. The limits of their receptive fields are often difficult to determine.

Most recordings of motion-detecting neurons in cats were made with curarized eye muscles. We know from experiments with man that paralyses of eye muscles causes various motion illusions when the subject tries in vain to move his eyes. Of course we have no way of obtaining such data in our cat experiments. Some changes in the direction of effective motion, mostly 180°. to the opposite side, which may occur when we make lengthy recordings of motion-detecting neurons, may be related either to such motion attempts by the curarized eye, or to moving afterimages.

Although direction-specific neurons occur in frog and rabbit retina, no such motion-detecting neurons were found in cat retina or lateral geniculate body. The cat's motion detectors depend upon intracortical neuronal transformations, but their coordination with tectomesencephalic mechanisms requires investigation.

Observations of human optokinetic nystagmus and on velocity perception have shown that visual motion detection involves both eye-following movements and moving retinal images, and that attention modifies the relation of both mechanisms in favor of eye-following and efferent motion detection [9, 21]. In the curarized cat, the most effective stimulus velocities for cortical neurons are rather low, below 5°/sec; these low velocities cause automatic eye-following in man without special attention.

A survey of the various transformations of neuronal organization in the visual system from retina to cortex is shown in Fig. 4. This wiring diagram is not an exact reconstruction of synaptic connections, which are mostly unknown. It shows only the most probable order of visual neuronal chains that may cause the reorganization of receptive fields on several levels.

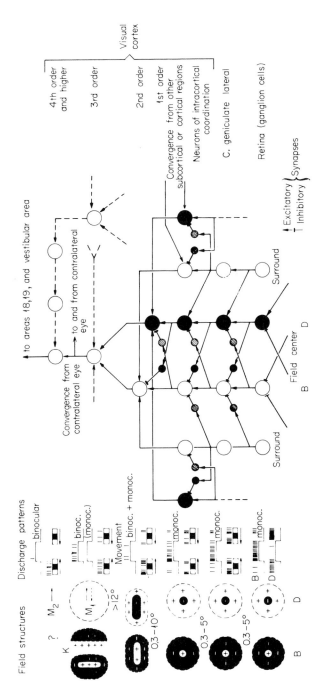

FIG. 4. Schematic survey of neuronal organization in the visual system. From Jung and Baumgartner [23]. Left: forms of receptive fields and their transformation from retina to cortex. The corresponding neuronal responses to diffuse light and moving stimuli at different levels are drawn schematically. Right: wiring diagram of possible intracortical connections for both antagonistic systems for brightness (B) and darkness information (D), located in the same field center with reciprocal inhibition. In the left column is shown the lateral inhibition for the B system, in the right column, organization of neighboring receptive fields occurs separately for B and D. In the following level, further convergence is established resulting in larger receptive fields and binocular interaction (3rd order). At this stage, a light–dark-antagonism of B versus D is lost in favor of special information for motion detection (M) of contour enhancement (K), elaborated further in areas 18 and 19. Motion direction is signaled in the 4th-order system.

Subjective Estimation of Visual Receptive
Field Diameters in Man

Baumgartner [2] first showed that one may use Hermann's grid to estimate the diameter of human receptive field centers in foveal and extrafoveal retinal regions [Fig. 5(a)]. Using this method, others obtained similar or slightly different results [13, 26]. Sindermann and Pieper [35] used the optimal brightness reduction of the "Binnenkontrast" between black bars, presented at various distances for estimation of the total receptive fields including the surround [34] [Fig. 5(b)].

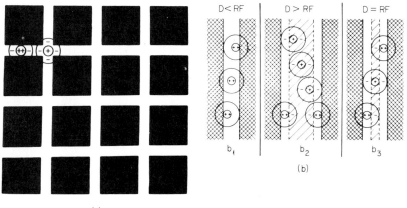

(a)   (b)

FIG. 5. Estimation of receptive fields in man by brightness contrast. The Hermann grid (a) and the scheme of dark bars of various distances (b) are modified drawings from experiments of Baumgartner [2] and Sindermann [34, 35]. (a) In the Hermann grid, gray spots are seen at cross intersections of the white stripes, except in the central foveal region of fixation. In the fovea, the neuronal receptive fields are much smaller and their inhibitory surrounds have similar effects in both white stripes and intersections. Therefore, the field-center-signal "brighter" receives the same lateral inhibition in nearly all positions, except in very small border regions similar to b_2. The size difference between foveal receptive fields and white bars is still larger than in b_2. Examples of larger receptive fields of extrafoveal regions are shown in critical positions at the left upper part. ++ marks stronger activation of on-center by diminished area of lateral inhibition. (b) Schematic relation of receptive field positions of the fovea with varying distance of two black bars. b_1 Demonstrates maximal brightness by activation of on-center neurons (++) which occurs in the white area when the distance is smaller than the diameter of the receptive field (D < RF), and lateral inhibition is diminished by black parts. In b_2, which the middle part of the larger white stripe has parallel gray lines which appear with diminished Binnencontrast. This corresponds to those regions where on-center B neurons receive full lateral inhibition of their inhibitory surround (D > RF). In b_3, when the diameter of the receptive fields equals the distance of the black stripes (D=RF), the gray line is smaller. This may also be seen in the Hermann grid (a). To see the phenomenon of a gray illusion (Binnenkontrast) in the white lines, one should look at Fig. 5(a) from various distances, e.g., at about 10 to 60 cm from the eye.

It has long been known that the grayish spot appearing at the cross points in Hermann's grid is a function of contrast vision and that no such spot appears at the fixation point corresponding to foveal vision. By comparing the grid at different distances from the eye, an appropriately smaller image of this contrast picture can be obtained in which a darker spot appears in the fixed foveal region. This can be explained as follows: The gray spot occurs at the intersection when the diameters of the receptive fields are of a size so that lateral inhibition from the surround becomes stronger at the intersection than between the black stripes. If the inhibitory surround is cut off by the margins of the black stripes, the on-center discharge is increased. In the white intersecting parts additional lateral inhibition occurs because of the illumination of the surround which results in a diminishing of the on-center discharge.

The diameter of the receptive field centers estimated with Hermann's grid is somewhat larger than 25 μ in the fovea [2, 8], and the total field diameter with surround, about 40-50 μ [35]. This would agree with the foveal field center of 28 μ, obtained by sinusoidal stimulation [8]. Of course one cannot measure the field of one single unit by this method but only the net response of a local population of neurons with similar field organizations. By comparing grids in black and white, one finds similar diameters for neurons of the B system and the D system. Temporal alterations of the foveal Hermann illusion at different angles, observed by Ronchi [31, 32] and the phenomena studied by MacKay [28, 29], suggest other interactions between widely separated areas of the visual field.

A neuronal correlate of the Hermann-grid effects in man can be demonstrated in visual neurons of the cat. Receptive fields of visual neurons are stimulated by a grid of black or white stripes in different positions for B and D neurons, respectively. Figure 6 demonstrates the responses of an on-center B neuron with a concentric receptive field. All of these neurons (retinal ganglion cells, geniculate neurons, and first-order neurons in the cortex) show strong activation when their field center is exposed between two black borders and when their field center corresponds to the width of the white stripe [Fig. 6(a) and (b)]. The responses are diminished to less than half of the spikes if the field center is exposed to the cross intersection of the stripes [Fig. 6(c)]. Schepelmann et al. [33] recently made a special study of the Hermann-grid effect on the oblong "simple field" neurons of Hubel and Wiesel [15]. When their receptive field axis is exposed to similarly orientated stripes of the Hermann grid, the neuronal activation is maximal. These responses are diminished when the field is shifted to cross the intersection of two stripes, one of which lies in the optimal axis orientation. The neuronal responses are further diminished or disappear if the receptive field is stimulated by the other stripe in rectangular orientation to the field axis. Thus, the neuronal interpretation of the Hermann effect is more complex for specialized cortical neurons, although diminished responses at the grid intersections are preserved in simple field neurons.

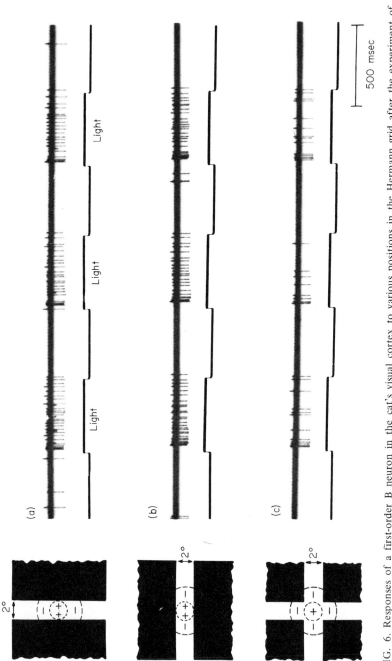

FIG. 6. Responses of a first-order B neuron in the cat's visual cortex to various positions in the Hermann grid after the experiment of Baumgartner *et al.* [33]. The neuron's receptive field has a diameter of about 6° and is located 20° paracentral. In (c) the on-response to light is minimal at the white cross intersection because of a larger area of surround illumination which is causing stronger lateral inhibition. The on-response drops in (c) to less than half of (a) and (b) at the same luminosity. The responses of this neuron are typical only for concentric fields of geniculate and first-order cortical B neurons. In the oblong "simple field neurons" of Hubel-Wiesel, the responses are maximal in stimulus condition (a) only when the receptive field axis is orientated in the same direction as the light bar. It would be minimal in the 90°-turned orientation (b) and intermediate in the cross field intersection (c).

Glezer reported other psychophysical and electrophysiological correlations of receptive field organization in man and frog [11]. They are concerned for the most part with adaptation processes which are difficult to investigate with the Hermann grid. Glezer's balance functions in the receptive fields may have some relationship to temporal changes of the Hermann effect.

Spillmann [26, 36] has obtained subjective estimates of human field sizes responsible for apparent motion. Receptive field size was studied as a function of retinal eccentricity by determining the spatial thresholds of Wertheimer's optimal beta movement and phi phenomenon. The receptive fields for apparent movement were 20 to 30 times larger in diameter than the field centers measured by simultaneous contrast of the Hermann grid. The diminution of field size from the retinal periphery toward the fovea showed a 50% linear decrease between 60° to 20° retinal projection, and a still greater decrease between 20° and the fovea. These psychophysical measurements of human receptive field size for brightness and motion perception agree well with neuronal recordings in animals.

It seems possible that some of the visual illusions of motion and depth perception studied by MacKay [28, 29] and others may also offer useful evidence on higher-order neuronal processes. They suggest a number of hypotheses about neuronal correlates of higher motion sensations and of stereoscopic depth perception which invite physiological investigation.

Our correlation of brightness contrast with receptive field organization is valid only for concentric or simple oblong receptive fields with lateral inhibition or activation. Since concentric forms are always constantly found in retinal and geniculate neurons and only rarely in the higher-order cortical neurons [6], determination of the receptive field diameter, made with the Hermann grid, seems to depend chiefly upon neurons of the lower visual system. If this were so, these neurons would have to project into the final neuronal stage of brightness discrimination with little change or with slight linear reorganization into Hubel's oblong fields. One may conclude that brightness sensation remains relatively independent of pattern vision in higher information processing. The neuronal explanation might be either that higher-order cortical neurons with complex and hypercomplex fields or motion-detecting M neurons have little influence on brightness sensation, or that receptive fields of human cortical neurons may be different from those in the cat. However, some influence of complex visual transformations in higher-order K neurons is suggested by subjective vision in man, since Ehrenstein [10] demonstrated similar illusions to those with the Hermann grid in more complex linear conditions of Gestalt stimulation. The resulting brightness illusions of these linear patterns are less constant and show more individual differences than the rather massive brightness illusions of the classic Hermann grid. Ehrenstein's linear brightness illusions seem to be partly dependent upon previous experiences, e.g., visual learning and conditioning. Further studies are necessary to elucidate the neuronal interaction in brightness and pattern vision with motion detection.

Conclusions

This chapter demonstrates that neurophysiological and psychophysiological research in vision can be combined. Coordinated studies of visual perception in man and physiological experiments in animals are mutually stimulating in three ways. First, neuronal investigations in the visual system can be better planned if we make use of subjective psychophysical data of vision. Second, hitherto unexplainable visual phenomena in man may be formulated in neuronal terms. Third, some properties of visual neurons can be predicted from analysis of human perception.

Of course the conditions of human perception and animal experiments are not strictly comparable. Species differences and restraint-procedure differences in experimental animals complicate our correlations. Hubel's successful neuronal recordings from unrestrained cats [14] could not be analyzed precisely for receptive fields and motion detection because of head and eye movement. Most animal experiments are made under abnormal conditions such as stimulation with fixed pupils and exclusion of eye movement by barbiturate narcosis [15-18] or curare [2-7]. In spite of these limitations, several correlations of neuronal activity in cats with subjective visual phenomena in man can be proposed.

Brightness-contrast phenomena of the Hermann grid and apparent motion of the Wertheimer type may be described in neuronal terms and can be used for quantitative estimation of receptive fields. Subjective apparent movement and motion aftersensations appear to be related to direction specific and opposite responses in motion-detecting neurons.

Both psychophysical and neuronal investigations show that pattern vision is facilitated and prepared by contrast enhancement but that higher-order processes of pattern abstraction and directional motion detection are guided by new processes, superimposed on basic neuronal processes of enhancement contrast. Since we see both contours and luminance differences in one subjective image, we may assume that in addition to cortical contour-abstracting processes in higher-order K neurons, the primary information of local surface brightness and darkness is signaled in parallel neuronal systems B and D to other structures which synthesize our perception. For brightness and darkness, the original retinal mosaic of concentric fields of the lower B and D subsystems seems to reach the neuronal substrate of the perceived image unchanged. This has been shown subjectively by the Hermann-grid illusion.

More complex visual phenomena and optical illusions allow only tentative correlations of neuronal transformations with pattern vision and motion detection. Many higher visual functions which are of greater interest to the psychologist cannot yet be formulated in quantitative neuronal terms. Neuronal recordings allow only limited insight into some mechanisms of the complex and well-organized higher visual systems. Unsolved problems of neuronal correlations with perception and behavior include multisensory integration, which has only been touched upon by neuronal recordings [25], the correlation of motion detection and eye movement, and last, but not least, visual learning and conditioning.

Summary

Pattern and motion detection are organized in the cat's visual system by successive stages of neuronal integration and specialization. Visual information is carried from the retina to the cortex in two parallel neuronal channels of antagonistic subsystems reciprocally related: B *system* (on-center neurons) signaling "brighter," and D *system* (off-center neurons) signaling "darker." Cortical neurons transform these messages into special signals of form and movement.

The neuronal basis of pattern vision is prepared by contour enhancement of simultaneous contrast. *Contrast coding* begins in the retina with two antagonistic receptive field organizations: the B system, which is on-center with lateral inhibition, and the D system, which is off-center with lateral activation by illumination of the surround. These neuronal signals of contrasting bright and dark surfaces are abstracted to specialized information on visual contours and direction of movement in higher-order cortical neurons by means of convergence of receptive fields.

Cortical neurons in areas 17, 18, and 19 are predominantly stimulated by moving contours of specific form, orientation, extent, and motion direction. Two main types of responses may be distinguished. *Contour-signaling neurons* (K) show optimal responses to specific contours and forms (space-oriented edges, lines, angles, curves, etc.), and *motion-detecting neurons* (M) respond predominantly to moving patterns in definite directions and possess large receptive fields with binocular summation.

Selective neuronal responses to contours in the cortex involve reduction of information about brightness and darkness of surfaces. This may be compared to similar abstract accentuation of contours, which is used in line drawings.

In man, the diameter of receptive field centers and their surrounds from the neuronal subsystems B and D can be estimated subjectively by brightness-contrast stimuli of various dimensions (white or black bars and Hermann's grid). In cats, contrast stimulation by Hermann's grid elicits neuronal responses of cells with concentric and simple fields which correspond well to subjective vision in man.

A neuronal scheme is proposed to explain the organization of visual transformations from the retina to the visual cortex.

Acknowledgments

I am grateful to Professor Baumgartner, now in Zürich, for many years of experimental work in Freiburg and to Dr. Spillmann and Dr. Sindermann for their perceptive field estimations.

REFERENCES

1. Barlow, H. B. Three Points about Lateral Inhibition. *In* "Sensory Communication" (W. A. Rosenblith, ed.), pp. 782-786. Wiley, New York, 1961.
2. Baumgartner, G. Indirekte Grössenbestimmung der rezeptiven Felder der Retina beim Menschen mittels der Hermann'schen Gittertäuschung. *Pfluegers Arch. Gesamte Physiol. Menschen Tiere* **272**, 21 (1960).
3. Baumgartner, G. Die Reaktionen der Neurone des zentralen visuellen Systems der Katze im simultanen Helligkeitskontrast. *In* "Neurophysiologie und Psychophysik des Visuellen Systems" (R. Jung and H. H. Kornhuber, eds.), pp. 296-313. Springer, Berlin 1961.
4. Baumgartner, G. Neuronale Mechanismen des Kontrast-und Bewegungssehens. *Ber. Deut. Ophthalmol. Ges.* **66**, 111-125 (1965).
5. Baumgartner, G., Brown, J. L., and Schulz, A. Visual motion detection in the cat. *Science* **146**, 1070-1071 (1964).
6. Baumgartner, G., Brown, J. L., and Schulz, A. Responses of single units of the cat, visual system to rectangular stimulus patterns. *J. Neurophysiol.* **28**, 1-18 (1965).
7. Baumgartner, G., and Hakas, P. Reaktionen einzelner Opticusneurone und corticaler Nervenzellen der Katze im Hell-DunkelGrenzfeld (Simultankontrast). *Pfluegers Arch. Gesamte Physiol. Menschen Tiere* **270**, 29 (1959).
8. Bryngdahl, O. Grössenschätzung des rezeptiven Feldzentrums der menschlichen Retina. *Pfluegers Arch. Gesamte Physiol. Menschen Tiere* **280**, 362-368 (1964).
9. Dichgans, J., Körner, F., and Jung, R. Retinale Bildwanderung und Augenfolgebewegung als zwei Mechanismen des Bewegungssehens: Abhängigkeit von visueller Zuwendung, optokinetischem Nystagmus und Fixation. *Pfluegers Arch. Gesamte Physiol. Menschen Tiere* **297**, R84 (1967).
10. Ehrenstein, W. "Probleme der ganzheitspsychologischen Wahrnehmungslehre," 3rd ed. Barth, Leipzig, 1954.
11. Glezer, V. D. The receptive fields of the retina. *Vision Res.* **5**, 497-525 (1965).
12. Grüsser, O. J., and Grüsser-Cornehls, U. Periodische Aktivierungsphasen visueller Neurone nach kurzen Lichtreizen verschiedener Dauer. *Pfluegers Arch. Gesamte Physiol. Menschen Tiere* **275**, 292-311 (1962).
13. Hommer, K., and Schubert, G. Die absolute Grösse der fovealen rezeptorischen Feldzentren und der Panumareale. *Graefes Arch. Ophthalmal.* **166**, 205-210 (1963).
14. Hubel, D. H. Single unit activity in striate cortex of unrestrained cats. *J. Physiol. (London)* **147**, 226-238 (1959).
15. Hubel, D. H., and Wiesel, T. N. Receptive fields of single neurons in the cat's striate cortex. *J. Physiol. (London)* **148**, 574-591 (1959).
16. Hubel, D. H., and Wiesel, T. N. Receptive fields, binocular interaction and functional architecture in the cat's visual cortex. *J. Physiol. (London)* **160**, 106-154 (1962).
17. Hubel, D. H., and Wiesel, T. N. Shape and arrangements of columns in cat' striate cortex. *J. Physiol. (London)* **165**, 559-568 (1963).

18. Hubel, D. H., and Wiesel, T. N. Receptive fields and functional architecture in two nonstriate visual areas (18 and 19) of the cat. *J. Neurophysiol.* **28**, 229-289 (1965).

19. Jung, R. Neuronal discharge. *EEG Clin. Neurophysiol. Suppl.* **4**, 57-71 (1953).

20. Jung, R. Neuronal integration in the visual cortex and its significance for visual information. *In* "Sensory Communication" (W. A. Rosenblith, ed.), pp. 627-674. Wiley, New York, 1961.

21. Jung, R. Korrelationen von Neuronentätigkeit und Sehen. *In* "Neurophysiologie und Psychophysik des Visuellen Systems" (R. Jung and H. Kornhuber, eds.), pp. 410-434. Springer, Berlin, 1961.

22. Jung, R., Baumgarten, R. von, and Baumgartner, G. Mikroableitungen von einzelnen Neuronen im optischen Cortex der Katze. Die lichtaktivierten B-Neurone. *Arch. Psychiat. NR.* **189**, 521-539 (1952).

23. Jung, R., and Baumgartner, G. Neuronenphysiologie der visuellen und paravisuellen Rindenfelder. *Proc. 8th Int. Congr. Neurol. Wien Sept.*, 1965. **III**, 47-75 (1965).

24. Jung, R., Creutzfeldt, O., and Grüsser, O. J. Die Mikrophysiologie corticaler Neurone und ihre Bedeutung für die Sinnes und Hirnfunktionen. *Deut. Med. Wochenschr.* **82**, 1050-1059 (1957).

25. Jung, R., Kornhuber, H. H., and da Fonseca, J. S. Multisensory convergence on cortical neurons. Neuronal effects of visual, acoustic and vestibular stimuli in the superior convolutions of the cat's cortex. *In* "Progress in Brain Research" (G. Moruzzi, A. Fessard, and H. H. Jaspers, eds.), Vol. 1, pp. 207-240. Elsevier, Amsterdam, 1963.

26. Kornhuber, H. H., and Spillmann, L. Zur visuellen Feldorganisation beim Menschen: Die receptiven Felder im peripheren und zentralen Gesichtsfeld bei Simultankontrast, Flimmerfusion, Scheinbewegung und Blickfolgebewegung. *Pfluegers Arch. Gesamte Physiol. Menschen Tiere* **279**, R5-6 (1964).

27. Kuffler, S. W. Discharge patterns and functional organization of mammalian retina. *J. Neurophysiol.* **16**, 37-68 (1953).

28. MacKay, D. M. Interactive processes in visual perception. *In* "Sensory Communication" (W. A. Rosenblith, ed.), pp. 339-355. Wiley, New York, 1961.

29. MacKay, D. M. Visual noise as a tool of research. *J. Gen. Psychol.* **72**, 181-197 (1965).

30. Ratliff, F. "Mach Bands: Quantitative Studies on Neural Networks in the Retina." Holden-Day, San Francisco, Amsterdam, 1965.

31. Ronchi, L., and Bottai, G. On the visual effects produced by a test-object consisting of two stripes darker than the background, intersecting with one another. *Atti Fond. Giorgio Ronchi* **18**, 47-70 (1963).

32. Ronchi, L., and Bottai, G. Simultaneous contrast effects at the center of figures showing different degrees of symmetry. *Atti Fond. Giorgio Ronchi* **19**, 84-100 (1964).

33. Schepelmann, F., Aschayeri, H., and Baumgartner, G. Die Reaktionen der "simple-field"-Neurone in Area 17 der Katze beim Hermann-Gitter-Kontrast. *Pfluegers Arch. Gesamte Physiol. Menschen Tiere* **294**, 57 (1967).

34. Sindermann, F., and Deecke, L. Psychophysische Studien an visuellen rezeptiven Feldern beim Menschem (In preparation).

35. Sindermann, F., and Pieper, E. Grössenschätzung von fovealen Projektionen receptiver Kontrastfelder (Zentrum und Umfeld) beim Menschen im psychophysischen Versuch. *Pfluegers Arch. Gesamte Physiol. Menschen Tiere* **283**, R47 (1965).

36. Spillmann, L. Personal communication.

2

Functional Organization of the Receptive Fields of the Retina

V. D. Glezer, A. V. Bertulis, V. A. Ivanov, N. B. Kostelyanets, and N. F. Podvigin

The present chapter reviews a number of studies carried out in the Visual Laboratory of the Pavlov Institute of Physiology and presents some general conclusions based on this work. The methodological aspects of these studies have been described in detail in a number of articles referred to below.

We shall consider here data obtained in investigations of the functional organization of the retinal receptive fields. The studies were done with microelectrode technique and pertain to the retina of the frog. During the experiments, responses of ganglion cells and the ERG from the vitreous body were recorded, and after the insertion of the microelectrode into the retina, the IERG was recorded as well. The electrophysiological data were compared with the results of psychophysical experiments.

Studies of the Receptive Fields of the Frog's Retina

In experiments on the isolated frog's eye [4, 14, 23], responses of the ganglion cells to light spots of different luminance (from 0.0001 to 900 lx) and size (from 0.10 to 4.2 mm in diameter) were studied. The microelectrode was either a platinum wire or a glass pipette filled with Wood's alloy (tip diameter 10 to 20 μ), or with 2.75 M KCl (tip diameter about 1 μ).

The duration of the light stimulus was 500 to 800 msec. Before the presentation of each stimulus, the retina was at the same level of dark adaptation, since the stimuli were presented after an interval of 1 min in the dark and control experiments showed that this interval was sufficient to prevent any influence of the preceding stimulus on the response to the subsequent flash.

Figure 1 illustrates for the responses of a ganglion on-cell (a) and an off-cell (b) the relation between the number of impulses and the area of the spot of light. The stimulus luminance varies for different curves. For a low luminance, the number of spikes in the response increases with an increase of the area of the light spot; thus, summation occurs over a large area of the receptive field. In the middle range of luminance, the spike counts increase at first with an increase of the stimulus area; however, with its further increase, the spike counts begin to decline. For high intensities, the spike counts decrease when the area of the spot of light increases. These results indicate that, when the luminance of the stimulus increases, an inhibitory ring develops at the periphery of the receptive field; it extends toward the center with an increase of the luminance and the area of the stimulus. The result of such a reorganization of the field is shown in Fig. 2(a). According to this interpretation, the receptors

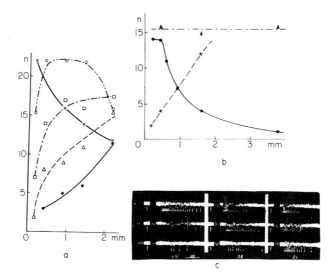

FIG. 1. Relation between the number of impulses in the response and the diameter of the light stimulus at different intensities. On-neuron: (a) and (c); off-neuron: (b). Abscissa for (a) and (b): diameter of the light spot. Ordinate: number of impulses in the response. Duration of the stimuli: 800 msec. Luminance of the stimuli: (a) 11 lx (crosses), 1.1 lx (circles), 0.11 lx (squares), 0.01 lx (triangles), 0.001 lx (filled circles); (b) 900 lx (filled circles), 9 lx (triangles), 0.9 lx (crosses); (c) numbers on the left indicate the luminance in lux; numbers below each column of records indicate the diameter of the stimulus spot in millimeters. Onset of stimulus is indicated by an arrow. Duration of the stimulus: 50 msec. Latency of each response is reduced by the time (in milliseconds) indicated in each record above the dotted line. Time mark: 100 msec.

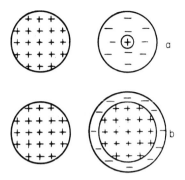

FIG. 2. Schemes illustrating two interpretations of the results presented in Fig. 1. See text for explanation.

subserving the periphery of the field, whose excitation eventually leads to spike discharges, send inhibitory signals when the illumination increases. Consequently, the on- and off-fields of the retina undergo a functional reorganization depending on the energy of the stimulus.

However, another interpretation of the data is also possible. It could be assumed [17] that the summation zone of the receptive field does not change but that an inhibitory ring arises around it with an increase of the luminance [Fig. 2(b)]. Concurrently, with an increase of the area of the spot of light, when the luminance is high, there is, also an increase in the intensity of the stray light which acts upon the peripheral inhibitory fringe. Thus, a decline in the spike counts resulting from an increase of the stimulus area, when the luminance is high, would not be due to inhibition prevailing over excitation in the central zone, but would rather be explained by an increase of the inhibitory effect in the periphery of the field due to a greater intensity of the stray light. The structure of the field itself would remain invariant. This interpretation is of particular interest, since work on the receptive fields in the cat's retina [3] indicates that the functional organization of the receptive field, during a transition from dark to light adaptation, is changed according to the scheme in Fig. 2(b). It should be noted, however, that Barlow *et al.* [3] were concerned with the receptive field under different conditions of adaptation, while we studied the organization of the field which results from an action of a stimulus at a given intensity.

In order to decide which of the two interpretations discussed is preferable, we compared the results of the electrophysiological experiments with the characteristics of the stray light caused by applied stimuli. The characteristics of the stray light were determined by means of a photomultiplier. Let us examine Figs. 1(a) and 3. Figure 1(a) presents experimental results concerning spike counts produced by a ganglion on-cell. Figure 3 illustrates the distributions of the luminous flux for the light spots applied [(a) shows the distribu-

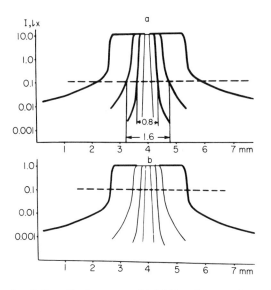

FIG. 3. Estimate of the effective zone of inhibition for experimental data shown in Fig. 1(a). Intensity of the direct light: (a) 11 lx, (b) 0.1 lx.

tions for intensity of 11 lx; (b) that for 1.1 lx]. The dashed lines in Fig. 3 correspond to the maximal illumination for which an increase of the stimulus area always led to an increase in spike counts, i.e., to that level at which no inhibition was demonstrable. For the neuron in question, this intensity was 0.1 lx. The thin lines indicate stimuli that did not produce any inhibitory effect, the thick lines the stimuli that provoked such an effect. From Fig. 3 it may be seen that, when the intensity of the direct light is 1.1 lx, inhibition arises only in responses to a stimulus with a diameter of 2.4 mm. At an intensity of 11.0 lx, inhibition is provoked by stimuli having diameters of 0.8 and 0.4 mm, respectively. Assuming that inhibition may arise at an intensity of more than 0.1 lx, the effective diameters of these stimuli must be taken as equal to 1.6 and 0.8 mm; this may be seen in the graph of Fig. 3. Since these effective areas lie within the summation zone of 2.4 mm, it must be concluded that the inhibition is evoked not by the stray, but by the direct light. Consequently, inhibition due to an increase of the illumination is determined not by stray light acting in the periphery of the field, but by the direct light acting inside the area within which only summation was observed under conditions of low illumination. Similar data were obtained for all cells studied. These data may be regarded as a proof for the reorganization of receptive fields by light stimuli. The reorganization takes place when the relations of the inhibitory and excitatory processes change during the action of the stimulus.

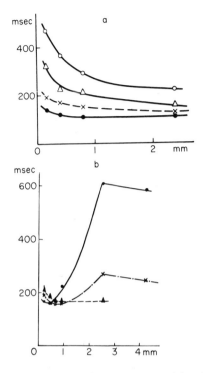

FIG. 4. Dependence of the latency of an on-response (a) and an off-response (b) on the diameter of the stimulating spot of light at different intensities. Abscissa: diameter of the spot. Ordinate: latent period in milliseconds. Luminance of the stimuli: (a) 11 lx (filled circles), 1.1 lx (crosses), 0.11 lx (triangles), 0.01 lx (circles); (b) 900 lx (filled circles), 90 lx (crosses), 9 lx (triangles).

Let us now consider in greater detail the development in time of the functional reorganization of the receptive field. Figure 4(a) shows the relation between the latency of an on-response and the area of the stimulus for several stimulus intensities. The latency decreases with increase of the diameter for all intensities. The inhibitory process does not manifest itself in the same way here as it did when the dependent variable was the number of impulses in the response. This observation suggests that the occurrence of the first impulses is a function of excitatory processes which are summated over the whole receptive field at any intensity and area of the stimulus. Therefore, it may be concluded that inhibition does not appear immediately, but is delayed in regard to the excitatory process.

The development of the inhibitory process in time can be better traced in graphs (Fig. 5) which illustrate for an on-cell the relation between the number of impulses in the response and the area of the stimulus for three intensities

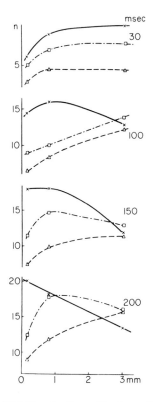

FIG. 5. Development of inhibition in time. Abscissa: diameter of the spot of light. Ordinate: number of impulses. Luminance of the stimuli: 110 lx (crosses), 11 lx (squares), 0.1 lx (triangles). For further explanations see text.

and four different periods of time. The graphs present, as it were, sections made at different times after the beginning of the process. Thus, during the first 30 msec of the response time, the number of impulses increases with an increase of the diameter of the stimulus for all intensities. No inhibition is demonstrable. For a period of 100 msec, the number of impulses also increases with the increase of the diameter of the light spot for all except the maximal intensity of 110 lx. For this intensity, an increase in the diameter of the spot causes an inhibitory effect. The inhibitory effect becomes gradually more pronounced and finally, for a period of 200 msec, it is fully developed.

Other observations also suggest that the inhibitory process is delayed in relation to excitation. In a number of experiments, in which the intensity and the area of the stimulus varied, the duration of the stimulus was also made a variable. Figure 6 indicates that for a stimulus of short duration even the most intense light does not produce any inhibition. The spike counts increase with

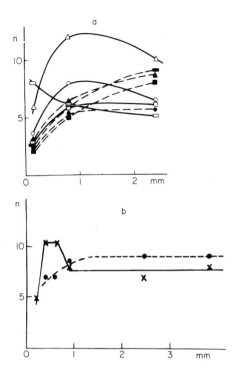

FIG. 6. Relation between the number of impulses in an on-response (a) and an off-response (b) and the diameter of the spot of light at different intensities of the stimulus. Stimulus duration: (a) 880 msec (solid lines) and 10 msec (dashed lines); (b) 240 msec (dashed line) and 30 msec (solid line). Luminance of the stimulus: (a) 110 lx (rectangules), 11 lx (triangles), 1.1 lx (circles), 0.11 lx (squares); (b) 90 lx (crosses), 900 lx (filled circles).

an increase of the area of the stimulus. Calculations reveal that these results are not caused by a decrease in the energy of the stimulus when the stimulus duration decreases. The data in Fig. 6(a) show that, for a duration of 880 msec, an inhibitory effect is present in response to a spot of light 2.4 mm in diameter and 1.1 lx in intensity. The amount of luminous energy was in this case 0.0044 lx msec/m^2. For a duration of 10 msec, the inhibitory effect is absent in responses to stimuli at an intensity of 110 lx and a diameter of 2.4 mm, i.e., when the amount of luminous energy was 0.0049 lx msec/m^2. The result is still more striking if one considers that the summation time is of the order of 50 to 150 msec. Hence, the amount of luminous energy in the first calculation should be reduced approximately ten times.

From Fig. 6(b), it is also obvious that the energy of a brief stimulus may be larger than that of a long-lasting one, and yet no inhibition occurs for the brief stimulus. Consequently, the effect is determined by the duration of the stimulus, i.e., inhibition arises only if the stimulus acts for a sufficiently long time. It follows that the inhibitory process in the receptive field is not an all-or-none process, but arises during the action of the stimulus.

The development of an on-response in time as a function of the area and intensity of the light spot is shown in poststimulus histograms in Fig. 7. The

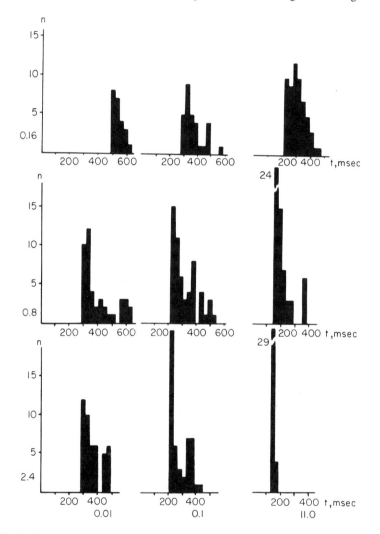

FIG. 7. Poststimulus histograms for discharges of a ganglion on-cell plotting the number of spikes against the time of their occurrence for various intensities and areas of a spot of light. Abscissa: time in milliseconds. Ordinate: number of impulses. Numbers on the left designate the diameter of the spot of light in millimeters; numbers below each column indicate luminance in lux.

figure illustrates once more that the response may decrease with an increase of the intensity and the area of the stimulus. Moreover, it also shows that an increase of stimulus intensity may lead to a shorter duration of an on-response, since the response may develop in time more rapidly. Similarly, an increase of the area of the stimulus may shorten the duration of the response. With an increase of the stimulus area, which, as shown above, intensifies the inhibition, a "compression" of the impulses in the response takes place.

If the structure of the response is determined by the summation of the excitatory and inhibitory processes, which develop in time, then a decrease of response duration signifies that, with an increase of the luminance and the area of the stimulus, the rate of growth for the excitatory and the inhibitory components is not the same. The development of the inhibitory process is more rapid in time (its time constant decreases), and inhibition balances the excitatory process more rapidly. As a result, the period of excitation for the output element of the receptive field becomes shorter [14, 16]. Thus, with an increase of luminance, the "compression" of the impulses in the response is due to an increased rate of growth of the excitatory process, as a result of which the spike counts increase in the initial segment of the response. Simultaneously, however, there occurs an increase in the rate of growth of the inhibitory process and, since this increase develops more rapidly, the spike train becomes shorter (Fig. 8).

Investigations of the Receptive Fields in Man

Let us compare the results of experiments on the on- and off-fields of the frog with psychophysiological experiments in man [18]. The latter were

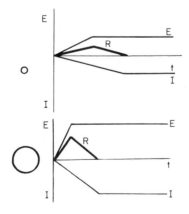

FIG. 8. Scheme for an interaction in time of the excitatory and inhibitory processes in the receptive field for different areas of the stimulus. The two circles represent the area of the stimulus. See text for explanation.

carried out with the aid of an optic set which made possible a simultaneous presentation of two stimuli, whose form, brightness, and duration could be varied independently. The subject saw the matching field as a ring of a given luminosity [B_m in Fig. 9(a)]. His task was to match the brightness of the light spots of different sizes seen in the center with that of the matching field. It is assumed that the brightness of the matching field and of the light spot seem equal to the subject when the respective receptive fields produce similar numbers of spikes. Therefore, the brightness of the matching field represents an estimate of the spike response. From Fig. 9(a) it may be seen that an increase of the brightness of the matching field results in a decrease of the area on the retina within which Ricco's law operates. In other words, the summation zone of the receptive field decreases with an increase of luminance. The slopes of the curves beyond the summation zone attest to the appearance of an inhibitory ring at high illuminations. We may replot the graphs assuming that a certain number of impulses (n) corresponds to a given level of illumination, and that, when the brightness of the ring and of the light spot are matched, the number of impulses produced in the respective receptive fields is equal.

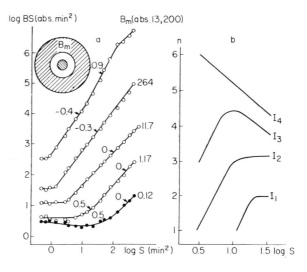

FIG. 9. Cone receptive fields of the human retina. (a) Change in the zone of complete summation of the human cone receptive fields and in the summation coefficient beyond this zone, depending on the brightness of the matching field. Abscissa: area of the stimulus. Ordinate: magnitude of the luminous flux. Numbers on the right designate the brightness of the matching field. Numbers on the curves indicate the coefficient n for IS^n = const. (b) Calculation of the dependence of the conventional value of the response of the human cone receptive field on the area of the stimulus at different intensities of the latter for data shown in Fig. 9(a).

The ordinate in Fig. 9(b) indicates the level of the perceived subjective brightness (brightness of the matching field), expressed as a number of impulses occurring in the receptive fields excited by the test spot. The abscissa shows the logarithm of the area of the test spot. The intensity of the test spot serves as a parameter. Graphs in Figs. 1(a), 1(b), and 9(b) are similar. Thus, experiments both on the frog and human retina indicate that for low stimulus intensities the response increases with an increase in the area of the stimulus until a maximal increase is reached for moderate intensities; for high stimulus intensities, the number of impulses in the response declines with an increase of the area of the stimulus. Hence, psychophysiological experiments demonstrate that inhibitory processes develop as a result of increased illumination of the retina.

The experimental curves based on discharges of the frog's ganglion cells and the experimental data in man were concordant only if the number of impulses in the on- and off-response was taken as a criterion of the response of the ganglion cells. Calculations based on the initial or final discharge rate or on the magnitude of an average interval between impulses did not reveal any concordancies. Hence, it may be assumed that the level of excitation (information about brightness) is coded by the number of impulses in the response.

Hypothesis Concerning the Functional Organization of the Receptive Field

The following conclusions may be drawn on the basis of all available data. (1) The inhibitory process in the receptive field develops more slowly than the excitatory process. (2) With an increase of the area and intensity of the stimulus, the time constant of the inhibitory process decreases. This leads to a decrease in the number of discharges and a decrease in the spike-train duration. (3) The excitatory process is balanced by the inhibitory process. (4) The level of excitation of a receptive field is signaled by the number of impulses in the on- or off-responses.

The hypothesis expressed in these four conclusions [14, 15] explains all the experimental data and above all the fact that for a receptive field summation occurs when the stimulus intensity is low, and inhibition when the intensity is high. This hypothesis is further corroborated by experiments with an electronic model of the receptive field which reproduces the correlations and changes in the time constants of the excitatory and inhibitory processes and in the weights to be given to them under different conditions [28].

Apparently, the mechanisms which are responsible for the functional organization of the on-field are similar to those of the off-field. It follows from Figs. 1(a) and 1(b) that both the on- and the off-fields are capable of functional reconstruction depending on the illumination and area of the stimulus.* Data in Fig. 6 show that, when the retina is excited by light stimuli of short duration, no inhibitory process is demonstrable in the on- or off-fields in terms of spike counts. On the other hand, data in Fig. 4 demonstrate some differences in the latent periods of the on- and off-responses. Although the latency of the on-response [Fig. 4(a)] suggests that only excitation occurs, irrespective of the area and luminance of the stimulus, the latency of the off-response reveals considerable inhibitory influences for high intensities and large areas of the stimulus [Fig. 4(b)]. It should be noted that the inhibitory process influences the latency of the off-response also when brief stimuli are presented to an off-field, although the effect is substantially less pronounced than is the case for long-lasting stimuli [Fig. 10(b)]. The latency of the on-responses does not reveal any inhibitory influence for either brief or long-lasting stimuli [Fig. 10(a)]. This difference in the behavior of the latencies for the on- and off-responses is, apparently, due to different mechanisms of their origin† and does not contradict the conclusion that the inhibitory process is delayed in comparison with the excitatory process and that it does not develop for stimuli of short duration.

Thus, the receptive field is not at all preformed. The functional interaction of its elements is subject to change depending on the level of illumination of the retina when a stimulus is applied. The resulting change, due to an increase in the energy of the stimulus, is expressed in a reduction of the effective area of the receptive field (i.e., of the summation zone) and in its extension at the expense of the peripheral inhibitory zone.

According to Barlow *et al.* [3], a reorganization of the receptive field occurs during the transition from dark to light adaptation [see Fig. 2(b)]. When dark-adapted, all the receptors of the field send excitatory signals to the ganglion cell; with light adaptation, an inhibitory ring appears at the periphery of the field.

However, it may also be supposed that the functional organization of the field is given not so much by the level of adaptation as by the intensity of the stimulus. Our data show that the more intense the stimulus, the more powerful the inhibition and reorganization of the field when stimuli are applied to the dark-adapted retina. Since the threshold is higher for the light-adapted retina than for the dark-adapted, the threshold stimulus presented against a light background provokes an inhibitory effect. Such a supposition explains both the data of Barlow *et al.* [3] and those presented in this chapter.

---

* We especially examined Barlow's statement [2] concerning the absence of inhibition in the receptive off-field and came to the opposite conclusion [22, 23].

† There are some reasons to assume that direct excitatory influences provoke an on-response, whereas postinhibitory activity [20, 32] takes part in the organization of an off-response.

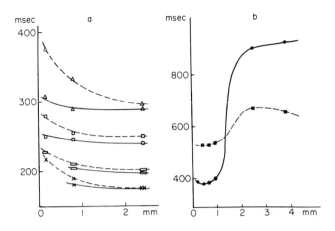

FIG. 10. Dependence of the latency of the on-response (a) and off-response (b) on the diameter of the stimulus at different intensity and duration of the latter. Duration of the stimulus: (a) 880 msec (solid lines) and 10 msec (dashed lines); (b) 240 msec (solid line) and 30 msec (dashed line). Luminance of the stimulus: (a) 110 lx (crosses), 11 lx (rectangles), 1.1 lx (squares), and 0.1 lx (triangles); (b) 900 lx (filled circles) and 90 lx (squares).

The Role of Functional Reorganization of the Receptive Field in the Processing of Visual Information

If the organization of the field is such, as discussed above, the receptive field of the retina may be viewed as a polyfunctional unit, performing a number of operations in the processing of visual information. At low levels of the light signal, summation occurs over a large area of the field. For such stimuli, the resolution of the retina is limited, but the light sensitivity due to spatial summation is great. At high intensity levels of the signal, summation occurs only over a small area of the field; however, the resolution capacity is great, since around the summation zone, there exists an inhibitory ring, and because of its presence, the contrasts are emphasized and the contours of the image are detected. The on- and off-responses and the detection of the contours are, from the point of view of information theory, highly important; they reduce the redundancy in the visual signals, since only those which change in time and space are transmitted.

Let us examine more closely the mechanism that is responsible for emphasizing the contours in the retina. Figure 11 suggests that in the region where the illumination begins to increase (field 2) there appear more inhibitory events than in field 1. This inhibition is caused by a stronger stimulation of

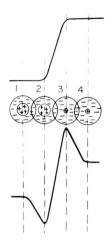

FIG. 11. Effect of emphasizing the illumination shifts in the response of the retinal receptive fields. Upper curve: distribution of illumination on the retina; lower curve: magnitude of the response of the receptive fields located in the regions where illumination changes occur.

the receptors located in the right peripheral inhibiting zone of this field. Field 3, which is located in the region where the illumination reaches a maximum, will be more excited than the right neighboring field (field 4). This is so since the left part of the field, lying in the region where the illumination is lower, exerts a weaker inhibitory influence. As a result, changes of the illumination are emphasized by dark and white Mach bands.

Experiments with a photic stimulus of short duration suggest that, for emphasis and detection of contours in man, the described mechanism is significant. It will be recalled that in the frog the response always increases with an increase of the intensity and area of a photic stimulus, if its duration is short. No inhibition is demonstrable under those conditions. In psychophysiological experiments in man [14], it was also found that the inhibitory process in the cone receptive fields is the less pronounced the shorter is the duration of the light stimulus. Our interpretation implies that the absence of inhibition in the receptive field, for stimuli of short duration, prevents emphasis of the contours. Psychophysiological investigations of the contour effect are concordant with such an interpretation. Thus, according to Thomas [31], the threshold intensity for perception of a white band declines with an increase of the exposure. Furthermore, Fiorentini [13] found that the white Mach band was subjectively well perceived when the duration of the stimulus exceeded 0.5 sec, and was not perceived at all when the exposure was less than 0.1 sec. Moreover, Matthews [25] and Novak and Sperling [26] showed that the contouring effect is pronounced when the time of exposure is 500 msec; this effect is less pronounced for a shorter duration (50 msec) and is absent for a duration of 10 msec.

Thus, there are some reasons to assume that the described interactions of the excitatory and inhibitory processes in the receptive fields of the retina are actually significant for the mechanism that is responsible for emphasizing contours.

Investigation of the Mechanisms Determining the Functional Reorganization of the Retinal Receptive Field

We still know very little about the locus at which the inhibitory regulation of the excitatory process occurs. Our data imply that this regulation takes place at different levels in the retina—both in the cells which are located peripherally to the second neuron and at the level of that neuron. Let us first consider the facts that attest to the existence of inhibitory regulation at the level of the first neuron.

We studied the positive a-wave of the IERG (Fig. 12) recorded from the receptor layer. In these experiments, we used glass micropipettes, filled with 2.75 M KCl with a tip diameter of about 1 μ. It was possible to show that

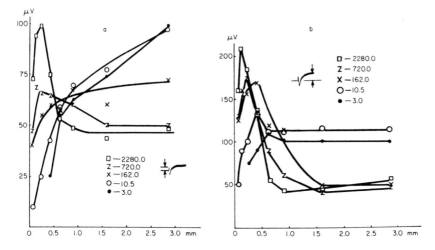

FIG. 12. Dependence of the a-wave of the IERG on the area and intensity of a light spot. Ordinate: amplitude of the response. Abscissa: diameter of the light spot. Luminance in lux is given with each symbol. Differences between graphs a and b are explained in text. The insets illustrate the method of measuring the parameters of the responses.

the area and the intensity of the photic stimulus are related in a very similar manner: to the amplitude of the IERG response, to the spike counts produced by the ganglion cells, and to the brightness estimates in psychophysiological experiments.

Figure 12 shows the relations between the *a*-wave and the area and intensity of the stimulus. The amplitude of the *a*-wave is plotted on the ordinate in Fig. 12(a). The ordinate in Fig. 12(b) plots the amplitude of the positive potential measured after the *b*-wave subsided. Both measurements apparently reflect the activity of the same cells since with a decrease in luminance, when the *b*-wave is no longer identifiable in the response, there remains a component of positive polarity whose onset corresponds to the *a*-wave of the IERG [1, 27]. However, there are some differences between the curves shown in Figs. 12(a) and 12(b). Thus, in Fig. 12(a), the amplitude of the response increases for any increase of the stimulus area for stimuli at low intensities. This is not so in Fig. 12(b), since an increase of the diameter of the photic stimulus above 0.6 mm does not lead to any further increase of the response. The curves in Fig. 12(b) presumably reveal the actual relationships. The continued increase of the amplitude with an increase of the stimulus area, as seen in Fig. 12(a), may be due to the fact that, when the area of the light spot is already large, the latency of the *b*-wave does not change, while the latency of the *a*-wave continues to decline [27]. This leads to an apparent growth of the response of the cells which generate the *a*-wave. Thus, the response of these cells is similar to that of the ganglion cells.

At present, it seems impossible to state with assurance which cells generate the *a*-wave (5, 7–10, 19, and others). It is probable that this wave reflects the activity either of the receptor cells or of the horizontal cells, or, what is most likely, of both. Of critical significance, in our view, is the fact that the inhibitory effect manifests itself at the level of the first neuron, i.e., peripheral to the bipolar cells.

Let us now turn to some other facts which imply the existence of an inhibitory process at the level peripheral to the bipolar cells, and to some time characteristics of this process. It is well known that there exists a linear relation between the amplitude of the *a*- and *b*-waves of the ERG and the logarithm of the light intensity. For IERG, such a relation is not always in evidence since for intraretinal records it is the area of the stimulus which is the essential parameter determining the amplitude of the response.

It may be shown that a semilogarithmic relation is present during the development of the response. Figure 13 shows records, at high sweep speeds, of *a*- and *b*-waves. Each wave consists of two components with different rates of growth. This implies that a new factor affecting the course of the reaction develops during the response. It must, however, be noted that two components in the *b*-wave are not observed in all experiments. This may probably be accounted for by the consideration that during summation of responses from

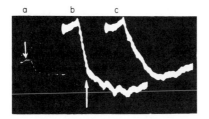

FIG. 13. Forms of the a-waves (a) and the b-waves (b, c) of the IERG. The arrows indicate the site of sharp change in the development of the response. See text for explanations.

a substantial number of cells, desynchronization may occur which would tend to smooth out the bends in the a- and b-waves.

Let us now analyze the relation of the first and the second segment of the response to the intensity of the stimulus. This can hardly be done for the a-wave, since this wave is overlapped by the b-wave. We shall therefore limit ourselves to considerations of the b-wave assuming that it follows the course of the a-wave with a certain delay. Figure 14(a) illustrates that, as a result of the action of the additional factor mentioned above, there occurs a transition from an exponential to a semilogarithmic relation. It is of interest to compare these data with the results of Brown and Watanabe [8], who showed that, when the cells of the internal nuclear layer are affected by clamping the retinal circulation, the late receptor potential markedly increases, as well as

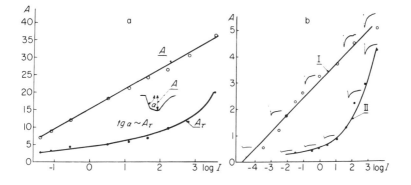

FIG. 14. Relation between b-wave and luminance. (a) Graph A_T plots the relation between the magnitude of the first phase of the b-wave and the luminance of the stimulus; graph A plots the relation between the latter and the magnitude of the second phase of the b-wave. (b) Relation between the amplitude of the b-wave and the luminance when the diameter of the light spot was 2.86 mm (I) and 0.07 mm (II), respectively. Oscillograms on which the measurements, used in the plot, were made are shown along the curves. The indifferent electrode was located in the vitreous body.

with the findings of Maffei and Svaetichin [12, 24], that under similar conditions there exists a linear relation between the receptor potential and the intensity of illumination.

A transition from an exponential to a semilogarithmic relation reflects a nonlinear transformation implying that the growth of the response slows down with an increase of illumination. Since the experiments in which spike discharges from the ganglion cells (Fig. 5) were studied indicated that there is a delayed development of an inhibitory process, we may conclude that the logarithmic transformation considered is connected with the development of the inhibitory process.

The role of the spatial factor may be analyzed in a similar way. Figure 14(b) shows the relation of the response amplitude to luminance for large and small areas of the stimulus. When the area of the stimulus is small, there exists an exponential dependence; it becomes a logarithmic one when the area of the stimulus increases. Figure 13(c) illustrates that for a small area of the spot of light, no sharp bends occur as the response develops.

Another series of experiments likewise suggests the existence of an inhibitory interaction at the prebipolar level, although in the course of these experiments, it was the *b*-wave of the ERG or IERG, the response of the

TABLE 1

Inhibitory Influence of Spot B upon the
b-Wave Produced by Neighboring Spot A[a]

Experiment No.	No. of responses of each type	A μV	B μV	A_B μV	$A - A_B$ μV
1	11	36	36	20	16
2	9	48	36	32	16
3	21	56	55	35	21
4	8	47	39	24	23
5	10	51	47	34	17
6	5	38	45	30	8
Average:		46	43	29	17

[a] Spot B was illuminated earlier

bipolar cells, which was studied. We recorded the b-wave of the ERG in response to the illumination of the retina by two light spots A and B. The recording was done with a fluid-filled microelectrode or with a platinum electrode placed in the vitreous body. We shall designate the response to the first stimulus by A and the response to the same stimulus, when a second stimulus was presented 30 sec earlier, by A_B. In order to eliminate the influence of diffused light, two light conductors with blackened side walls were placed close to the retina. The diameter of their luminous ends was 370 μ; the distance between the centers of the light spots was 2.500 μ. From Table 1, it may be seen that A is larger than A_B.

In order to make certain that the decrease of the response, when stimulus B was presented earlier, is not due to stray light from spot B reaching the part of the retina illuminated by stimulus A, the following experiment was performed. After recording the A and A_B responses, the segment of retina between both illuminated spots was resected. After such a resection, A equals A_B (Table 2). This indicates that the effect $A > A_B$ is determined by an inhibitory process.

For the purpose of recording responses from the inner nuclear layer (b-wave of the IERG), the usual light spots with a diameter of 50 μ were applied. As will be shown later, the application of such small spots reduces substantially stray light produced when a stimulus is presented. In this case also A was larger than A_B.

TABLE 2

Responses after Resection of the
Retina between Spots A and B

Experiment No.	No. of responses of each type	A μV^a	B μV	A_B μV
1	7	68	48	68
2	4	75	24	75
3	5	78	70	72
Average:		74	47	72

[a] The small deviation from the equality $A = A_B$ is not significant, since in each experiment $p > 0.1$.

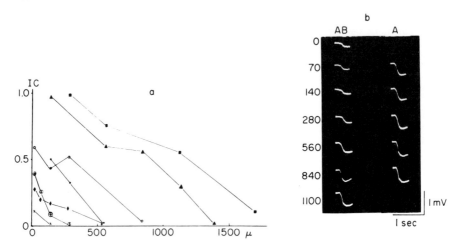

FIG. 15. Inhibitory interaction between a retinal test spot A and a background spot B illuminated 30 sec earlier. (a) Relation between the coefficient of inhibition (based on data of the b-wave of the A_B response) and the distance between spots A and B at different intensities of the spots. Intensity of the spots: A and B: 1000 lx (circles), 100 lx (filled circles), 10 lx (crosses in circle); A: 100 lx, B: 1000 lx (triangles); A: 10 lx, B: 1000 lx (squares); A: 1000 lx; B: 100 lx (diamonds); A: 1000 lx; B: 10 lx (crosses). Measurements based on microelectrode records of the b-wave from the bipolar layer of the frog's retina. (b) Relation between the amplitude of the b-wave of the A_B response and the distance between the illuminated spots. Intensity of the spots: 1000 lx.

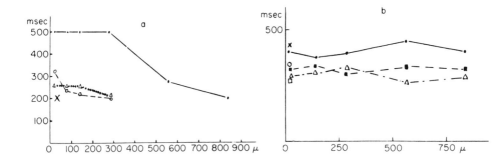

FIG. 16. Relation between the latency of the response and the distance between two retinal spots. (a) Ordinate: latency of the A_B response. The intensity of the background illumination varies. No background illumination: 1 lx (triangles); 10 lx (circles). Latency of the response to illumination of spot A alone is marked by an "X"; intensity of 1000 lx for both spots A and B (filled circles). (b) Ordinate: latency of the AB response at different intensities for spots A and B; 10 lx (filled circles), 100 lx (squares), 1000 lx (triangles). Latency of the response to illumination of spot A alone is marked by a cross for 10 lx, by a circle for 100 lx, and by a square for 1000 lx.

In our further exposition we shall use the expression "coefficient of inhibition" and define it as $IC = (A - A_B)/A$.

Figure 15 shows that the IC declines with an increase of the distance between the spots. For the intensity of the light spots of 1000 lx, the radius of the inhibitory zone was 840 μ. This zone decreased with a decrease of the intensity of both spots or only of spot B. The latency of the A_B response declined with an increase of the distance between the spots [Fig. 16(a)].

It can be shown that the influence of spot B (which was illuminated before spot A) does not result from stray light acting upon the receptors lying underneath spot A. With the aid of a photomultiplier we ascertained the characteristics of stray light caused by a spot with a diameter of 50 μ (curves 1, Fig. 17). When a foil with an opening in it (100 μ diameter) was placed in the light beam near the cathode of the photomultiplier, the characteristics of the stray light were as shown in curves 2 in Fig. 17. In order to explore the effect of stray light in the transparent media of the retina, an isolated retina was placed on the cathode of the photomultiplier. The characteristics did not show any essential changes.

Let us define the effective area of the light spot, i.e., that area of the retina under the spot which substantially contributes to the response. With this aim in view, we carried out the following experiments. We recorded responses from spot A which was illuminated through an opening 100 μ in diameter in a piece of foil placed in the vitreous body. We compared such responses when the light spot with or without a mask was at different distances from the

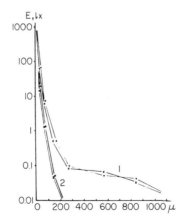

FIG. 17. Intensity of diffused light at different distance from the edge of a light spot 50 μ in diameter. 1, curves obtained without a mask; 2, curves obtained with a mask. Curves obtained when no retina present (filled circles); with the retina (crosses). For measurements of the intensity of diffused light with a mask, the latter was placed on the retina.

microelectrode. In either case, the magnitudes of the responses were equal. This indicates that stray light from a spot with a diameter of 50 μ at an intensity of 1000 lx, when blocked by a mask, does not contribute to the response. But what contribution to the response is made by the stray light under the mask (curves 2, Fig. 17)? In other words, what is the actual effective area of the light spot?

In order to determine the effective area, it is necessary to know the threshold intensity for it. Since this is not known, we shall determine first the threshold intensity for a light spot, 840 μ in diameter (Fig. 18), which obviously exceeds the effective area. The latter cannot be larger than a retinal disc 400 μ in diameter, since the contributing stray light from a ring, whose inner diameter is over 100 μ, is cut off by the mask. For a spot with a diameter of 840 μ, the threshold intensity is 0.1 lx. At this intensity (curves 2, Fig. 17), the diameter of the effective area is 250 μ. The above considerations make it clear that this size is substantially overstated. Still, for the sake of argument, we shall accept it.

Knowledge of the effective area of the test spot permits determination of whether it is the inhibition caused by the neighboring spot or the stray light that causes the decline of the response.

Special experiments were performed in which the relation between the amplitude of the response A (*b*-wave of the IERG) and the diameter of the background spot was ascertained (Fig. 19). We recorded responses to illumination of spot A with photic stimuli 50 μ in diameter and 1000 lx intensity when the background spot was illuminated earlier. The center points of the test and background spots coincided and the tip of the microelectrode was

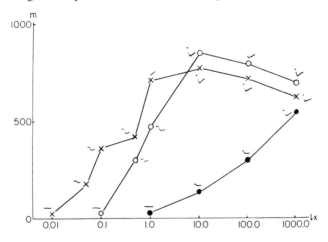

FIG. 18. Relation between the amplitude of the response and the intensity of test spots of different sizes. Diameter of the test spot: 50 μ (filled circles), 840 μ (circles), 2000 μ (crosses).

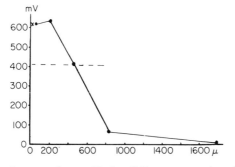

FIG. 19. Relation between the amplitude of the response A and the diameter of a background spot. Dashed line: amplitude of the A_B response; cross indicates response A with no background illumination; solid line: response A when the background spot is illuminated before spot A.

also placed in the center. The intensity of the background spot was 0.5 lx i.e., it was equal to the intensity of the diffused light which was generated by light spot B at a distance of 150 μ from spot A. We chose this distance because the maximal inhibitory effect was observed precisely under these conditions. The diameter of the background spot varied between 50 and 2000 μ. As can be seen from Fig. 19, a background spot with a diameter of 300 μ does not practically change the response A.

Table 3 contains data from three experiments (the diameter of the background spot corresponded to 220 and 310 μ), similar to those which are shown in Fig. 19. From these data, it follows that $A = A_{back}$ ($p > 0.1$), while $A > A_B$ ($p < 0.001$).

Another important consideration, which indicates that the observed effects are not due to the action of stray light, is as follows. If the decrease of the response were due to the action of stray light, then, with an increase of the background spot until that spot becomes equal to the effective area of spot A, no further decrease of the response should occur. But the data in Fig. 19 show that, with an increase of the diameter of the background spot to 300 μ and over, the response sharply declines. This is another convincing proof of adaptation which is caused by the action of inhibitory influences originating in the neighborhood of the bipolar cells, and not by the influence of the stray light from spot B acting on the receptors lying under spot A.

It is of interest to compare our data with the results of Westheimer [35] and Teller et al. [30] in their psychophysiological experiments. In these experiments, they projected a small test light on the retina and determined its threshold intensity as a function of the dimension of the background spot. Teller et al., unlike Westheimer, performed their experiments on an immobilized eye. They found that an increase of the background spot to 40 - 45 min

TABLE 3

Influence of Background Light and
Neighboring Spot upon Response

Experiment No.	No. of responses of each type	A μV^a	A_B μV	A_{back} μV
1	14	730	570	700
2	6	860	700	800
3	12	545	385	490

[a] A: Amplitude of the responses to illumination of spot A with a stimulus 50 μ in diameter of 1000 lx intensity. A_B: Amplitude of the responses to illumination of spot A when spot B, at a distance of 150 μ from the edge of spot A, was illuminated earlier. The intensity and area of the stimulus are the same for spots B and A. A_{back}: Amplitude of the response to the illumination of spot A when the background spot was illuminated earlier. Diameter of stimulus for background spot B was in the first experiment 220 μ; in the second and third experiment 210 μ. Intensity was approximately 0.5 lx. The difference between responses A_B and A_{back} is highly significant, since $p < 0.001$.

resulted in a rise of the threshold, while its further increase led to a decline of the threshold values. According to their experiments, the rise in threshold was due to the adaptation of the summation zone of the receptive field. With further increase of the background spot, the inhibitory ring was stimulated by the background light, the adaptation influence of the background spot was thus suppressed and the threshold of the test spot declined.

In our experiments, an increase of the background spot resulted only in a decrease of the response to the illumination of the test spot; in other words, we recorded the response not from one receptive field but from several overlapping fields.

Our data show that there exists inhibition which spreads from a constantly illuminated part of the retina to the neighboring nonilluminated parts. If the inhibition were to occur on the bipolar cell level (from bipolar to bipolar), then the inhibitory influence of the light spot, upon the response provoked by the neighboring spot, would manifest itself only during the development of the response of the bipolars and would disappear upon completion of the response. In reality, however, the inhibition acts as long as the light is on. Consequently, it develops in those cells where the response is sustained during the entire period of illumination (receptors and horizontal cells).

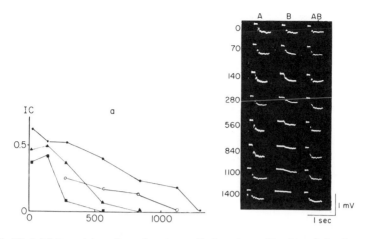

FIG. 20. Inhibitory interaction when two retinal spots are illuminated simultaneously. (a) Relation between the coefficient of inhibition and the distance between spots A and B at different intensities. A and B: 1000 lx (filled circles), 100 lx (triangles), 10 lx (squares); A: 1000 lx; B: 100 lx (circles). (b) Relation between the amplitude of the *b*-wave of the *AB* response and the distance between the spots. Intensity of the spots: 1000 lx.

Nonetheless, it is well known that lateral inhibition exists on the level of the bipolar cells [6, 21, 27, 34]. A characteristic feature of this inhibition is that it persists during the development of the response of the bipolar cells [33].

Experiments were performed in which spots A and B were illuminated simultaneously. The results are presented in Fig. 20. The plot graphs the value of the coefficient of inhibition (*IC*) [calculated according to the formula $IC = (A + B - AB) / (A + B)$ against the distance between the spots. The radius of the zone of inhibitory interaction is 1400 μ when stimuli were 50 μ in diameter at an intensity of 1000 lx. This zone decreases with the decrease of the intensity of the stimuli. In contrast to the A_B response [see Fig. 16(b)], the latency of the *AB* response did not change as a function of the distance between the spots.

Let us now summarize the basic results obtained.

1. The inhibitory influence produced by a light spot which is turned on earlier than the other spot persists during the whole period of illumination. This influence can be exerted only by cells whose response lasts as long as the retina is illuminated. Since the horizontal and receptor cells are such cells, it is assumed that the inhibitory influence considered originates at that level of the retina. However, when both light spots are presented simultaneously, inhibition arises which manifests itself only during the response of the bipolar cells. It is concluded that this type of inhibition develops at the bipolar cell level.

2. When the light spots are presented simultaneously, the zone of inhibition is considerably larger (its radius equals 1400 μ) than the zone of inhibition when one photic stimulus spot precedes the other (its radius equals 800 μ). This indicates that the two inhibitory processes considered are produced by different mechanisms.

3. Since the latency of the response A_B changes as a function of the distance between the spots, while the latency of the response AB shows no change at all, the following is assumed. When one of the light spots is presented earlier, inhibition develops at the level of the receptors and horizontal cells. If this is so, potentials of different values impinging upon the bipolar cell determine different values of the latency of the response. However, inhibition originating in one bipolar cell and acting on another does not change the latency of the response AB, since the inhibitory signal from a neighboring bipolar cannot arrive before the response begins.

All the observations indicate, in our view, that the inhibitory regulation of the excitatory process is controlled by different mechanisms at different levels of the retina. The organization of the inhibitory processes is shown in a hypothetical scheme (Fig. 21).

Excitation, arising in the neural segments of the receptors and transmitted to the bipolars, is regulated by an inhibitory influence generated by the horizontal cells. Some authors have advanced different hypotheses concerning this mechanism [11, 29]. It is supposed that excitation of the horizontal or glial cells hampers, in a metabolic or an electrical way, the transmission of excitation from the receptor to the bipolar cell.

Thus, a response, which is a resultant of two opposite processes, arises in the first link of the chain [Fig. 21(b)]. This reaction develops according to the on-response type, although it is actually formed by two responses, each of which is sustained during the whole period of illumination. The responses are the late receptor potential and the S potential (or response of the horizontal cells). The character of the response transmitted from the receptor to the

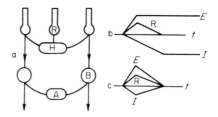

FIG. 21. Scheme illustrating the interaction of the excitatory (E) and inhibitory (I) processes in the retina. (a) Scheme of the junction of neural elements in the retina. R, Receptors; H, horizontal cells; B, bipolar cells; A, Amacrine cells. (b) Scheme of interaction at the level of the receptors and horizontal cells. (c) Scheme of interaction at the level of the bipolar cells.

bipolar cells is determined by the time constants of the excitatory and inhibitory processes. The latter, in turn, are determined by the intensity of the light stimulus as well as by its area and duration.

The response formed on the level of the first neuron arrives at the bipolar cells, where it may be transformed by signals from the neighboring bipolar cells [Fig. 21(c)].

It is of interest to compare these conclusions with that of Barlow and Andrews [2a] made on the basis of psychophysiological data. The authors conclude that the "adaptation pool" was smaller in magnitude than the "summation pool" and that it was located peripheral to the latter.

REFERENCES

1. Arden, G. B., and Brown, K. T. Some properties of components of the cat electroretinogram revealed by local recording under oil. *J. Physiol. (London)* **176**, 429-461 (1965).
2. Barlow, H. B. Summation and inhibition in the frog's retina. *J. Physiol. (London)* **119**, 69-88 (1953).
2a. Barlow, H. B., and Andrews, D. P. Sensitivity of receptors and receptor "pools." *J. Opt. Soc. Amer.* **57**, 837-838 (1967).
3. Barlow, H. B., Fitzhugh, R., and Kuffler, S. W. Change of organization in the receptive fields of the cat's retina during dark adaptation. *J. Physiol. (London)* **137**, 338-354 (1957).
4. Bertulis, A. V. Functional reorganization of the receptive fields of the frog's retina as a result of changes in the intensity and area of the light stimulus. *Biophysics (USSR)* **11**, 314-320 (1966) (in Russian).
5. Bortoff, A. Localization of slow potential responses in the necturus retina. *Vision Res.* **4**, 627-635 (1964).
6. Brindley, G. S. Responses to illumination recorded by microelectrodes from the frog's retina. *J. Physiol. (London)* **134**, 360-384 (1956).
7. Brown, K. T., and Murakami, M. A new receptor potential of the monkey retina with no detectable latency. *Nature (London)* **134**, 360-384 (1956).
8. Brown, K. T., and Watanabe, K. Isolation and identification of a receptor potential from the pure cone fovea of the monkey retina. *Nature (London)* **193**, 958-960 (1962a).
9. Brown, K. T., and Wiesel, T. N. Localization of origins of electroretinogram components by intraretinal recording in the intact cat eye. *J. Physiol. (London)* **158**, 257-280 (1961).
10. Byzov, A. L. Origin and some properties of the P. III component of the frog's electroretinogram. *Sechenov Physiol. J. USSR* **49**, 440-448 (1963) (in Russian).
11. Byzov, A. L. Horizontal cells of the retina as regulators of synaptic transmission. *Sechenov Physiol. J. USSR* **53**, 1115-1124 (1967) (in Russian).
12. Fatehchand, R., Laufer, M., and Svaetichin, G. Retinal receptor potentials and their linear relationship to light intensity. *Science* **137**, 666-667 (1962).
13. Fiorentini, A. Influence d'un gradient d'ecloirment retinen et de ses variations sur la sensation. "Problems in Contemporary Optics," pp. 600-603. Arcetri, Florence, 1955.

14. Glezer, V. D. The receptive fields of the retina. Dissertation, Leningrad, 1962 (in Russian).
15. Glezer, V. D. The receptive fields of the retina. *Vision Res.* 5, 497-525 (1965).
16. Glezer, V. D. "Mechanisms of Identification of Visual Images." Nauka, Leningrad, 1966 (in Russian).
17. Glezer, V. D., and Bertulis, A. V. On the functional reorganization of the retinal receptive field. *Probl. Physiol. Opt.* 14, 5-9 (1967) (in Russian).
18. Glezer, V. D., Zyazina, Z. N., and Smolenskaya, L. N. Concerning changes in the human foveal fields. *Biophysics (USSR)* 7, 486-488 (1962) (in Russian).
19. Granit, R. The components of the retinal action potential and their relation to the discharge in the optic nerve. *J. Physiol. (London)* 77, 207-239 (1933).
20. Granit, R. "Sensory Mechanisms of the Retina." Oxford Univ. Press, London, 1947.
21. Granit, R., Rubinstein, B., and Therman, P. O. A new type of interaction experiment with retinal action potential. *J. Physiol. (London)* 85, 34-36 (1935).
22. Kostelyanets, N. B. Investigation of receptive off-fields of frog retina by means of dark moving stimuli. *Fed. Proc.* 25 (Part 2), 377-380 (1966).
23. Kostelyanets, N. B. Inhibition in the receptive off-field of the frog's retina. *Probl. Physiol. Opt.* 14, 10-19 (1967) (in Russian).
24. Maffei, L., and Poppele, R. E. Frequency analysis of the late receptor potential. *J. Neurophysiol.* 30, 993-999 (1967).
25. Mathews, M. L. Appearance of Mach bands for short duration and at sharply focused contours. *J. Opt. Soc. Amer.* 56, 1401-1402 (1966).
26. Novak, S., and Sperling, G. Visual threshold near a continuously visible or a briefly prevented lightdark boundary. *Opt. Acta* 10, 187-191 (1963).
27. Podvigin, N. F. Analysis of the IERG of the frog's retina. *Probl. Physiol. Opt.* 13, 5-29 (1966) (in Russian).
28. Shetalov, I. N. Electronic model of the retina. *Probl. Physiol. Opt.* 13, 142-149 (1966) (in Russian).
29. Svaetichin, G., Laufer, M., Mitarai, G., Fatehchand, R., Vallecalle, E., and Villegas, J. Glial control of neuronal networks and receptors. *In* "The Visual System: Neurophysiology and Psychophysics." (R. Jung and H. Kornhuber, eds.), pp. 445-456. Springer, Berlin, 1961.
30. Teller, D. Y., Andrews, D. P., and Barlow, H. B. Local adaptation in stabilized vision. *Vision Res.* 6, 701-706 (1966).
31. Thomas, J. P. Threshold measurement of Mach bands. *J. Opt. Soc. Amer.* 55, 521-524 (1965).
32. Tomita, T., Murakami, M., Hashimoto, I., and Sasaki, S. Electrical activity of single neurons in the frog's regina. *In* "The Visual System: Neurophysiology and Psychophysics." (R. Jung and H. Kornhuber, eds.), pp. 24-30. Springer, Berlin, 1961.
33. Zenkin, T. M., and Maksimov, V. V. Investigation of the horizontal interaction on the level of slow bipolars of the frog's retina. *Biophysics (USSR)* 9, 718-725 (1964) (in Russian).
34. Zenkin, T. M., Maksimov, V. V., and Byzov, A. L. Investigation of the horizontal interaction on the level of slow bipolars of the frog's retina. *Biophysics (USSR)* 9, 612-620 (1964) (in Russian).
35. Westheimer, G. Spatial interaction in the human retina during scotopic vision. *J. Physiol. (London)* 181, 881-894 (1965).

3
Cyclic Changes in the Activity of Neurons in the Visual Cortex after Brief Stimulation

I. N. Kondratjeva*

Following transient stimuli, whose duration is about 1 msec, a series of events may develop in a cortical neuronal chain that may last scores and even hundreds of milliseconds. Excitation spreads along the neurons—possibly within the limits of the functional columns of neurons situated along the vertical plane—and is transmitted to other cortical zones [15, 24, 27]. Simultaneously, in the visual area of the cortex, the primary evoked potential is followed by a series of subsequent oscillations of the potential [3, 29, and others]. For many neurons, the initial spike activity is followed in a cyclic manner by a pause, then by a subsequent activation and a new inhibition [4, 12, 14, 18, 30, 33, and others]. It has been shown that the excitability of the cortex passes through several stages—an initial increase is followed by a depression, and this by a new increase [2, 6, 19, 29, 30, and others].

The purpose of the present work was to explore whether there exists a relation between the excitability changes of the cortex, the evoked potentials, and the impulse activity of the cortical neurons following the stimulus, and, if so, what mechanisms cause these events. The experiments were carried out on unanesthetized animals since some authors [28] believe that certain changes (e.g., the phase of depression) following a stimulus are due to anesthesia.

Methods

The experiments were performed on gently restrained unanesthetized rabbits. We studied impulse activity and evoked potentials in an intact visual area

*Deceased.

of the cortex and in a neurally isolated cortical slab, 5×10 mm in size, prepared according to the method of Cholodov [9]. The micromanipulator of Melechova and Dyakonov was attached during the experiment to the exposed bone of the skull, and a microelectrode (a glass capillary with a tip diameter of 1 to 2 μ, and resistance of 1 to 15 MΩ) was inserted into an opening made in the bone underlying the visual area. The microelectrode was connected in parallel to two cathode followers and two amplifiers. One of them with a bandpass of 0.1 to 80 Hz registered evoked potentials; the other with a bandpass of 150 to 5000 Hz registered unit activity. The potentials were displayed on the tube face of the oscilloscope for photography. A flash of a phototube with a duration of about 1 msec (energy of the flash, 0.4 J) served as a stimulus. Flashes were presented singly or rhythmically once per second, or as double flashes at intervals of 20 to 150 msec. The neurally isolated slab was stimulated through a bipolar nichrom electrode (diameter, 100 μ; interelectrode distance, 150 μ) which was inserted to a depth of 1800 μ. Stimuli of 0.05 to 0.5 msec in duration (7 to 20 V) were generated by a "Physiovar" stimulator with an attachment which prevented the occurrence of artifacts. The stimulation frequency was one stimulus per 1 or 5 sec, or once every 2 min. In some cases, a pair of stimuli was applied at intervals of 20 to 2000 msec. Studies on the cortical slab were carried out for some 8 to 24 hr after the isolation. The success of the isolation of the slab was checked by histological studies.

The data pertain to studies on 70 rabbits. In the course of the study, the activity of 500 neurons was examined.

Results and Discussion

A number of oscillations may be recorded from the surface of the visual cortex of a wakeful rabbit in response to a flash of light—a primary response (an early positive wave and a negative oscillation) and a secondary or late response [a fast positive wave (FPW), a slow negative oscillation (SNW), and a slow positive wave (SPW)]. These events may be followed by another series of SNW and SPW. All these waves invert in the depth of the cortex. What is the cause of these oscillations of the potentials?

Following a flash one can observe, apart from neurons which do not react to the stimulus, cells which react initially with inhibition of discharges or neurons which become initially active (a detailed description of spike activity in unanesthetized rabbits was presented by Kondratjeva [18], Polyansky [30], and Kondratjeva and Volodin [21]). The latent periods for activity of most neurons fluctuate between 20 and 80 msec. For many neurons a period of activity is followed (25 to 120 msec later) by a silent pause; this pause is followed after 120 to 240 msec by a new activation with subsequent inhibi-

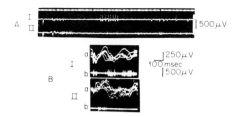

FIG. 1. Various reactions of neurons of the visual cortex and evoked potentials in response to a flash of light. (A) I: discharges of a neuron at depth of 1030 μ; II: discharges of a neuron at depth of 2030 μ. Each oval spot: 10 msec. Arrows indicate the time of flash occurrence. (B) Ia and IIa: surface-evoked potentials (negative deflection is up); Ib: discharges of a neuron at depth of 1350 μ; IIb: discharges of a neuron at depth of 1470 μ. Flash starts the sweep on the oscilloscope.

tion, and so on. Some cells (about 2%) have a longer latent period to the first activation (about 50 to 100 msec), and a high discharge rate occurs for them [Fig. 1(aII, bII)] precisely at a time at which a silent pause is observed for most other neurons [Fig. 1(aI, bI)]. It is possible that these cells are internuncial inhibitory neurons which are responsible for the occurrence of the inhibitory pause (see below). For most neurons the response periods occur at definite intervals after the application of the stimulus. Because of that, an average poststimulus histogram for many neurons in the visual cortex clearly reflects all phases of the response, namely, activation, diminished activity, and activation again [18].

If one compares average poststimulus histograms of many neurons with the oscillations of the evoked potentials, it transpires that the primary response and the FPW coincide in time with the first activation of the neurons; a diminution in spike activity—for many neurons a silent pause—occurs during a slow surface-negative oscillation, while the resumption of activity takes place during a slow positive wave. These correlations are particularly clear when impulse and slow activity are recorded simultaneously by the same microelectrode. Primary spike activity may be observed during the primary response and during a fast depth-negative wave of the secondary potential. For most responsive neurons (except for those which have been related by us to inhibitory neurons), a pause in spike activity is observed during a slow depth-positive wave and a slow surface-negative oscillation [Fig. 1(BI)].

Application of paired stimuli indicates that, when a test stimulus is applied during the silent pause, especially during its first half, which corresponds in time to the time at which the ascending part of a surface-negative wave occurs, there is no reaction to a test stimulus (Fig. 2). With an increase of the interval between the stimuli, a response to a test stimulus appears, and, when this interval is 120 to 180 msec (in Fig. 2, it is 135 msec), the response begins to exceed the values for the response to the conditioning stimulus. It is

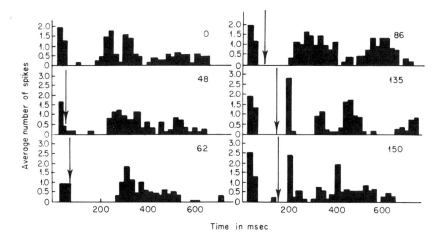

FIG. 2. Histograms showing the distributions of spikes for neurons (depth: 1150 μ) in the visual cortex in response to a flash or a pair of flashes. Ordinate: average number of spikes in the stated bin. Abscissa: time in milliseconds; each bin = 20 msec. Histograms based on responses to 10 flashes. Time of application of the first flash coincides with the origin of the ordinate; arrows indicate the time of presentation of the second flash. Numbers on the right indicate intervals between the stimuli in milliseconds.

noteworthy that for an interval of 60 to 70 msec (in Fig. 2, it is 62 msec) no spike activity occurs in response to a test stimulus, but the inhibitory pause becomes longer. This observation implies the existence of two different pathways that respectively, affect the activation and the impulse pause of a neuron. For the case considered, the excitatory pathway appears blocked, while the inhibitory one is still active; thus, a summation of the inhibitory processes can occur. We have shown that the recovery cycles for the spike responses after a conditioning stimulus and those for evoked potentials are very similar (29).

Since during the silent pause neurons are less excitable and since the activity of the neuron and the silent pause are influenced by separate pathways (the latent periods to the first activation and to the pause [18] are not correlated and the two pathways are not blocked simultaneously), we assumed that the silent pause is caused by an inhibitory process. It was likewise assumed that the slow (depth-positive) wave, which coincides in time with the pause, reflects a hyperpolarization of the membranes of the cell bodies, and that this hyperpolarization is an inhibitory postsynaptic potential (IPSP). Using intracellular electrodes, it was recently established that the silent pause after afferent stimuli corresponds to an IPSP [13, 32, 34].

Thus, in the activity provoked by a stimulus a relation exists between the impulse activity of the neurons, the oscillations of the evoked potential, and the fluctuations in the excitability of the cortical neurons. This becomes particularly clear when certain drugs are used. When, for example, small doses of sodium pentobarbital (25 to 30 mg/kg) are administered to rabbits, there occurs a marked diminution of the slow surface-negative (depth-positive) wave evoked by a flash; at the same time, the silent pause and the period of depression in the recovery cycle after a conditioning stimulus become shorter [20].

The following questions may be asked: What factors determine the fluctuations in activity of the cortical neurons after afferent stimuli? What role may be played by the cortical processes themselves and what may be the influence of the subcortical formations?

A neurally isolated cortical slab makes it possible to exclude any extracortical influences. While working with such a slab, we stimulated electrically the deep cortical layers (1800 μ) and recorded the evoked potentials and responses of cortical neurons. In records from the surface, the evoked potential consisted of a positive or a positive-negative wave; in records from depth, the potential was a negative or a negative-positive wave. These findings agree with those of Susuki and Ochs [31]. After the initial complex, we observed also another series of waves which differed in sign.

In an isolated slab of the cortex, in addition to nonreactive neurons, there were cells which were initially inhibited by the stimulus and cells which were initially activated. In most cases, the cells were silent. The state of the responsive neurons in the isolated slab changed after the stimulus application for a considerable period of time and the character of these changes depended on the time that passed after the operation. During the first 6 to 7 hr after the isolation, the reaction of the neurons which responded with initial excitation consisted only of the activation phase. However, after an initial excitation of the neuron its excitability did not return to the original level. This was clearly shown by application of test stimuli. The excitability was substantially increased for 100 to 200 msec after the stimulation. The neuron responded to a second stimulus with a shorter latent period and with a larger number of spikes (Fig. 3). Six to 12 hr after the isolation, and sometimes even 24 hr after it, a second burst of activity was recorded following an initial phase of activation; it was separated from the first one by a silent pause. In contrast to observations during the first hours after isolation, the neurons did not react now to the test stimulus for some 200 to 400 msec (in Fig. 4, 342 msec). As is the case in the intact cortex in response to a flash, one could observe a summation of the inhibitory processes when the stimuli were delivered at specific intervals (in Fig. 4, 32 and 50 msec). A decline or absence of the response to a test stimulus was observed also for the evoked potentials (Fig. 5); the descending part of a depth-positive wave corresponded to the silent pause and to the period of ineffectiveness of the test stimulus. In most cases we observed reactions 24 hr after isolation, in which the initial phase of activation was followed by a protracted time during which there was no spike,

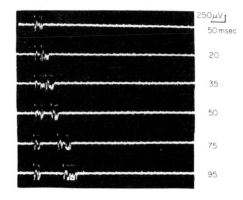

FIG. 3. Responses of a neuron at a depth of 920 μ in an isolated slab of the cortex in a state of heightened excitability after the first phase of activation. Stimulus artifact identified by a white dot. Numbers on the right indicate time intervals in milliseconds between two stimuli.

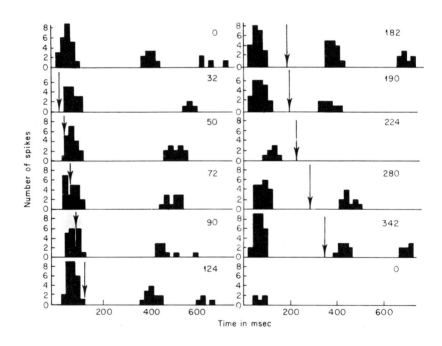

FIG. 4. Poststimulus histograms for polyphasic unit responses in an isolated slab of the cortex (depth: 1230 μ). Responses to two electric stimuli at various intervals. Ordinate: number of spikes in a bin; bin = 20 msec. See legend for Fig. 2 for further explanations.

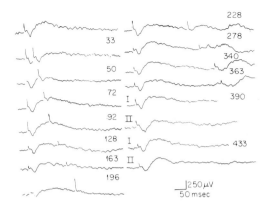

FIG. 5. Modifications of evoked potentials (depth: 900 μ) in response to two electrical stimuli at various intervals. Spike activity for this preparation is shown in Fig. 4. Stimulus artifacts indicate the time of stimulation. Positive deflection is up. See legend for Fig. 3 for further explanations.

or slow potential, response to the test stimulus (about 1.3 sec in Fig. 6). The absence of any response after the stimulus was not accompanied by distinct slow oscillations.

Thus, changes in the state of the neurons after a stimulus in the isolated slab of the cortex persist for a long time just as they do in the intact cortex.

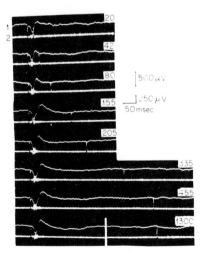

FIG. 6. Neural activity in an isolated slab of the cortex and modifications of the evoked potential (depth: 1020 μ) with protracted inhibition after activation. Curve 1: evoked potential (positive deflection is up); curve 2: impulse activity of the neuron. Stimulus artifacts indicate the time of stimulation. Numbers on the right indicate time intervals between the stimuli.

However, the excitability differs depending on the time which elapsed after isolation. The presence of polyphasic unit responses [1] in the neurally isolated slab, 6 to 12 hr after the operation, probably indicates that in the cortex itself there are some cells which cause inhibition. This conclusion is in agreement with the data of Burns [7], Creutzfeldt and Struck [10], and Krnjević et al. [22, 23].* It is probable that the inhibition is provoked by those neurons which are activated during the silent pause of other neurons (Fig. 1). Some workers failed to observe these presumably inhibitory cells [23, 34]. It is likely that the internuncial inhibitory neurons are small and hence difficult to isolate with the microelectrode. During the surgical isolation of the cortex, these neurons possibly suffer most from the operative trauma. In any case, a postexcitatory inhibition is absent during the first hours after isolation and there is even a protracted increase of excitability. The prolonged absence of spike responses to a test stimulus, in an isolated slab of the cortex 24 hr after the operation, and the lack of any oscillations in the slow potential are very similar to the inhibition which occurs after large doses of barbiturates [5, 16, 26]. It is possible that this inhibition is determined by metabolic changes.

In the intact cortex, the postexcitatory inhibition is followed by a second period of spike activity and by a surface-positive slow wave of the evoked response. Two interpretations have been proposed regarding the origin of this activity. Some authors believe that it is determined by afferent inflow from the thalamus [8, 11]. It may be assumed, however, on the basis of work on thalamic neurons [1], that this period of activity is determined by a postanodal rebound which occurs after hyperpolarization of the membrane. In the responses of neurons in an isolated cortical slab, the second period of activation was observed only when the first activity period was followed by an inhibition, whose duration was not more than 400 msec and by a depth-positive wave. If after the primary response the excitability was increased, or if the inhibitory period was protracted and was not accompanied by oscillations of the slow potential, the second period of activation did not occur at all. Consequently, it may be supposed that a synaptic inhibitory process plays a role in the genesis of the second period of activation. However, the influence of subcortical formations cannot be excluded since sometimes it could be observed in the isolated slab that the slow surface-negative wave in the evoked response was not followed by a positive oscillation (Fig. 5).

What is the significance of these prolonged reactions in the functioning of the central nervous system? As is known, these reactions are most pronounced when the stimulus is very intense [20, 22, 30]. Hence, it may be assumed that the postexcitatory inhibition limits the avalanche-like spread of excitation

---

* Experiments, with stimulation of deep layers and intracellular recordings, on the intact cortex are needed in order to compare the inhibitory processes in an isolated slab with those in the intact cortex. No such data are available at present.

in the cortex [17, 25]. However, this problem requires further experimental work pertaining to the postexcitatory states of the neurons during the behavioral reactions of animals.

REFERENCES

1. Andersen, P., Eccles, J. C., and Sears, T. A. The ventrobasal complex of the thalamus: types of cells, their responses and their functional organization. *J. Physiol. (London)* 174, 370-399 (1964).
2. Bartley, S. H. Temporal and spatial summation of extrinsic impulses with the intrinsic activity of the cortex. *J. Cell Comp. Physiol.* 8, 41-62 (1936).
3. Bartley, S. H., O'Leary, J., and Bishop, G. H. Differentiation by strychnine of the visual from the integrating mechanisms of the optic cortex in the rabbit. *Amer. J. Physiol.* 120, 604-618 (1937).
4. Baumgartner, G. Reaktionen einzelner Neurone im optischen Cortex der Katze nach Lichtblitzen. *Pflueger's Arch. Gesamte Physiol. Menschen Tiere* 261, 456-469 (1955).
5. Berry, C. A., and Hance, A. J. Patterns of excitability in the cat cerebral cortex. *Electroencephalogr. Clin. Neurophysiol.* 18 124-130 (1965).
6. Bishop, G. H. Cyclic changes in excitability of the optic pathway of the rabbit. *Amer. J. Physiol.* 103, 213-224 (1933).
7. Burns, B. D. "The Mammalian Cerebral Cortex." Arnold, London, 1958.
8. Chang, H. T. The evoked potentials. *In* "Handbook of Physiology" (J. Field *et al.*, eds.), Vol. I, Sect. 1, pp. 299-313. Amer. Physiol. Soc., Washington, 1959.
9. Cholodov, J. A. "Effects of Electromagnetic and Magnetic Fields on the Central Nervous System." Nauka, Leningrad, 1966 (in Russian).
10. Creutzfeldt, O. D., and Struck, G. Neurophysiologie und Morphologie der chronisch isolierten Cortexinsel der Katze: Hirnpotentiale und Neuronentätigkeit einer isolierten Nervenzellpopulation ohne Afferente Fasern. *Arch. Psychiatr. Z. Gesamte Neurol.* 203, 708-731 (1962).
11. Eccles, J. C. Inhibition in thalamic and cortical neurones and its role in phasing neuronal discharges. *Epilepsia* 6, 89-115 (1965).
12. Fromm, G. H., and Bond, W. Further observations on the correlation between slow changes in the EEG and cortical neuron activity. *Electroencephalogr. Clin. Neurophsiol.* 18, 520[A] (1965).
13. Fuster, J. M., Creutzfeldt, O. D., and Straschiel, M. Intracellular recording of neuronal activity in the visual system. *Z. Vergl. Physiol.* 49, 605-622 (1965).
14. Grützner, A., Grüsser, O.-J., and Baumgartner, G. Reaktonen einzelner Neurone im optischen Cortex der Katze nach elektrischer Reizung des Nervus opticus. *Arch. Psychiat. Z. Gesamte Neurol.* 197, 377-404 (1958).
15. Hubel, D. H., and Wiesel, T. N. Receptive fields and functional architecture in two nonstriate visual areas (18 and 19) of the cat. *J. Neurophysiol.* 28 229-289 (1955).
16. Jarcho, L. W. Excitability of cortical afferent systems during barbiturate anesthesia. *J. Neurophysiol.* 12, 447-457 (1949).
17. Jung, R., and Baumgartner, G. Hemmungsmechanismen und bremsende Stabilisierung an einzelnen Neuronen des optischen Cortex. *Pflueger's Arch. Gesamte Physiol.* 261, 434-456 (1955).
18. Kondratjeva, I. N. On the inhibition of neurons in the visual cortex. *J. Higher Nervous Activity (USSR)* 14, 1069-1078 (1964) (in Russian).

19. Kondratjeva, I. N. On inhibition in the neuronal systems of visual cortex. *In* "The Problems of Neurocybernetics," Abstr. Rep. 2nd Int. Conf. Neurocybernetics, p. 52. Rostov State University Press, 1965 (in Russian).

20. Kondratjeva, I. N. Cyclic changes in cortical neuronal activity after short-duration stimuli. *In* "Contemporary Problems of Electrophysiology of Central Nervous System," pp. 148-159. Nauka, Moscow, 1967 (in Russian).

21. Kondratjeva, I. N., and Volodin, B. I. Recovery cycles of neuron responses to flashes in the visual area of the cerebral cortex in rabbits. *J. Higher Nervous Activity (USSR)* **16**, 874-881 (1961) (in Russian).

22. Krnjević, K., Randić M., and Straughan, D. W. An inhibitory process in the cerebral cortex. *J. Physiol. (London)* **184**, 16-48 (1966).

23. Krnjević, K., Randić, M., and Straughan, D. W. Nature of a cortical inhibitory process. *J. Physiol. (London)* **184**, 49-77 (1966).

24. Livanov, M. N. Neurokinetics. *In* "The Problems of Contemporary Neurophysiology," pp. 37-72. Nauka, Leningrad, 1965 (in Russian).

25. Livanov, M. N. Inhibition in neuronal systems of the cerebral cortex. *In* "Brain Reflexes." Int. Conf. Dedicated to the Centenary Celebration of I. N. Sechenov's Book, pp. 64-71. Nauka, Leningrad, 1966 (in Russian).

26. Morin, G., Gastaut, H., Naquet, R., and Roger, A. Variations du cycle d'excitabilité des aires réceptrices visuelles du chat, sous l'effet d'agents pharmacodynamiques. *J. Physiol. (Paris)* **43**, 820-824 (1951).

27. Mountcastle, V. B. Modality and topographic properties of single neurons of cat's somatic sensory cortex. *J. Neurophysiol.* **20**, 408-434 (1957).

28. Mountcastle, V. B. Some functional properties of the somatic afferent system. *In* "Sensory Communication." Contributions to the Symposium on Principles of Sensory Communication. (W. A. Rosenblith, ed.), pp. 403-436. M. I. T. Press, Cambridge, Massachusetts, 1961.

29. Pearlman, A. L. Evoked potentials of rabbit visual cortex: relationship between a slow negative potential and excitability cycle. *Electroencephalogr. Clin. Neurophysiol.* **15**, 426-434 (1963).

30. Polyansky, W. B. On the connection between spike discharges and evoked potentials in the visual cortex of the alert rabbit. *J. Higher Nervous Activity (USSR)* **15**, 903-910 (1965) (in Russian).

31. Suzuki, H., and Ochs, S. Laminal stimulation for direct cortical responses from intact and chronically isolated cortex. *Electroencephalogr. Clin. Neurophysiol.l.* **17**, 405-413 (1964).

32. Skrebitsky, V. G., and Voronin, L. L. Intracellular records of the single unit activity of the visual cortex in nonanaesthetized rabbits. *J. Higher Nervous Activity (USSR)* **16**, 864-873 (1966) (in Russian).

33. Tolkunov, B. F. Relationship between periods of activation and depression in responses of cortical neurons to electrical pulse and photic stimulation. *Sechenov Physiol. J. USSR* **51**, 286-292 (1965) (in Russian).

34. Watanabe, S., Konishi, M., and Creutzfeldt, O. D. Postsynaptic potentials in the cat's visual cortex following electrical stimulation of afferent pathways. *Exp. Brain Res.* **1**, 272-283 (1966).

4

Characteristics of Temporal Summation at Different Levels in the Visual System of the Cat

I. A. Shevelev and L. H. Hicks*

Investigations of the capacity of a sensory system to accumulate in time information about an external signal are a prerequisite for the understanding of the physiological mechanisms concerned with signal detection and discrimination. Such studies make use of sensory and electrical stimuli and utilize different criteria in evaluation of the temporal summation. Thus, many authors [2, 4, 5, 7, 8, 15, 19, 23-25] studied temporal summation in the visual system in psychophysical experiments in man, while others [1, 6, 16, 21, 28, 37] used electrophysiological criteria. As was shown for the auditory system [11-14, 18, 38], electrophysiological data permit description of some functional properties of large pools of neurons in the first moments after stimulation.

The present study compares characteristics of temporal summation at different levels of the visual synaptic chain (retina, optic tract, dorsal nucleus of the lateral geniculate body, and primary visual cortex) using threshold responses for the primary evoked potentials in anesthetized cats and single unit activity in the dorsal lateral geniculate body in unanesthetized animals.

Methods

The study of the evoked potential thresholds was done on 17 adult cats anesthetized with sodium amytal (initial dose was 70 mg/kg, given intraperito-

* Present address: Department of Psychology, Howard University, Washington, D. C.

neally). Metal electrodes were stereotaxically inserted into the optic tract and
the dorsal nucleus of the lateral geniculate body contralaterally to the stimulation; the cortical electrode was placed on the surface of the primary visual
cortical area in the posterior part of the lateral gyrus. The retinal electrode for
the electroretinogram recordings was applied to the cornea of the stimulated
eye. The positions of the deep electrodes were determined during the experiment by the evoked responses in the optic tract and the dorsal lateral
geniculate body. These positions were checked histologically after the experiment, when the brain was perfused with 10% formalin.

In 25 experiments, devoted to studies of single units, a tungsten microelectrode was stereotaxically inserted into the dorsal nucleus of the contralateral
lateral geniculate body of the unanesthetized cats relaxed by d-tubocurarine.
Neuron activity was recorded extracellularly.

For the photostimulation, a R1131C Sylvania modulation tube was used
which produced white light. Flashes were presented to the entire retina
through an opaque screen. The stimulated eye was atropinized, the other was
closed with sutures. Since the rise- and decay time of the flash were about
0.32 msec, it was necessary to introduce an intensity correction for flashes
shorter than 1 msec. Duration of the flashes was controlled by a Phisiovar
(Alvar-electronic) stimulator which had a range from 100 μsec to 250 msec.
Intensity of flashes was changed by neutral, calibrated glass filters placed in
the light beam. For convenience of calculation and display of the data, the
light intensity was expressed in relative logarithmic units (decibels).* We used
eight intensity levels which differed in steps from 3 to 8 dB. The total range
was 50 dB (1 to 100, 000).

Evoked potentials and unit activity were photographically recorded from
the screen of a four-channel Biophase-IY-2-4 (Alvar-electronic) amplifier system with a frequency band between 10 and 4000 Hz.

During the experiments, the thresholds of the evoked response in the
various regions of the visual system were determined preliminarily from the
monitor screen. A flash intensity giving a response probability near 0.7 was
taken as the threshold. The final thresholds were determined from the oscillograms independently by three observers using a ciphered code. For all data,
the curves plotting the relation of the threshold intensity for the primary
evoked potential to the duration of the flash were drawn by the least-squares
method. The reliability of the data was determined by the t-test.

Poststimulus-time histograms (PST) for different flash durations and different intensities were used to determine the threshold response of single units in
the dorsal lateral geniculate body. A stimulus was considered to be at threshold intensity for a given unit if it produced a reliable increase in the number
of its discharges.

* A change by 10 dB or by one log unit corresponds to a tenfold change in light
intensity.

During the experiment, the temperature of the animal was held constant and anesthesia was maintained at a level at which only occasional spindles occurred in the electrocorticogram. In the experiments, in which units were examined, artificial respiration was used. During the experiment, control responses to a stimulus of constant brightness and duration were recorded every 15 to 20 min. As a rule, such control responses did not substantially change with time and, thus, the desired extensive measurements on evoked responses or unit spikes could be carried out.

Results

With an increase of the signal duration from 100 μsec to 250 msec the thresholds for the evoked response at first diminished, but then stabilized at all explored levels of the visual system. However, as seen in Fig. 1, not only do the absolute thresholds differ in the various regions, but the amount of threshold decrease and the range of stimulus durations, for which this decrease occurs, differ as well. The highest thresholds for all durations were found for the retina, the lowest for the cortex; intermediate threshold values occurred for the optic tract and the dorsal lateral geniculate body responses. These differences were seen very clearly both for the first [Fig. 1(b)] and the second [Fig. 1(c)] deflection of the response.

Table 1 assembles the relevant data for the shortest flash (100 μsec). The threshold for the initial deflection in the response is 1350 times higher for the retina than for the visual cortex. The optic tract threshold, under the same conditions, is 25 times higher than that for the visual cortex; the dorsal lateral geniculate body threshold is 3.2 times higher. For flashes of 100-msec duration, the threshold differences persist, but they become smaller. Thus, threshold for the a-wave of ERG is 100 times higher than that for the cortical response; for the optic tract, it is ten times and for the dorsal lateral geniculate body only 2.2 times higher than the cortical response threshold.

The decrease in the differences between the threshold values (ΔI_t) in the various regions, when the flash is made longer, results from marked decreases in thresholds in the more peripheral regions of the analyzer, as shown in Fig. 1(b). Thus, when the flash duration was lengthened from 100 μsec to 100 msec, the threshold (for the a-wave) became 100 times lower in the retina; 45 times lower for the optic tract; 16 times lower for the dorsal lateral geniculate body; and 14 times lower for the visual cortex. Accordingly, the steepness of the sloping part of the intensity-duration curve is maximal for the retina and minimal for the visual cortex. It is possible to estimate the rate of threshold decrease by the tangent of the angle ($n = tg\alpha$) that is formed by the linear part of the curve with the abscissa. The slope of the linear part of the threshold intensity-duration curve characterizes the degree of the temporal

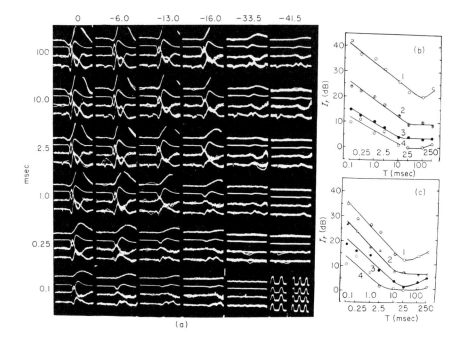

FIG. 1. Relation of the threshold of the evoked response to the intensity and duration of light flashes at different levels of the visual system in an anesthetized cat. (a) Oscillograms from experiment NC-80. Each block of four oscillograms shows successively 15 superimposed responses of retina, optic tract, dorsal lateral geniculate body, primary visual cortex. For all traces, except those for the retina, the positive deflection is down. Numbers on left indicate the duration of the flash in milliseconds. Numbers above the oscillograms indicate the intensity of light in relative log units (decibel attenuation). The maximal intensity of light available was taken as 0 dB. Calibration: 100 μV, 50 Hz. (b) and (c) Relation of the threshold intensity to the duration of the flash for the first deflection of the evoked response (b) and for the second (c). Ordinate: threshold intensity in decibels (dB). Threshold intensity for the evoked response of the visual cortex for stimuli 100 msec in duration was taken as 0 dB. Abscissa: duration of the light flash in milliseconds. Notice the logarithmic scale. Curve 1: retina; curve 2: optic tract; curve 3: dorsal lateral geniculate body; curve 4: visual cortex. Mean results for all experiments on anesthetized animals.

summation in the system. As is known [29], on a log-log scale such a curve must have a slope of 45° (and $n = 1.0$), if the threshold stimuli of various durations are of equal energy, i.e., if there is a complete exchange between intensity and duration and vice versa. A more abrupt decrease of thresholds ($n > 1.0$) may indicate that some energy of the short signals is not used effectively by the system for a synchronous response generation. This occurs, for example, when the optic nerve is electrically stimulated [35]. By contrast,

TABLE 1

Relation of Threshold Intensity for the Evoked
Response to the Flash Duration in Various Regions of the Visual System[a,b]

Region	Deflection of evoked response	Flash duration							
		100 μsec	250 μsec	1 msec	2.5 msec	10 msec	25 msec	100 msec	250 msec
Retina	A_1	41.1 ± 4.7	36.8 ± 3.8	35.0 ± 3.6	31.0 ± 4.2	26.0 ± 3.1	21.7 ± 3.5	20.0 ± 3.9	23.5 ± 3.4
	A_2	24.2 ± 4.7	18.0 ± 4.8	16.0 ± 3.8	13.0 ± 2.4	4.0 ± 3.5	1.8 ± 5.6	3.5 ± 4.7	5.0 ± 3.5
Optic tract	A_1	23.8 ± 5.6	22.1 ± 4.2	20.0 ± 4.3	17.0 ± 3.3	12.5 ± 3.3	8.8 ± 2.9	10.0 ± 3.0	8.5 ± 5.9
	A_2	16.0 ± 4.3	13.0 ± 5.1	6.5 ± 7.0	5.5 ± 3.2	-3.3 ± 3.9	-3.0 ± 5.3	-4.5 ± 3.5	-4.0 ± 5.3
Dorsal lateral geniculate body	A_1	14.8 ± 2.6	12.5 ± 2.4	10.0 ± 1.3	7.7 ± 2.6	4.0 ± 3.3	4.0 ± 2.4	3.3 ± 2.5	3.5 ± 2.4
	A_2	8.0 ± 2.4	5.2 ± 2.5	3.5 ± 3.9	-2.5 ± 2.4	-7.0 ± 3.8	-9.5 ± 2.5	-7.0 ± 3.1	-5.5 ± 2.6
Visual cortex	A_1	9.8 ± 2.2	11.1 ± 3.2	5.5 ± 2.1	6.2 ± 1.8	1.0 ± 2.3	0.0 ± 1.7	0.0 ± 2.3	1.3 ± 2.3
	A_2	0.0 ± 1.7	3.0 ± 3.8	-3.5 ± 2.4	-9.0 ± 2.1	-9.8 ± 1.8	-10.5 ± 2.0	-9.5 ± 1.9	-9.3 ± 2.1

[a] Data given in decibels.

[b] The threshold for the first deflection of the evoked response in the visual cortex to a light flash of 100-msec duration was taken as 0 dB.

a less steep course of the curve ($n<1.0$), when stimuli are adequate (Table 2), may indicate that the system possesses some mechanisms which use more effectively the energy of the brief signals or less effectively the energy of the long ones. The successive intensity-duration curves from the retina to the visual cortex show a tendency to gradual transition from the law of complete summation to the Pieron law (from $n = 1.0$ to $n = 0.5$).

One important index of the temporal summation is its critical duration (T_{cr}), which makes it possible to estimate the time up to which a change in the energy and temporal configuration of the stimulus at near-threshold intensity can influence the response. In this way, it is possible to judge the information value of the response or of its part [11]. However, it is possible to analyze this index unequivocally only for very much simplified situations. Thus, if all inputs of a single unit or of a pool of units with similar properties are synchronously excited, T_{cr} may approximately correspond to the maximal time constant of EPSP growth for a near-threshold stimulation [31]. For most of the actual situations—when the synaptic bombardment is more or less desynchronized and the properties of the neurons vary (mainly as regards the

TABLE 2

Main Characteristics of the Temporal
Summation at Various Levels of the Visual System

| Region of the visual system | Deflection of evoked response | Decrease in threshold intensity ΔI_t (dB); | | | | Slope of the summation curve ($n=tg\alpha$) | Critical summation time T_{cr} (msec) |
| | | Duration range (msec) | | | | | |
		0.1-1	1-10	10-100	0.1-100		
Retina	A_1	7.0	7.0	6.0	20.0	0.7	25.6
	A_2	10.0	10.0	3.0	23.0	1.0	8.8
Optic tract	A_1	6.75	6.75	3.0	16.5	0.67	9.3
	A_2	9.5	9.5	2.0	21.0	0.95	7.5
Dorsal lateral geniculate body	A_1	5.5	5.5	1.0	12.0	0.56	4.7
	A_2	8.5	8.5	2.0	19.0	0.83	8.0
Visual cortex	A_1	5.0	5.0	1.5	11.5	0.5	6.6
	A_2	7.5	5.5	0.5	13.5	0.8	2.4

number and weight of excited inputs)—T_{cr} will be an integrative index, determined by the degree of synchronization of the excitatory afferent volley.

In practice, we used for T_{cr} determination a previously proposed [14] graphical estimate which determines a duration that gives a reliable (by the Fischer-Student criterium) threshold difference in comparison with the threshold level for long-duration stimuli. Under our conditions, the threshold difference of about 3 dB, i.e., a twofold intensity change, was found to be reliable.

A comparison of the critical summation times in all regions of the visual system shows (Table 2) that this time became successively shorter from retina to cortex. It is noteworthy that a T_{cr} shortening must cause a steeper slope of the summation curve. Our data indicate that at higher levels of the visual system the log T_{cr} decreased somewhat more slowly than log ΔI_t; this probably causes less steep curves.

Findings for the second deflection of the evoked response are at all levels essentially the same as for the first. Figure 1(c) shows that the threshold differences between various levels become slightly smaller with prolongation of the flash. It is interesting that in the retina, the slope of the curve (for b-wave of ERG) is $45°$ ($n = 1.0$), which indicates a perfect summation.

The basic characteristics of the temporal summation, as established by the evoked potential criteria for the lateral geniculate body, are well enough substantiated by studies of single units (Fig. 2). The intensity-duration curves in the temporal summation range practically coincide. Different threshold levels for stimuli of long duration may be accounted for by including into the data high-threshold neurons with longer summation times, and also by the difficulty in detecting the evoked response when stimuli are of long duration,

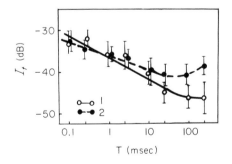

FIG. 2. Relation of threshold intensity to the duration of the flash. Ordinate: stimulus intensity in decibels (*re* maximal intensity available). Abscissa: time in milliseconds. Curve 1: for single unit responses in the dorsal lateral geniculate body (mean value and standard error for 14 neurons); curve 2: for the primary evoked potential (first deflection) in the dorsal lateral geniculate body (mean value and standard error for all experiments in unanesthetized cats).

since the responses of single elements at threshold intensity are less synchronized. For a number of low-threshold units, summation characteristics completely coincide with those obtained in the dorsal lateral geniculate body for slow evoked responses in experiments on unanesthetized cats (Fig. 3). A more detailed analysis of the temporal summation processes for the geniculate units will be made in another paper.

Discussion

Our determinations of thresholds of the primary evoked responses reveal reliable differences in temporal summation characteristics at various levels of the visual system in anesthetized cats. The threshold intensity, for a light flash of various durations, successively decreases from retina to cortex; the critical summation time and the degree of summation diminish. It may be assumed that all these indices are related to some common mechanisms which process the primary afferent inflow in the visual system.

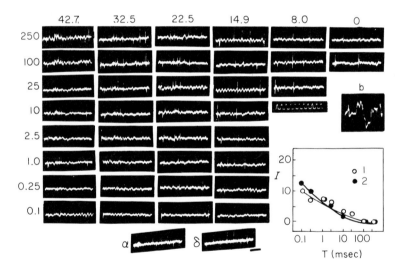

FIG. 3. Graph, curve 1: threshold intensity-duration curve for a low-threshold unit in the dorsal lateral geniculate body (35-LG) in an unanesthetized cat (UC-103); curve 2: mean threshold data for the evoked response in this body in unanesthetized cats. See legend for Fig. 1 for further explanations. Oscillograms: spike activity of the same unit. Negative deflection is up. Small positive deflection at the beginning of each sweep is a stimulus artifact indicating the start of the flash. Numbers above oscillograms indicate flash intensity in decibels (threshold intensity of a flash 100 msec in duration was taken as 0 dB). Numbers on left indicate duration of the flash (in milliseconds). Time calibration: 50 Hz. (a) Response; δ, background activity at a slower speed of the sweep (time calibration: 100 msec). (b) Focal evoked response and spikes of the same unit.

We shall not consider here the cause for the differences in absolute thresholds for the evoked responses at various levels of the system since this question was discussed previously in detail [34, 36]. It seems, however, relevant to discuss here the shortening of the T_{cr} and the decrease of ΔI_t at the higher levels of the visual system.

As already mentioned, T_{cr} for evoked potential thresholds may reflect the dispersion of the latent periods of the discharges of single elements and the temporal density of their afferent inputs rather than actual differences in the summation capacity of the neurons at various levels. Accordingly, at the higher levels, synchronization of the initial afferent inflow is higher than in the peripheral regions of the system. It has been previously shown that, at the higher levels of the visual system, the temporal density of the inflow can increase due to simple net properties of the structures and initial desynchronization of the signal in the retina [34]. Suggestions about a possible connection between the degree of synchronization of unit activity and the effectiveness of the temporal summation were made by Chang [9] and Gersuni [11]. Data regarding a shortening of summation time with an increase in intensity and area of light flashes indirectly corroborate these suggestions [15, 19, 21, 24], because under such circumstances, the synchronization at the afferent input increases.

Nevertheless, these considerations give no answer to the question of why the synchronization of the initial afferent inflow leads, in the direct visual synaptic chain, to a less prominent decrease of thresholds for long rather than short signals. Theoretically, it seems reasonable to believe that in a system consisting of similar elements, where the afferent inflow is transmitted from one level to another without reorganization, all temporal summation characteristics at different levels should be equal and the summation should be complete. Actually, in the visual system the temporal summation is close to complete only for the threshold characteristics of the ERG. A gradual decrease of the temporal summation capacity, in the more central regions of the analyzer, is difficult to explain without invoking successive inhibitory processes. It appears that such processes are more pronounced at the upper levels of the system and/or are more synchronized. If it is true that in the central regions of the sensory system the prevailing elements are those with a phasic or a rapidly adapting type of discharge [10, 20, 22] and consequently with a short summation time [20, 32, 33], then an increase in temporal density of the initial afferent input may be most important for the responsiveness of these elements. On the other hand, the prolongation of the flash may be less effective owing to inhibition after the first discharge. In the cat's retina, the horizontal inhibition is more pronounced for stimuli of long duration than for brief ones [3]. However, it may be suggested that, in the neuronal populations of the more peripheral regions of the system, the units adapt more slowly on the average and, consequently, have a longer critical summation time and greater capacity for temporal summation owing to a less pronounced limiting inhibition. Hence, prolongation of a flash may be more effective here than for the more centrally situated units. Such assumptions seem supported by studies of the visual and auditory neurons at various levels [12, 16-18, 26-28, 30] where substantial differences were shown to exist between the units in the peripheral and the central regions of the analyzer as regards the properties important for temporal summation.

Thus, it appears that the changes in the critical summation time at different levels of the visual system are the result of synchronization of the initial afferent inflow, while differences in the summation capacity may be due to the intensity and synchronization of the successive inhibitory events.

It is important to stress that, considering an effective signal processing, a formal deterioration of the summation characteristics at high levels of the visual system provides a valuable finding because it implies a temporal sharpening of the afferent inflow which is essential for a reliable detection and recognition of the visual images.

Summary

1. Threshold intensities for the evoked potentials for various durations of a flash were determined in the retina, optic tract, dorsal lateral geniculate body, and visual cortex in anesthetized cats. Similar thresholds were measured for discharges of single units in the dorsal lateral geniculate body in unanesthetized cats.

2. It was shown that all characteristics of temporal summation (threshold level, threshold decrease with prolongation of flash duration, and the critical summation time) diminished successively and reliably as one proceeds from the peripheral to the central regions of the visual system.

3. The suggestion is made that the decrease in thresholds and the shortening of the critical summation time at the higher levels of the visual system are the result of synchronization of the initial afferent inflow, while differences in the degree of summation are due to the amount of synchronization of the successive inhibitory events.

REFERENCES

1. Adrian, E. D., and Matthews, R. The action of light on the eye, Part III. *J. Physiol. (London)* **65**, 273 (1928).
2. Barlow, H. B. Temporal and spatial summation in human vision at different background intensities. *J. Physiol. (London)* **141**, 337 (1958).

3. Barlow, H. B., Fitzhugh, R., and Kuffler, S. W. Change of organization in the receptive fields of the cat's retina during dark adaptation. *J. Physiol. (London)* **137**, 338 (1957).
4. Baumgardt, E. Les théories photochimiques classiques et quantiques de la vision et l'inhibition nerveuse en vision liminaire. *Rev. Opt.* **28**, 661 (1949).
5. Baumgardt, E. Visual spatial and temporal summation. *Nature (London)* **184**, 71 (1959).
6. Baumgardt, E., and Hillman, B. Duration and size as determinants of peripheral retinal response. *J. Opt. Soc. Amer.* **51**, 340 (1961).
7. Bloch, A. Expériences sur la vision. *C. R. Soc. Biol.* [8], **2**, 493 (1885).
8. Bouman, M. Peripheral contrast thresholds of the human eye. *J. Opt. Soc. Amer.* **40**, 825 (1950).
9. Chang, H.-T. An observation on the effect of strychnine on local cortical potentials. *J. Neurophysiol.* **14**, 23 (1951).
10. Creutzfeldt, O., Spehlmann, K., and Zehmann, D. *In* "Neurophysiologie und Psychophysik des Visuellen Systems" (R. Jung and H. Kornhuber, eds.), p. 351. Springer, Berlin, 1961.
11. Gersuni, G. V. The organization of afferent inflow and discrimination of signals of various duration. *J. Higher Nervous Activity (USSR)* **15**, 260 (1965) (in Russian).
12. Gersuni, G. V. On the time-place organization of the auditory system. 18 Int. Psychol. Congr., Publ. D-t Symp. 15 "Sensory Processes at the Neuronal and Behavioral Levels," Moscow, 1966, p. 105.
13. Gersuni, G. V., Gasanov, U. G., Zaboeva, N. V., and Lebedinsky, M. M. Evoked potentials of the auditory cortex and the time characteristics of the sound stimuli. *Biophysics (USSR)* **9**, 597-606 (1964) (in Russian).
14. Gersuni, G. V., Shevelev, I. A., and Lichnitsky, A. M. Dependence of the primary response of auditory cortex on the temporal characteristics of signal in alert cats. *J. Higher Nervous Activity (USSR)* **14**, 489 (1964) (in Russian).
15. Graham, C. H., and Margaria, R. Area and intensity-time relation in the peripheral retina. *Amer. J. Physiol.* **113**, 302 (1935).
16. Hartline, H. K. Intensity and duration in the excitation of single photoreceptor units. *J. Cell Comp. Physiol.* **5**, 229 (1934).
17. Ikeda, M. Temporal summation and negative flashes in the visual system. *J. Opt. Soc. Amer.* **55**, 1527 (1965).
18. Jonson, E. P., and Barlett, N. R. Effect of stimulus duration on electrical responses of the human retina. *J. Opt. Soc. Amer.* **46**, 163 (1956).
19. Karn, H. W. Area and the intensity-time relation in the fovea. *J. Gen. Psychol.* **14**, 360 (1936).
20. Katsuki, Y., Watanabe, T., and Maruyama, N. Activity of auditory neurons in upper levels of brain of cat. *J. Neurophysiol.* **22**, 343 (1959).
21. Kuchler, G., Pilz, A., and Sickel, W. Adaptations- und Reizwirkse amkeit des Lichtes im ERG des isolierten Froschauges. *Pfluegers Arch.* **263**, 577 (1956).
22. Li, C.-L., Ortiz-Galvin, A., Chou, S. N., and Howard, S. Y. Cortical Intracellular potentials in response to stimulation of LGB. *J. Neurophysiol.* **23**, 592 (1960).
23. Luizov, A. V. Inertia of the vision. *Priroda (Moscow)* **9**, 13 (1947) (in Russian).
24. Makarov, P. O. Study of the sensitivity of the human optical system to adequate stimuli of various intensities and durations. Physiol. Opt. Conf., Leningrad, 1936, p. 245 (in Russian).
25. Makarov, P. O. Study of the sense organs in microtime. *In* "Primary Processes in Receptor Elements of Sense Organs" (V. G. Samsonova, ed.), p. 64. Nauka, Leningrad, 1966 (in Russian).

26. Maruseva, A. M. On the temporal characteristics of the auditory neurons in the inferior colliculus of rats. *18th Int. Congress. Psychol. Symp. 15, Publ. D-t, Moscow, 1966,* p. 162.

27. Mkrticheva, L. I., and Samsonova, V. G. Sensitivity of neurons of the frog's tectum to changes in the intensity of light stimulus. *Vision Res.* **6**, 419 (1966).

28. Mkrticheva, L. I., and Samsonova, V. G. Importance of time for response information in units of visual center in frog. *J. Higher Nervous Activity (USSR)* **15**, 274 (1965).

29. Nasonov, D. N. "Local Protoplasm Reaction and Spreading Excitation," p. 277. Moscow, 1959 (in Russian).

30. Popov, A. V. This volume, Chap. 17.

31. Radionova, E. A. Reaction of units in cochlear nucleus to sounds of various duration. *J. Higher Nervous Activity (USSR)* **15**, 739 (1965).

32. Radionova, E. A. Correspondence of some characteristics of the auditory system neurons in their reaction to sound stimuli. *Biophysics (USSR)* **11**, 478 (1966) (in Russian).

33. Radionova, E. A. The temporal characteristics of the reaction of the cochlear nucleus neurons. *18th Int. Congr. Psychol. Symp. 15 Publ. D-t.* Moscow, 1966, p. 156.

34. Shevelev, I. A. Synchronization of the initial afferent inflow in the visual system. *J. Higher Nervous Activity (USSR)* **15**, 350 (1965).

35. Shevelev, I. A., and Leushina, I. P. Some characteristics of evoked potentials which are produced by electric stimulation of the optic nerve at various levels of the visual system. *In* "Electrophysiology of the CNS" (A. I. Roitbak, ed.), p. 327. Mezriereba Tbilisi, 1966 (in Russian).

36. Shevelev, I. A. and Hicks, L. H. Investigation of afferent inflow at various levels of the visual system by means of a mass evoked electrical response. *J. Higher Nervous Activity (USSR)* **15**, 148 (1965).

37. Shevelev, I. A., and Hicks, L. H. Temporal summation in the visual system as measured by primary evoked potentials. *18th Int. Congr. Psychol. Symp. 15 Publ. D-t.* Moscow, 1966, p. 74.

38. Vartanian, I. A. Quantitative characteristics of temporal summation in inferior colliculus and lateral lemniscus of the rat brain. *J. Higher Nervous Activity (USSR)* **16**, 103 (1966).

5
Sources of Information in the Perception of Visual Spatial Relations

L. I. Leushina

Eye Movements and Space Vision

The question of participation of the oculomotor system in the perception of visual spatial relations has been discussed in the literature since the times of Helmholtz, Hering, Sechenov, and Sherrington. Some investigators believe that the eye movements are a source of information about such spatial properties as the position of the objects in the visual field, their motion, size, remoteness, position relative to one another, relation of their sizes, etc. Other investigators consider that measurements of visual spatial relations are affected by the visual system without participation of eye movements.

On the basis of the data in the literature and our own experimental results, we tested the hypothesis that eye movements are a source of information about visual spatial relations. In the literature, the following factors are mentioned as possible indicators of the spatial properties of a visual stimulus: saccadic eye movements, as a source of information concerning two-dimensional space; convergence and accommodation, as a source of information concerning the remoteness of the object; and pursuit eye movements, as a source of information concerning the motion of the object. We have analyzed the time and amplitude characteristics of all the above-mentioned types of eye movements [17].

SACCADIC EYE MOVEMENTS

The development of a saccade in time has been thoroughly studied by numerous authors [22, 24, 26, and others]. The velocity of the eye movement increases quite rapidly, from zero to the maximal level; after that, it maintains an even level for a long time for large angles of turning, and then again declines more or less rapidly to the zero level. This form of the saccade is due to the application of an active force during the acceleration or inhibition of the eye movement [22].

According to data of numerous authors, the velocity of voluntary and involuntary saccadic eye movements increases with an increase of the amplitude of the movement. The velocity of the eye movements cannot be changed voluntarily; it remains relatively constant for the same subject for the same angle of turning of the eye; it does not depend on the initial position of the eyes or on the direction of the saccade; it changes only with the change of the angle at which the eye must turn. Figure 1 presents data [10, 24, 25] concerning the maximal angular velocities which are developed by the eye already at the onset of the saccade (after covering 10 to 15% of the whole path [24]). Similar results have been obtained by some other authors [13, 26]. A correlation between amplitude and velocity of the saccadic eye movement is observed not only when the maximal velocity developed by the eye is measured, but also for measurements of the average velocity of the movement during the saccade [2, 3, 5, 26, and others]. A linear dependence between the amplitude and the average velocity of the saccadic eye movement was recorded also in children 1 year old and older [4].

The unquestionable correlation between the velocity of the saccadic eye movement and the angle of turning is of great interest when considering the problem of perception of spatial relations. This correlation permits prediction at the very onset of the saccade—on the basis of the velocity of the movement—of the position of the eye after the saccade, the point in space to which the gaze will be directed. Consequently, at the moment of the onset of

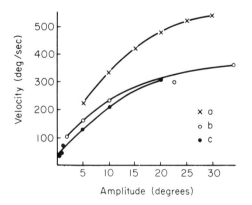

FIG. 1. Relation between maximal angular velocity and amplitude of a saccadic eye movement according to: (a) Westheimer (25); (b) Gurevich (10); and (c) Vossius (24).

the saccade, not only is the point of the new fixation already chosen, but the distance to it is measured and an appropriate muscular effort selected, which accelerates the eye movement and imparts to it a velocity appropriate to the amplitude of the future movement. Thus, the distance between the objects (or the size of the object) is already measured before the beginning of the saccadic eye movement.

However, is not the visual estimate of the distance preliminary in character? Is it not ascertained more precisely after the end of the movement on the basis of proprioceptive signals? What do we know about the accuracy of measurement of the distance prior to the saccadic eye movement and about the accuracy of its estimate on the basis of the "muscular sense"?

Glezer [7] showed that a saccadic eye movement toward a new point of fixation arises only if the retinal visual image is displaced from an initial point of fixation to a distance of not less than 4 to 6 angular minutes; within these limits lies the zone of retinal insensitivity. We know that a saccadic eye movement, once started, cannot be changed [24-26]. Consequently, the accuracy of the saccadic eye movement toward a new point of fixation characterizes the estimate of the distance which has been determined before the onset of the eye movement. Lauringson and Shchedrovitsky [15] measured the amplitude of saccades for different angles, up to $10°$, and found that the movements are performed with the same accuracy—of the order of 4.5 to 6 angular minutes.

The possibilities of the "muscular sense" are more limited. According to Merton and Brindly [20], a passive stretch of the eye muscles to a value which corresponds to a turn at an angle of $20°$ does not elicit any sensation of movement or any reflex changes in the position of the other eye.

Cornsweet [1] pointed out that the eye "wanders" in the dark within the limits of $1°$, when the attempt is made to retain the direction of fixation; he regards the zone of this "wandering" as an index showing the accuracy of the proprioceptive estimate of the position. Gippenreiter [6] obtained similar results in experiments with fixation and pursuit of a contour in a relatively homogeneous field, under daylight conditions. She found that the zone of proprioceptive insensitivity has a diameter of $1°10'$ to $1°20'$. Although the author's statement that these values characterize the accuracy of the proprioceptive (but not of the innervational) estimate of the position and movement of the eyes is open to question, there is no doubt that it is impossible to measure the distance by means of the oculomotor system with an accuracy higher than $1°$.

Thus, the visual system performs a preliminary measurement of the distance with an accuracy of 4 to 6 angular minutes, whereas the accuracy of the allegedly "more precise" measurement with the help of the oculomotor system is only about $1°$.

It could be assumed that the eye movements do not correct the measurements of the visual system but only perform parallel measurements which raise the reliability of the spatial perception. But this hypothesis, too, is contradicted by the available facts.

We have carried out an investigation [16] in which the dependence of the reaction time on the amount of obtained information, a relationship well known in information theory (11, 14, and others), was used to explore the participation of eye movements in the estimation of distance. We recorded eye movements when the subject was estimating the distance between two points (Fig. 2). The subject was fixating on a luminous point and, when a second luminous point appeared, he shifted his gaze to it and signaled the distance between the two points by disconnecting an appropriate electrical button [Fig. 2(a)]. Two distances were used in a series: a larger one, which was always 20°, and a smaller one. The difference between them was varied in different series of experiments. The smaller the difference, the more precise had to be the estimate made by the observer.

With the increase of the needed measuring accuracy, the latency of the saccadic eye movement became longer [Fig. 2(b)]; that is in accord with the idea that the reaction time increases with an increase in the amount of information received by the subject. The time interval between the onset of the saccadic eye movement and the subject's response remained unchanged [Fig. 2(c)]; however, it is precisely this time interval in which information about the movements of the eyes and their new position would have to be transmitted by the proprioreceptors of the eye muscles and to be processed. Consequently, no information concerning the distance between two points is received by the subject as a result of the eye movements. It was also found that in 30% of all cases the subjects estimated the stimulus prior to the end of the eye movement, i.e., before the occurrence of proprioceptive signals about the new position of the eye [Fig. 2(d)].

These facts demonstrate convincingly that the distance between the stimuli is estimated by the visual system before the onset of a saccadic eye movement and that the oculomotor system does not perform any additional measurement during the saccade.

A similar analysis of the convergence, accommodation, and pursuit movements of the eyes indicates that the eye movements do not participate in the measurements of the remoteness of objects nor of their motion in the visual field.

Thus, the hypothesis that eye movements are a source of information about visual spatial relations is not confirmed. The position of an object in the visual field, its size, remoteness, motion in space, and other spatial properties are estimated by the visual system with high accuracy before the onset of eye movements.

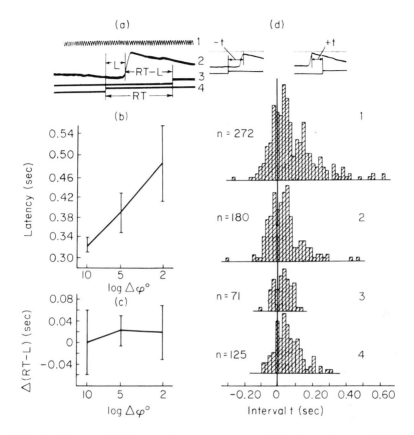

FIG. 2. Estimate of distance and eye movements. (a) Electrooculogram (EOG): (1) time marks, 20 msec; (2) EOG; (3) subject's signal concerning the distance between two points of fixation; (4) stimulus occurrence. (b) Dependence of the latency of a $20°$ saccadic eye movement on the difference ($\Delta\varphi$) between two distances (in degrees). (c) Graph plotting the interval between the eye movement and the signal of estimate against $\Delta\varphi°$. (d) Histograms plotting the intervals between the end of the saccadic eye movement and the time when the subject's signal occurs ($+t$, $-t$) against the frequency of occurrence of such intervals; graphs 1, 2, 3, and 4 are for individual subjects.

Estimation of Spatial Properties of an Image in the Visual System

By measuring the time that is required for identification of an image [8, 21] in man, we studied the identification of some spatial properties of an image as well as the relationships between the processes of form identification and the estimate of spatial properties of an object.

When investigating the mechanisms of information transmission in the visual system, Glezer and Nevskaya [9] established two types of identification of visual images. The amount of information received by the observer during the identification of the images of objects depends on the time of observation, and therefore, the longer the time required for the identification of an image, the greater the number of possible images, i.e., the greater the information content of the presented stimulus. The authors believed that this type of identification can be described as a system of successive choices from a multitude of expected visual images (alphabet of images). Naturally, the program for such successive choices is elaborated anew when the identified alphabet is changed. The amount of information received by the observer during the identification of simple configurations (for example, the slope of a line) is not determined by the time of observation—during the same exposure, the probability of proper identification does not depend on the number of possible alternatives; in other words, the more information the subject receives, the more information is presented. According to the authors, this manner of identification attests to the existence, in the human visual system, of specialized automatic mechanisms of the type of complex receptive fields, found by Hubel and Wiesel [12], which act according to some predetermined sets.

We studied the identifications of the following spatial signs of images: the position of an object in the visual field, the length and the slope of a line, and the size of an object. Figure 3 presents the results of estimates by the subject of the position of an object in the visual field. The time of such estimation did not depend on whether the object could appear in one of two, or in one of four or in one of eight sites of the visual field, i.e., it was not determined by the information content of the stimulus. During the same exposure, the more information the subject received, the more information was presented [Fig. 3(b)]. When choosing from two, four, or eight possible positions, the subject correctly estimated the position of the object in the visual field within the same period of time and in the same percentage of cases [Fig. 3(c)]. Consequently, time was of equal significance for the probability of a correct estimate of the object position irrespective of the amount of information received by the subject. The same phenomenon was regularly observed by us during the estimation by the subject of the size of an image, as well as of the length and orientation of a line [19]. Thus, it was shown that the studied spatial properties of the images are perceived by the human visual system with the aid of a set of specialized detectors automatically reacting to the appearance of a corresponding property in the visual field.

We also studied the detectors of the position of an object in the visual field by analyzing errors committed by the subject in estimating the position when the time of the exposure of the object was insufficient for faultless identifica-

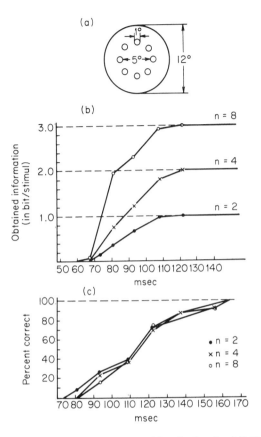

FIG. 3. Identification of the position of the object in the visual field. Positions of the objects in the visual field used in the experiment (a). Dependence of the amount of information obtained (b) and of the percentage of proper identifications (c) on the time of presentation; n, number of sites at which the image may appear.

tion. The subjects committed systematic errors in the estimates of an object's position ($p < 0.01$). These errors were different, depending on whether the object was presented to the right or to the left eye. The scheme in Fig. 4 illustrates an example of errors committed by one of our subjects. If an object located in the upper part of a 12° visual field was presented to the right eye, the subject perceived it as an "upper" (more often) or a "left" one. If it was presented to the left eye, the subject perceived it as an "upper" or "right" one. It may be assumed that, when binocular vision is used, the errors of the right and left eye will cancel each other out and that the subject will perceive the object as an "upper" one. This assumption was confirmed.

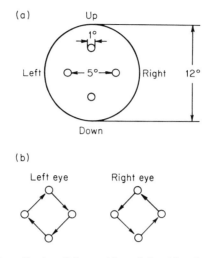

FIG. 4. Errors in the estimates of the position of the object in the visual field. Subject E.A. (a) Positions of the objects in the field of vision used in the experiment. (b) Systematic errors in the estimates of the position by the subject during the exposure of the objects to the left or the right eye.

The detectors may be conceived of as filters specialized in detecting definite properties of an image. From this point of view, the systematic errors in the estimates of the position of an object in the visual field suggest that the detectors which ascertain this position are not filters with a very narrow bandwidth. However, when the detectors of the right and left eye are both utilized and converge to a common output, this may create a more precise system than is provided by the initial elements.

Relations between Identification of the Form and Estimation of the Spatial Properties of an Image

As already mentioned, two types of identification of images have been described in the visual system: identification of the form of the image and identification of its spatial properties [9, 19]. But the different types can exist only if the subject's decisions concerning the form of the object and its spatial properties are separated from each other, i.e., if the visual system possesses separate channels for identifying the forms of objects and for estimating their spatial properties [8]. Studies of the relationship between the identification of the form of an image and the identification of its size indicate that such separate channels do exist and that they function independently of each other [8, 18, 23].

The relationship between the identification of the form of an image and the estimate of its position in the visual field was also studied. Let us suppose that the form of the image is identified only after its position in the visual field has been ascertained. In such a case, the subject will be unable to identify the form of an object properly if his estimate of the position of that object has been wrong. Now, let us assume that it is the form of an object which is identified first (which seems to us unlikely); in such a case, the subject will be able only to guess the position of that object if its form has been identified erroneously. Finally, let us suppose that the form and position of an object are ascertained independently of each other through parallel channels. If this is the case, a proper estimate of the position of an object is possible even if the identification of its form is wrong; and vice versa, if the estimate of the position of an object is erroneous, it is possible to identify properly its form with a probability which exceeds the probability of accidental correct guessing.

Drawings of geometrical figures were presented to a subject tachystoscopically for a time that was insufficient for faultless identification. Single drawings appeared in a random order in one of four sites of the visual field. The subject had to name a given figure and indicate its position; the answer "I don't know" was not allowed. Cases of erroneously identified forms of images were selected from the subject's answers, and in these cases the estimates of the position of the drawing in the visual field were analyzed by the chi-square test. In cases of an erroneous estimate of the position of the drawing, the identification of the form was subjected to this test. Table 1 presents some examples of the distribution of the subjects' answers concerning the form of the graphic image in cases of erroneous estimates of its position, and data concerning the position of the object in cases of a wrong identification of its form. Table 2 shows the results of an analysis of the subjects' answers.

The data indicate that all the subjects were able to estimate correctly the position of the drawing in the visual field in cases of a wrong identification of its geometrical form ($p < 0.001$). Consequently, the position of an object in the visual field is ascertained irrespective of form identification. Somewhat different results were obtained from analysis of the form identification in cases when it was the position of the object which was erroneously estimated by the subject. The analysis indicates that at first (i.e., during the first experimental day), the subjects were unable to identify the form of a given image if their estimate of the position of that object in the visual field was wrong ($p \sim 0.5$ and $p > 0.70$), although—if all presentations made during the experiment are taken into consideration—they properly identified the form in 65% of all cases. However, after a short training period (during the second day of the investigation) the subjects began to identify the form correctly, even in cases when the position of an object was estimated by them erroneously ($p < 0.05$).

TABLE 1

Identification of Images when the Time of the Object
Exposure Was Insufficient for a Faultless Identification[a]

Set of images to be identified	Conditions of exposure	Total no. of tests	Identified erroneously	
			Form	Position
Two figures, each in four positions	Against a masking background	3120	865	1209

Distribution of the answers

Concerning the position of the image
(form has been identified erroneously)[b]

Image presented	Subject's answer				Total
	Above	On the right	On the left	Below	
Above	107	47	65	66	285
On the right	67	69	50	67	253
On the left	28	39	39	22	128
Below	59	41	39	60	199
	261	196	193	215	865

Concerning the form of the image
(position has been estimated erroneously)[c]

Form of image presented	Subject's answer		Total
	Square	Star	
Square	292	165	457
Star	414	338	752
	706	503	1209

[a]Subject A.N. [b]$\chi^2 = 30.3, p < 0.001$. [c]$\chi^2 = 9.05, p < 0.01$.

TABLE 2

Identification of the Form of an Image and Its Position in the Visual Field when the Time of the Object Exposure Was Insufficient for a Faultless Identification

Subject	Experimental conditions, session	Conditions of exposure of the drawing	Identification of the form (position has been estimated erroneously)[a]			Estimation of the position (form has been identified erroneously)[b]		
			No. of tests	χ^2	Significance confidence level (p)	No. of tests	χ^2	Significance confidence level (p)
E.A.	1st	In a light field	84	1.55	~0.5	78	36.2	<0.001
A.V.,A.N., E.A.,I.A., N.K., and N.M.	1st (summary data)	Against a masking background	2187	0.12	>0.70	1674	36.3	<0.001
A.N.,E.A., and N.M.	2nd (summary data)	Against a masking background	689	4.0	<0.05	478	28.0	<0.001
E.A.	1st to 5th	Against a masking background	711	8.2	<0.01	448	40.0	<0.001
N.M.	1st to 5th	Against a masking background	1160	6.70	<0.01	823	60.0	<0.001
A.N.	1st to 5th	Against a masking background	1209	9.05	<0.01	865	30.3	<0.001
I.A.	1st to 7th	Against a masking background	1616	15.0	<0.001	1152	19.7	<0.02
E.A.	30th to 35th	Against a masking background	1441	20.3	<0.001	1107	194.0	<0.001

[a] No. of degrees of freedom = one. [b] No. of degrees of freedom = nine. [c] Set of images presented for identification.

With further training, the subjects acquired the ability to identify the form regardless of whether their estimate of the position of the object was right or wrong.

Thus, the identification of the form of an object and the estimate of its position in the visual field take place in the visual system independently of each other, just as is the case for the estimation of the size of an object and identification of its form. It may be assumed that other spatial properties of an image are also estimated in the visual system independently of the processes of form identification.

Conclusions

1. The hypothesis that eye movements are a source of information about visual spatial relations is not confirmed by experimental facts. The position of an object in the visual field, its size, remoteness, motion, and other spatial properties are estimated by the visual system with a high accuracy before the onset of the eye movements.

2. The spatial properties of an image, such as the position of an object in the visual field, its size, the length of a line, and its slope are detected by specialized automatic mechanisms operating according to predetermined sets which do not depend on the information content of a stimulus.

3. Information concerning the position of an object in the visual field (as well as its size) is processed in the visual system in special channels, independently of the form of the image. It is supposed that other spatial properties of the image are also estimated independently of the processes of form identification.

4. It is assumed that the separate spatial properties of the image, perceived in the visual system by specialized detectors, serve as a source for the formation of notions concerning visual spatial relations.

REFERENCES

1. Cornsweet, T. N. Determination of the stimuli for involuntary drifts and saccadic eye movements. *J. Opt. Soc. Amer.* **46**, 987-993 (1956).
2. Ditchburn, R. W., and Ginsborg, B. Involuntary eye movements during fixation. *J. Physiol. (London)* **119**, 1-17 (1953).
3. Dodge, R. Five types of eye movements in the horizontal meridian plane of the field of regard. *Amer. J. Physiol.* **8**, 307-329 (1903).
4. Gatev, V. Electrooculographic studies on the biodynamics of the saccadic eye movements in normal children. *In* "Third National Conference of the Bulgarian Society for Physiological Sciences." Summary N 40. Varna, 1967.

5. Ginsborg, B. Small involuntary movements of the eye. *Brit. J. Ophthalmol.* **37**, 746-758 (1953).

6. Gippenreiter, Ju. B. On intrinsic noise of eye movement system. *Probl. Psychol. (USSR)* **4**, 69-82 (1964) (in Russian).

7. Glezer, V. D. The eye as a servo-system. *Sechenov Physiol. J. USSR* **45**, 271-279 (1959) (in Russian).

8. Glezer, V. D. "Mechanisms of Visual Image Identification." Nauka, Leningrad, 1966 (in Russian).

9. Glezer, V. D., and Nevskaya, A. A. Synchronous and consecutive information processing in the visual system. *Rep. Acad. Sci. USSR* **155**, 711-714 (1964) (in Russian).

10. Gurevitch, B. Kh. Role of proprioception in the mechanisms of the oculomotor fixation reflex and in the activity of the human visual analyzer. *Sechenov Physiol. J. USSR* **45**, 1308-1316 (1959) (in Russian).

11. Hick, W. E. On the rate of gain of information. *Quart. J. Exp. Psychol.* **4**, 11-26 (1952).

12. Hubel, D. H., and Wiesel, T. N. Receptive fields of single neurons in the cat's striate cortex. *J. Physiol. (London)* **148**, 574-591 (1959).

13. Hyde, J. Some characteristics of voluntary human ocular movements in the horizontal plane. *Amer. J. Ophthalmol.* **48**, 85-94 (1959).

14. Hyman, R. Stimulus information as a determinant of reaction time. *J. Exp. Psychol.* **45**, 188-196 (1953).

15. Lauringson, A. L., and Shchedrovitsky, L. P. On the accuracy of the eye turning during the change of fixation points. *Biophysics (USSR)* **10**, 369 (1965) (in Russian).

16. Leushina, L. I. On the estimation of light stimulus position and eye movements. *Biophysics (USSR)* **10**, 130-136 (1965) (in Russian).

17. Leushina, L. I. Eye movements and space vision. *In* "Problems of Sensory Systems Physiology" (Reviews) (G. V. Gersuni, ed.), pp. 53-83. Nauka, Leningrad, 1966 (in Russian).

18. Leushina, L. I. On separate channels for form and size identification of the visual image. *Probl. Fiziol. Opt.* **14**, 128-134 (1967) (in Russian).

19. Leushina, L. I., Turkina, N. V., and Kuznetzova, I. N. On the study of the estimation mechanisms of the visual spatial relations. *Probl. Fiziol. Opt.* **13**, 125-135 (1966) (in Russian).

20. Merton, P. A., and Brindly, O. O. Absence of conscious position sense in the human eyes. *In* "The Oculomotor System" (M. Bender, ed.), pp. 314-320. Harper, New York, 1964.

21. Nevskaya, A. A. Determination of channel capacity of the human visual analyser. *Sechenov Physiol. J. USSR* **49**, 892-896 (1963) (in Russian).

22. Shaknovich, A. R. On the study of the mechanism of optokinetic nystagmus. *Biophysics (USSR)* **10**, 304-308 (1965) (in Russian).

23. Stefanova, N. On the invariance of visual images. *In* "Second National Conference of the Bulgarian Society for Physiological Sciences." Summaries. Bulgarian Academy of Sciences, Sofia, 1964, p. 15:N 97.

24. Vossius, G. Das System der Augenbewegung. *Z. Biol. (Munich)* **112**, 27-57 (1960).

25. Westheimer, G. The mechanism of saccadic eye movements. *A.M.A. Arch. Ophthalmol.* **52**, 710-724 (1954).

26. Yarbus, A. L. Eye movements during the change of fixation points. *Biophysics (USSR)* **1**, 76-78 (1956) (in Russian).

II. Audition

6
Temporal Organization of the Auditory Function

G. V. Gersuni

Despite numerous investigations on hearing, basic problems of organization of the auditory function still remain unsolved. We conclude, as did Békésy [16], that thus far, no general theory of hearing has been proposed. There exists only a theory of frequency discrimination of stationary sound in the cochlea.

It is necessary to draw such a conclusion because as soon as one considers the mechanisms beyond the cochlea and examines the auditory system as a whole, thus no longer limiting the inquiry to the action of stationary pure tones, the contradictory character of the data obtained with different methods as well as serious gaps in basic knowledge immediately become manifest.

The inadequacy of a theory that evaluates the auditory phenomena solely from the point of view of the mechanism determining the spatial representation of the signal frequency, becomes obvious when we consider the structural design of the first synaptic regions of the auditory system, namely, the cochlear nuclei.

As is known, the auditory nerve fibers entering the cochlear nuclei are arranged in an orderly manner that maintains the spatial projection of the unfolded cochlea. Fibers from the apex of the cochlea are distributed to the lower parts of the nuclei; fibers from the base of the cochlea to their upper sectors.

The distribution of fibers in the cochlear nuclei may be electrophysiologically established by determining the frequency-threshold curves. A separate frequency projection exists for the three basic nuclei of the cochlear complex: the anteroventral, the posteroventral, and the dorsal [70, 71].

When entering the cochlear nuclei, the auditory nerve fibers divide into ascending and descending branches which reach the three basic divisions of the cochlear complex (Fig. 1). Thus, in the cochlear nuclei, the disposition of the fibers in the dorsoventral direction results in a projection of the length of the cochlea (i.e., a frequency projection), whereas the course of each fiber in the sagittal plane provides a projection of a limited part of the cochlear sensory surface which may be restricted to one to three inner hair cells. In Fig. 1, the latter projection has a regular, somewhat concave contour corresponding to the course of the nerve fiber after bifurcation. In contrast to the dorsoventral projection, which corresponds to the frequency scale, the sagittal projection can be conveniently designated as an isofrequency projection. The question is, what functional significance can be attached to it?

Licklider [50] assumed that the structure of the cochlear nuclei provides, besides a frequency axis, a time axis due to successive synaptic delays. Although Licklider's scheme was based on a model that provides an autocor-

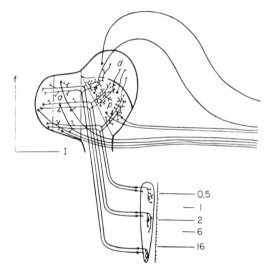

FIG. 1. Scheme of projection of the cochlear nerve fibers upon the cochlear nuclear complex in a sagittal plane. Bottom: schematic representation of unfolded cochlear partition. Dashes indicate scale in millimeters for the cochlear partition; corresponding frequencies in kilohertz on the right. *a*, Anteroventral cochlear nucleus; *p*, posteroventral cochlear nucleus; *d*, dorsal cochlear nucleus. Auditory nerve fibers from apex to base of the cochlea are shown to project in a ventrodorsal direction in the cochlear complex; *f* and *I* are the approximate orientation of the frequency and isofrequency axis, respectively (see text). (The scheme of the cochlear nucleus composed by Ratnikova is based on data of Cajal, 1909; Lorente de Nó, 1933; Harrison and Warr, 1962; and Sando, 1965.)

relation analysis (and the scheme was not meant to deal with actual functional and structural data), the model raised the question of the temporal and spatial principles that are significant in the organization of the auditory system and that must be dealt with on the level of the cochlear nuclei.

An investigation of this problem by studies of the temporal characteristics of single neurons in various divisions of the auditory system constituted the first part of the research program which was undertaken by our laboratory.

Another series of facts indicating important gaps in our knowledge in regard to events that take place in the auditory system pertains to the role played by the cortical auditory area in frequency discrimination. Here, the results obtained by electrophysiological and behavioral methods are highly contradictory. Thus, electrophysiological experiments using the method of evoked potentials implied that there exists a frequency projection along the surface of the auditory cortical area [48, 80, 81]. On the other hand, behavioral experiments [14, 57, 61] suggest that a complete bilateral ablation of this area does not cause any impairment in the discrimination of intensity and frequency of a sound. This striking contradiction prompted us to search for its causes.

The first results lead to the conclusion [23] that this contradiction is due to the use of markedly different time criteria in the electrophysiological and behavioral investigations. In the former, the effective duration of the signal could not exceed 10 to 15 msec (time of the development of the primary evoked response), while in the behavioral experiments the signals lasted for 1000 to 2000 msec. Subsequent work showed that, if in the behavioral experiments the duration of the signal varied, it was possible to detect considerable differences in the role played by the auditory cortex in the discrimination of brief (up to 10-15 msec) and of longer sounds (20 msec and longer). With lesions in cortical auditory areas, the discrimination only of brief sounds is impaired [8, 9, 11, 32]. This observation suggested that a cortical frequency projection is utilized predominantly for sounds of short duration.

This conclusion, which does not agree with the usual concepts of spatial frequency projection, suggests that different mechanisms may be employed in the discrimination of sounds of different duration.

In recent years, our laboratory started investigations of the activity of the auditory system both by electrophysiological methods (recording of responses of single elements and evoked potentials), and by behavioral methods (studies of animals and patients with lesions of the auditory cortical areas). The main aim was to evaluate the significance of the time parameters of sound signals and temporal characteristics of the responses for sound discrimination in different parts of the auditory system.

The following measurements, equally applicable to the electrophysiological and behavioral methods, were usually made: (1) measurement of threshold as a function of signal duration (temporal summation); (2) measurement of the latent period of the response as a function of signal intensity; (3) measurement of frequency selectivity as a function of signal duration; (4) evaluation of the responses that transmit information concerning the development of the signal in time.

Responses of Single Units in Two Divisions of the Auditory System (Cochlear Nuclei and Inferior Colliculus)*

COCHLEAR NUCLEI

The cochlear nuclei, which constitute the first central relays of the auditory system, were examined with the microelectrode technique (extracellular recording) by a number of researchers [31, 45, 49, 66, 67, 71]. We shall consider here the data obtained in our laboratory and relate them to the structural scheme presented in Fig. 1.

Each of the three pairs of fibers shown in this scheme, which arise from the apical, middle, and basal coils of the cochlea, must be characterized by a different optimal (best or characteristic) frequency since they derive from a separate and distinct part of the cochlear receptor surface.

When considering the structure, it is natural to assume that nerve impulses generated by a given part of the receptor surface and conducted by a single fiber to the various divisions of the cochlear complex undergo certain transformations after synaptic transmission along the isofrequency line. From a functional point of view, such an organization could be instrumental in producing information with different temporal criteria from the same sector of the receptor surface. For the evaluation of this assumption, investigation of responses of single units that have the same optimal frequency is of particular importance.

It is well known that different neurons in the cochlear nuclei may respond differently under similar conditions of acoustic stimulation [31, 46, 49, 67, 68, 71]. In our work, we established two types of responses that differ greatly from each other.

The first type is characterized by (1) a considerable decrease of threshold value when the duration of the signal increases, i.e., by a very marked temporal summation; (2) an appreciable decrease of the latent period when the intensity of a near-threshold sound is increased; (3) a sharpening of the frequency-threshold curve with an increase in signal duration (from 2 or 3 to

---

* This part of the article has been written jointly with I. A. Vartanian, with the participation of G. I. Ratnikova.

100 msec) which results from a striking fall in threshold for the optimal frequency; (4) discharges which occur during the whole period of the sound signal even at low intensities. The characteristics mentioned under 1, 2, and 4 are valid both for tonal signals at optimal frequency and for broadband noise.

The second type of response is characterized by (1) insignificant changes in thresholds when the signal duration increases, i.e., by absence of any marked temporal summation; (2) a latent period which varies little when the sound intensity changes from threshold to maximal values; (3) a similar frequency-threshold curve for stimuli of brief and long duration; (4) an initial discharge burst, which consists of a small number of impulses (1 to 2) and which often preserves its configuration when the sound intensity increases to considerable, and sometimes to maximal values.

Broadly speaking, the first response type may be characterized as a long-latent, slowly summating, tonic discharge and will be termed a *long-time constant response*; the second type is a short-latent, rapidly summating, phasic discharge and will be referred to as a *short-time constant response*.

The long-time constant response predominates in the cochlear nuclei. Of more than 500 neurons studied by Radionova [67, 68], 60% were of this type. The short-time constant response was present in less than 20% of all neurons. Intermediate characteristics of the responses were observed in the remaining 20% of the investigated population.

Both response types may be encountered in any division of the cochlear nuclei [67, 68]. The long-time constant neurons are rather evenly distributed throughout the entire extent of the cochlear nuclei. The short-time constant neurons, on the other hand, are apparently located mainly in some sectors of the dorsal cochlear nucleus as well as in the posteroventral and anteroventral nuclei in the region near the cone of the incoming fibers of the auditory nerve [49].

It is clear that the transformations which occur in the transmission of information concerning the signal, especially near-threshold, differ sharply for the two types of responses described. Of great significance is the fact that different neurons may respond optimally to the same frequencies, but may differ in the type of response. This suggests that the afferent flow from the same sector of the receptor surface may undergo different transformation, presumably due to the existence of various elements in a given isofrequency region. This is already demonstrable in the cochlear nuclei but is much more pronounced at the level of the inferior colliculus.

Figure 2 presents data showing the optimal frequencies and locations of individual neurons along the tracks of eight electrodes passing through the various divisions of the cochlear complex in the posteroanterior and dorsoventral direction. The following can be stated on the basis of these data: (1) There is a progressive sequence of the optimal frequencies—from high to

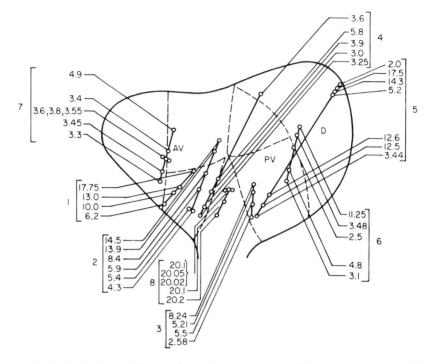

FIG. 2. Optimal (best) frequencies and response types of single neurons along eight electrode tracks in different parts of the cochlear complex (after Radionova and Ratnikova). Filled circles: short-time constant neurons; circles: long-time constant neurons. Tonotopical organization is seen in some penetrations (tracks 1, 2, 3, and 5). Progressive change in the optimal frequency from high to low along these tracks as the electrodes advance in dorsoventral direction. Neurons with similar optimal frequencies but different time characteristics are shown in tracks 2, 3, and 4.

low—along the tracks in a number of punctures (Fig. 2: tracks 1, 2, 3), and there is a jump in the optimal frequency sequences when the electrode passes from one division to another (Fig. 2: tracks 5, 6), data that agree with the results previously described [71]. (2) Neurons with different time characteristics may possess nearly the same optimal frequencies (Fig. 2: tracks 2, 4, 8). (3) An electrode may pass through regions where neurons respond optimally to similar frequencies (Fig. 2: tracks 4, 7, 8).

It should be pointed out that the presence of a group of neurons which display similar optimal frequencies along the tracks of some electrodes is as noteworthy as the tonotopical arrangement of neurons observed in other more numerous penetrations. A small number of electrodes passing along elements with very similar optimal frequencies is probably accounted for by the difficulty of advancing the electrode parallel to the supposed course of the fibers after bifurcation (see scheme in Fig. 1).

INFERIOR COLLICULUS

The inferior colliculus was extensively investigated in cats and white rats in a number of studies conducted in our laboratory.

A study of responses in the inferior colliculus showed that both the short-time constant neurons and the long-time constant neurons occur. However, the proportion of short-time constant neurons is greater here than in the cochlear nuclei. The short-time constant neurons constituted 40% of the population of 270 collicular neurons in the white rat [55, 56] and 50% in a sample of 108 neurons in the cat [25].

Figure 3 presents the frequency-threshold relations for several neurons in the inferior colliculus of the white rat when the sound signal had a duration of 100 and 2 msec, respectively. The frequency-threshold curves for the three

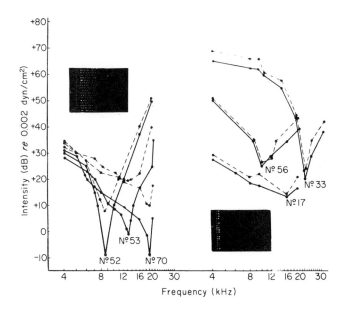

FIG. 3. Frequency-threshold curves for three long-time constant neurons (on left) and three short-time constant neurons (on right), obtained in experiments on inferior colliculus of the white rat for brief and long sound bursts. Broken lines: stimulus duration, 2 msec; continuous lines: stimulus duration, 80 to 100 msec. Typical discharge patterns of a long-time constant and a short-time constant neuron are shown in records obtained with Wall's [88] method. The first dot on the left in each line indicates the beginning of the stimulus, all other dots indicate the time of occurrence of the neural discharge. Each line corresponds to one stimulus presentation. Note the onset discharge in the record of the short-time constant neuron and sustained discharges for the long-time constant neuron. Interval between successive stimuli is 1 sec; duration of sound burst, 80 msec; stimulus intensity, 50 dB above threshold.

short-time constant neurons, which produced only one impulse per stimulus, are practically independent of the duration of the signal. Temporal summation, expressed in a fall of the threshold value when the signal duration increases, is insignificant (not more than 2 to 3 dB) even at the optimal frequency, a characteristic observation for neurons of this type. The frequency-threshold curves for the three long-time constant neurons, which produced sustained discharges (Fig. 3, left), greatly differ for signals of long and short duration. At the optimal frequency, the difference in threshold exceeds 20 dB (neuron 53), i.e., there is a marked temporal summation. At frequencies remote from the optimal one the threshold changes for signals of different durations are small (less than 5 dB) for most neurons.

It appears from such findings that the frequency sensitivity of a neuron in the inferior colliculus may be a function of sound duration. The data on rats are concordant with similar data on the cat which are presented in more detail elsewhere in this volume [25].

As is known, a common interpretation of the sharpness of the threshold tuning curves assumes the existence of lateral inhibition which was first described in the classical study on the eye of the limulus [36].

However, it is not at all clear what actual mechanisms are responsible for the sharpening of the tuning curves in different divisions of the auditory system. Possibly, such sharpening already occurs in the cochlea. The sharp tuning curves obtained for fibers of the auditory nerve [47] and the rapid development of sharpening phenomena in time [93] support this assumption [21]. Other observations, however, imply that sharp tuning curves are particularly pronounced in the central divisions of the auditory system and that some central mechanisms may be responsible for their occurrence [37, 46, 78].

Although our data do not reveal the actual mechanism that causes frequency sharpening, they suggest that marked differences exist in the development of this phenomenon between the short-time constant and the long-time constant neurons.

For the long-time constant neurons some frequency sharpening (in comparison with the cochlea) possibly occurs even for brief sounds; however, most characteristic is a considerable sharpening when the signal duration is increased. This sharpening is due to temporal summation taking place mainly at the optimal frequency (Fig. 3). In addition, at the optimal frequency, the response consists of a larger number of impulses than at nonoptimal frequencies for signals at the same intensities. The differences between the response patterns in the rat's inferior colliculus at the optimal and nonoptimal frequencies are shown in Fig. 4. Similar phenomena in the cat's inferior colliculus were described by Gersuni et al. [25], and in the cochlear nucleus by Radionova [68].

Both phenomena—a substantial temporal summation and a long duration of the discharges of the long-time constant neurons at the optimal frequency—

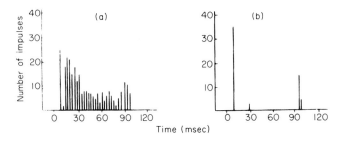

FIG. 4. Poststimulus histograms (PST) of a long-time constant neuron (No. 52, see Fig. 3) which were obtained when the stimulus was at its optimal frequency of 8.5 kHz (a) and at a nonoptimal frequency of 14 kHz (b). PST histograms were obtained with the aid of an automatic impulse counter. Abscissa: time of analysis in msec, each bin equals 3 msec. Ordinate: number of impulses in 30 presentations of the signal. Sound duration, 100 msec; intensity: 30 dB above threshold. Inferior colliculus of the white rat.

determine the expressiveness of the frequency sharpening when the signal duration increases.

For the short-time constant neurons the sharpening does not depend on the signal duration and reaches its final value during the action of a brief sound, i.e., there is no appreciable temporal summation. The temporal characteristics of the discharges suggest that the sharpening is probably due to a peripheral mechanism the existence of which is assumed by a number of authors [21, 93]. Thus, information concerning the frequency of the signal, available at the level of the first neuron, may be transmitted to the higher centers with a minimal delay due to the activity of the short-time constant neurons.

When broadband noise is the stimulus, the characteristics of the responses (temporal summation, latency shifts, impulsation pattern) tend to be similar to those that occur when the neurons respond to the optimal frequencies, especially at low sound intensities (see also 56a). Figure 5 presents poststimulus (PST) histograms of the impulse activity of the two types of neurons during the presentation of noise.

Of great significance is the fact that the presentation of sound signals with different temporal parameters often reveals marked differences in responses of neurons of the two types. Thus, for short-time constant neurons there is characteristically a considerable increase in the response threshold (up to 20 dB) when the risetime of the signal increases from 0.1 to 7-12 msec. By contrast, the threshold for a typical long-time constant neuron is not appreciably affected by a substantial increase in the risetime of the signal [66, 67]. The different sensitivity of the different neurons to risetime of the signals is obviously correlated with other characteristics of short-time constant and long-time constant neurons. We wish to emphasize the significance of these observations for determination of the frequency-threshold curves. Usually,

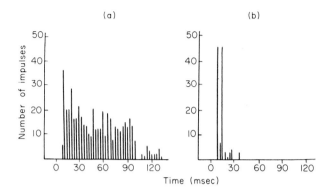

FIG. 5. PST histograms for a long-time constant neuron (a) and a short-time constant neuron (b) obtained when white noise was the stimulus. Stimulus duration: 100 msec; intensity: 50 dB above threshold. Inferior colliculus of the white rat.

such curves are determined by signals with a risetime of several milliseconds [47-49, 71, 72, and others].

Since we wished to apply signals of very short duration and make precise measurements of the latent periods, we determined the frequency-threshold curves of the neurons with rectangular signals [25, 56, 67].

Determinations of the frequency-threshold curves for signals with different risetime (the signal duration being not less than 50 msec) revealed significant differences between the short-time constant and long-time constant neurons. For the short-time constant neurons the shape of the frequency-threshold curves remained substantially unaffected, but there was a general increase of thresholds at all frequencies. For the long-time constant neurons, the sharpness of the frequency-threshold curves increased due to a rise in thresholds for the side frequencies (Fig. 6; see also Fig. 12 in the work of Radionova [68] in this volume).

The data of Maruseva [56a], pertaining to responses to pairs of clicks that were delivered at varying time intervals, suggest a substantial difference in the time of recovery of the response to a second click for different groups of neurons. Typically, the short-time constant neurons are characterized by a very short recovery time (up to 10 msec).

Characteristic differences between both groups of neurons in the responses to amplitude modulation are described in the work of Vartanian [86].

The data available leave no doubt that at the level of the inferior colliculus there are neurons that possess greatly differing temporal properties. Nonetheless, as in the cochlear nuclei, one may observe an orderly spatial, tonotopical arrangement of the elements.

A tonotopical organization, which reflects the projection of the cochlear length, has been described in the inferior colliculus of the cat [25, 72] and

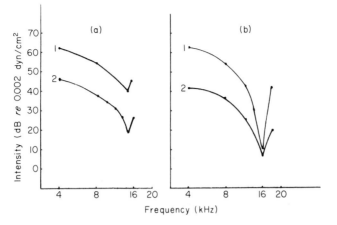

FIG. 6. Frequency-threshold curves for signals with different risetime for two collicular neurons (a and b). Records from white rat after Vartanian and Snetkov. (a) Short-time constant neuron. Curve 1: risetime of the signal, 5 msec; curve 2: rectangular signal. (b) Long-time constant neuron. Curve 1: risetime of the signal, 80 msec; curve 2: rectangular signal.

the white rat [87]. The work of Gersuni *et al.* [25] indicates that neurons with sharply differing time characteristics, but having a similar optimal frequency, may be located in proximity to each other along the track of the same electrode. Figure 5 in the work of Gersuni *et al.* [25] illustrates the following: (1) a regular distribution of the optimal frequencies from low to high when the electrodes were directed from above downward and from the front posteriorly (tracks 4, 5); (2) the presence of tracks [3, 6, 7] in which the optimal frequencies change only within a narrow range (from 0.5 to 1.5 oct) and which are characterized by a smaller angle of slope in the anteroposterior direction; (3) the presence in all tracks of neurons characterized by different temporal characteristics but similar optimal frequencies.

The tonotopical organization in the rat's inferior colliculus was investigated by Vartanian and Ratnikova [87] by the method of evoked potentials.

These workers determined the frequency-threshold curves at different points of the inferior colliculus when the electrode was advanced either rostrocaudally or dorsoventrally. The thresholds were estimated by observing the initially positive phase of the response in the inferior colliculus.

The scheme, which presents a sagittal section of the rat's brain at the level of the central nucleus of the inferior colliculus (Fig. 7), suggests that the frequency of 4 kHz is represented in the region of the posterior pole (which occupies approximately the caudal 1000 μ of tissue); the frequency of 8 kHz is represented in a segment extending between 1000 and 1800 μ from the caudal end; and frequencies of 12, 16, and 20 kHz are represented in the region of the anterior pole (1.800 to 2.600 μ from the caudal end of the

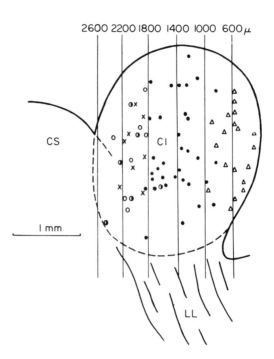

FIG. 7. Tonotopical organization and isofrequency columns in the inferior colliculus of the white rat. Schematic outline of sagittal section through the midbrain at the level of the central nucleus. ci: Inferior colliculus, cs: superior colliculus, *ll*: lateral lemniscus. Numbers at the top: distance in microns from the caudal pole of the inferior colliculus. Triangles, filled circles, half-filled circles, crosses, and circles indicate the loci at which the lowest thresholds for the indicated frequencies (4, 8, 12, 16, and 20 kHz, respectively) were registered in different evoked potential experiments (after Vartanian and Ratnikova).

inferior colliculus). The representations of different frequencies overlap to some extent.

Determinations of the frequency-threshold curves, when the electrode was advanced vertically from the surface of the colliculus, revealed that the optimal frequency does not change as the electrode advances. In cases when the electrode successively passed from the posterior to the anterior part of the colliculus the optimal frequency changed progressively from low to high [87].

The data on single neurons from the white rat's inferior colliculus are, at the present time, insufficient to form a judgment as regards the tonotopical organization of the region. However, an evaluation of a small number of electrode tracks which were made in the dorsoventral direction indicates that neurons with similar optimal frequencies but differing greatly in their temporal characteristics are often encountered along the same track. In general, the presented data show that there exist both a frequency projection, i.e., a projection of the cochlear length, and also (Fig. 7) isofrequency strips which extend in the dorsoventral direction perpendicularly to the rostrocaudal frequency projection.

There is no doubt that data obtained by the method of evoked potentials give a rather gross average picture and the more detailed tonotopical and isofrequency patterns are yet to be established with the help of the microelectrode technique. However, the data obtained by the method of evoked potentials are concordant with Morest's [58] description of the laminar structure of the inferior colliculus. His papers [58, 59] concerning the organization of the inferior colliculus and the medial geniculate body provide a further basis for a spatial scheme of organization of the auditory system.

A number of workers [39, 63, 78, 81] have concluded on the basis of evoked potentials or single unit data that the isofrequency elements in the auditory cortex are organized in an orderly way into strips and columns. (However, for a partly contradictory report see ref. 20).

The functional significance of this organization is far from clear and various interpretations have been proposed. Some models assume that the isofrequency elements produce temporal delay [50], others, that they act in detection of stimulus intensity [15, 53]. Clearly, more work is needed on the isofrequency elements at all levels of the auditory system since their functional significance may be different at different levels. Our own data pertaining to the cochlear nuclei and the inferior colliculus suggest that along an isofrequency line there are elements present which possess different time characteristics. Such an organization is particularly clear in the inferior colliculus.

Thus, a movement of the same segment of the cochlear partition excites many isofrequency cells which have different time characteristics. The information transmitted by a single fiber seems to be processed simultaneously in different ways by the isofrequency cells with different time constants in the cochlear nucleus and the inferior colliculus. The information transmitted is not equivalent. The system with a short-time constant presumably singles out the transient phenomena in the signal which develop within a very short time. Such an organization seems more probable than a monotonic growth of temporal delays caused by an increase in the number of synaptic relays as it is assumed, for example, in Licklider's scheme [50].

Classification of the Neural Responses and the Excitatory Inhibitory Phenomena

The types of neural responses established by us to sounds of short and long durations coincide to a considerable degree with the response types of neurons established by other workers. Thus, the typical group of neurons in the inferior colliculus, designated by us as short-time constant cells or "a" neurons [25] coincides with neurons which were described by Rose et al. [72] and Hind et al. [40] as "pure onset" neurons. These papers [40, 72] contain some essential data which further characterize the neurons with short-time constant; thus, these neurons display very precise latent periods which vary systematically in small steps for different frequencies and for different intensity levels [40].

The second group of neurons, which we designated as neurons with long-time constant, coincides in part with the group described by Rose et al. [72] as characterized by discharges which persist during the whole period of stimulus presentation ("neurons with sustained discharges"). However, we included in the group of the long-time constant neurons [25] only neurons with a latent period of not less than 20 msec, at threshold intensity of the optimal frequency. Whereas the first group of neurons is characterized by a relative constancy of the response, which is to a large extent independent of variation in such parameters of the stimulus as its frequency and intensity, it is characteristic for the long-time constant neurons to be highly sensitive to changes of these parameters. This sensitivity is emphasized in the quoted papers [40, 72] as well as by us in the work on the inferior colliculus [25, 55, 56a] and cochlear nuclei [66-68].

A change in the physical parameters of stimulus (e.g., a shift from the optimal to a nonoptimal frequency) determines the reaction of the long-time constant neurons. Thus, at the optimal frequency these neurons function under their characteristic long-time constant regime; at nonoptimal frequencies, they behave very nearly as neurons functioning under the short-time constant regime (see Fig. 4; also [25]). It is noteworthy that the ability of one and the same neuron to function, as it were, under different time constant regimes is observed not only in mammals (cats and rats), but also in invertebrates with a well-defined auditory function, as, for example, in the locust [64, 65].

There is no doubt that the evaluation of the inhibitory and excitatory processes as they develop and interlace following the delivery of the sound signal is of particular importance in the study of the neural response. Thus, Maruseva [56a], working on the inferior colliculus of the white rat on neurons whose discharges could be inhibited by increase of stimulus strength (nonmonotonic neurons of Rose et al. [72]), observed that the inhibitory effect was a function of signal duration. The spike-count functions were monotonic for sounds 1 to 2 msec in duration while they manifested a nonmonotonic decline with a relatively small rise in stimulus intensity for signals of longer duration (50 to 100 msec). The simplest explanation of these phenomena is that the inhibitory processes, which become manifest with increase of the signal duration,* develop more slowly in time than does the excitation.

---

* An evaluation of the curves of the spike-count functions for different durations leads to the conclusion that it is the time factor (t) of the signal, and not its energy ($t \times I$), which determines the inhibitory effect described by Maruseva [56a].

For some short-time constant neurons of the inferior colliculus (see [25]; neuron 17, Fig. 7) and for some neurons in the cochlear nuclei [67], the thresholds for brief sounds are lower than those for long-lasting signals. This can be accounted for by the same general mechanism if the inhibitory effects require more time for their development than do the excitatory events which cause a spike discharge.

It is of interest to point out that neurons with short- and long-time constants differ probably markedly in their temporal characteristics not only in regard to the excitatory but also in respect to the inhibitory events. It is often assumed that an onset discharge pattern of central neurons is due to inhibitory influences which originate in the marginal sectors of the receptive field. Such a concept is developed, for example, in Suga's scheme [78]. However, the usual concept of lateral inhibition, which may be valid for long-latency neurons, is insufficient when applied to the onset neurons which are characterized by a very short latent period, insignificant temporal summation, a short recovery period [56a], and sensitivity to high-frequency modulation [86]. If we accept that inhibitory influences play a role in the formation of the onset discharge and influence its characteristics, it is also necessary to accept that the inhibitory phenomena are very precise and that they develop within a very short time.

The data which were used for classification of neurons were obtained by monaural contralateral stimulation. If we assume that the neurons, which behave under those conditions as short-time constant neurons, are the same cells which under conditions of binaural stimulation cause very precise alternation in time of the excitatory and inhibitory events [1, 73], then one can assume that the characteristic short-time constant of these neurons may be significant also for the development of the inhibitory processes. That the inhibitory processes may differ in their time characteristics and that under some conditions of stimulation the inhibitory phenomena may develop very rapidly was described by Rose *et al.* [73] for binaural stimuli, and by Radionova [67a] for monaural stimulation. It should also be noted that the overall characterization of the short-time constant neurons, as functioning irrespective of the character of the stimulus, must be qualified. They actually act in this way only for certain monaural stimuli. When binaural stimulation, monaural volleys of impulses [3] and amplitude-modulated signals of different frequencies [86] are applied, the responses of these neurons display a dependence on the properties of the stimulus, which is, apparantly, connected with a fine temporal structure of the signals. In connection with these facts, the assumption that "pure onset" neurons (short-time constant neurons, which form a group of neurons highly specialized in short-time domain measurement) are connected with the auditory area of the cortex seems justified (see page 106).

The ideas developed in this discussion are based mainly on the consideration of data obtained in studies of the inferior colliculus although the division of neurons in long-time constant and short-time constant groups is already discernible in the cochlear nuclei, as shown by Radionova [66-68]. However, in contrast to the colliculus, the short-time constant characteristics in the cochlear nuclei neurons are well defined, as a rule, only near threshold.

It should be emphasized that all our data on which the classification of neurons is based were in response to signals not longer than 100 msec, and thus adaptation phenomena were not considered.

Slow Wave and Summated Spike Responses at Various Levels of the Auditory System

In the transmission of sensory information, the evoked potentials are important indices as to how responses of a large population of neurons [18] are locked in time to the stimulus.

In the cochlear complex, slow waves of high amplitude are recorded in the ventral nuclei [6, 60] where the cellular elements (especially in the anteroventral nucleus) are densely packed [69]. Three components are described in this response. The last of them was regarded as a postsynaptic potential whose latency shift ranges from 3.6 to 2.0 msec as the intensity rises from a near threshold to a maximal value. The intensity-dependent latencies are close to the values which are observed for the spike activity of the short-time constant neurons of the cochlear nuclei [66, 67].

Threshold of the slow potentials is not dependent on the duration of the signal in the cochlear nuclei. Some properties of the slow wave response are similar to the characteristics of the short-time constant neurons in the cochlear nucleus.

In the lateral lemniscus, the most pronounced component of the slow wave may be regarded—on the basis of its duration—as a presynaptic response in the incoming fibers. The response of the fibers in the lateral lemniscus is characterized by insignificant latency change for signals of varying intensity and by small threshold change, not exceeding 2 dB, as a function of the signal duration. In the central nucleus of the inferior colliculus, the latency of the postsynaptic response changes to a somewhat greater degree [85]; the threshold changes, depending on the duration of the signal, amount on the average to 11 dB at the optimal frequency, and in some cases even to 15-18 dB.

In the records from the surface of the cat's auditory cortical area (zone A_1), an initially positive wave is typically registered which is generally regarded as being of a synaptic origin. Its latency shifts within the range of 8 to 11 msec with variations in the intensity of the signal from maximal to minimal levels [5]. The thresholds, as a function of signal duration, become lower (on the average by 9 dB) when the duration of the noise pulses becomes some 7 to 9 msec [27, 28, 82]. When pure tones are employed, the temporal summation is particularly pronounced at the optimal frequency [91].

One more characteristic feature of the slow wave is noteworthy; it appears when the risetime of the stimulus varies. A transition from rectangular signals to signals with an increasing risetime leads in all divisions of the auditory system to changes in the responses. These changes manifest themselves in a decline of the amplitude and in a rise of the threshold when the time constant of the signals increases [29, 90, 92]. It is possible to determine for each synaptic region of the auditory system the risetime constant of the signal at which a given component of the response disappears—the so-called limit of disappearance [90]. This limit increases sharply as one examines the successive regions in the auditory synaptic chain. Thus, the limits of disappearance for the most typical components of the action potential in the auditory nerve (N_1 and N_2) are expressed (for exponentially growing signals) by the values of 4 and 10 msec; for the typical components of the cortical response—initially negative, initially positive, and subsequently negative—the mean values are 170, 270, and 300 msec, respectively [23, 24a, 24b, 29, 90, 92].

A marked increase of the limit of disappearance occurs during a transition from responses of the auditory nerve to those of the cochlear nucleus. Thus, the slow component of the response of the cochlear nucleus (A_3) is characterized by a limit of disappearance of more than 100 msec [6].

The disappearance of the typical action potential in the auditory nerve by no means signifies the disappearance of the discharges in the auditory fibers. As shown [30, 90], a redistribution in time of the discharges of numerous nerve fibers takes place under these conditions. When stimulated with a rectangular signal, many fibers discharge simultaneously, and thus cause the emergence of N_1 and N_2. Owing to differences in thresholds for various fibers, the number of simultaneously excited fibers greatly decreases during stimulation by slowly growing signals and the synchronized responses become reduced; concurrently, the desynchronized impulse activity, which is evidenced during the entire period of the action of the signal, increases.

Thus, during the action of either a rectangular or a slowly rising signal there is a flow of impulses in the fibers of the auditory nerve towards the cochlear nuclei; in the first case, the discharges are initially highly synchronized; in the second, initial synchronization is absent.

The fact that the short-time constant neurons of the cochlear nuclei are highly sensitive to a change in the risetime of the signal whereas the long-time constant neurons are relatively insensitive to such changes, is a natural consequence of different reactions of the rapidly and slowly summating neurons to the initially synchronized or desynchronized flow of the impulses that bombard them.

Properties peculiar to both types of neurons in the cochlear nuclei manifest themselves in various degrees in responses of the higher divisions of the auditory system. They are particularly clear in the cortical responses, especially in the most thoroughly investigated initially positive wave.

These properties make it possible: (1) to transmit information about the signal within a short time, which, in the case of rectangular signals, does not exceed 8 to 10 msec and, in the case of slowly rising signals, is not more than 20 to 25 msec; (2) to signal the beginning of the sound despite a considerable increase in the risetime of the sound when the peripheral afferent flow is completely desynchronized.

Responses of Neurons in the Primary Auditory Cortex (A_1)

An investigation of single unit responses in the A_1 zone of the auditory cortex (extracellular recordings) was carried out in our laboratory by Vardapetian [83, 84].

His data show that a group of neurons, defined by him as the "stable" group, exhibited the same characteristics of temporal summation and the same latency-intensity relationships which were described for the initially positive wave of the primary response in the cortical auditory areas.

In respect to spike activity, the responses of "stable" neurons resemble in some aspects those of both the short-time constant and the long-time constant neurons. On the one hand, spike responses arise at the onset of the sound signal; on the other hand, the number of impulses produced varies from one to five or six, depending on the intensity of stimulation. Temporal summation—a decline in the threshold values with increase of stimulus duration—was of the order of 6 to 9 dB, which is a higher figure than that usually seen for the short-time constant neurons, but lower than for the typical long-time constant neurons.

Thus, the characteristics of the short-latency response of the cortical neurons in the primary auditory area are a combination of properties of the two types of neurons encountered in the lower divisions of the auditory system. Because of that, the relatively short latent period of such neurons tends to remain short for signals of different forms. This makes it possible first, to respond fast both to rectangular signals and to those with a slow risetime; second, to ensure the processing of information regarding the spectrum of the signal within a short time (from 6-8 to 20-25 msec, depending on the form of the signal).

It should be emphasized that the characteristics considered refer to the initial response of these neurons, which corresponds in time to the primary evoked response [27, 28, 82]. However, as described by Vardapetian [83], there occurs for these neurons also a late response, separated from the initial response by an interval of not less than 150-200 msec. This late response is probably associated with the late components of the slow wave which were investigated by some authors, in particular by Gasanov [22]. The late response reflects events quite different from those produced by the early one.

In a neurophysiological scheme, the neurons of the auditory cortex may be viewed as elements upon which the short-time constant and the long-time constant neurons (seen in lower divisions) converge. (The characteristics of neurons in the medial geniculate body are now being examined to determine whether this assumption is valid.) In addition, these neurons respond also after prolonged delay which may last thousands of milliseconds. However, it would be premature, at the present time, to suggest a neurophysiological mechanism which could account for such late components of the response.

It is noteworthy that Oonishi and Katsuki [63] described neurons in the auditory cortical area, whose threshold tuning curves showed discontinuous frequency bands at some intensity levels. They interpreted such findings to indicate that several neurons of the medial geniculate body, with different optimal frequencies, converge on such neurons. Consequently, it would be of interest to examine whether there is convergence of neurons of the lower divisions with different, both temporal and spectral, characteristics upon a single cortical neuron.

Besides the group of "stable" neurons, Vardapetian [83] described several other cortical groups. The neurons of these groups must be of great importance for further processing of the incoming sensory information. There exists, thus, neurons whose activity pattern, in response to a stimulus, may last up to 10 min [83, 84] as well as neurons which respond only to novel sounds (i.e., not presented previously) and neurons which respond only to frequency-modulated signals [78, 89] and amplitude-modulated sounds [86]. There further exist rare neurons which curiously enough display an alternating type of response to the presentation of clicks at intervals of 10 min or longer [2].

All such responses require further thorough studies since without them the mechanisms of the auditory functions will remain incomprehensible. However, rather little is known about these highly important phenomena [84] and little could be gained by speculations about them at the present time.

Detection and Discrimination of Sounds of Different Duration after Lesions of the Cortical Auditory Region

In order to understand the mechanisms of the auditory function it is necessary to investigate the detection and discrimination of sounds in the intact organism. As is known, such investigations in man are carried out with psychophysical methods and these are also applicable, within limits, to animals.

Determination of the threshold intensity and measurements of frequency selectivity as a function of the duration of the sound signal were performed on dogs, in which various parts of the cortical auditory region had been ablated—unilaterally or bilaterally. The avoidance method was used; the animal had to withdraw its paw when the signal was sounded and could thus avoid an electric shock [12].

Determination of the threshold intensity for sounds of different spectral composition (broadband noises and pure tones of different frequency) indicated that after unilateral ablation of the cortical auditory region, there was a rise in thresholds when the contralateral ear was stimulated by brief sounds of 1 to 10-16 msec in duration [9, 23]. No threshold changes were observed for longer sounds. Typical findings are shown in Fig. 8.

Such findings were obtained with extensive ablations of the temporal region (both unilateral and bilateral) as well as with more limited lesions which affected mainly the medial ectosylvian gyrus. The data are convincing that lesions of the auditory cortex affect the thresholds of detection for very short sounds only (Baru, [12]).

A study of tone discrimination (in the course of establishing the differential frequency thresholds) demonstrated that lesions in the cortical auditory region

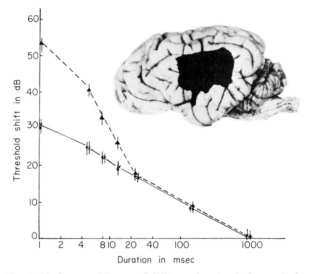

FIG. 8. Thresholds for sound bursts of different duration before and after ablation of the left temporal cortex (regions AI, AII, Ep, and SS) in the dog. Abscissa: duration of the sound signals in msec. Ordinate: threshold shift in dB in relation to the threshold value for a signal 1000 msec in duration which was taken as a zero reference point. Solid line: thresholds for the left and right ear signals before ablation of the cortex (filled circles) and for left ear signals after cortical abalation (crosses). Dashed line and triangles: threshold for the right ear signals (contralateral to the lesion) after cortical ablation. A rise of thresholds for brief sounds is evident. Length of the vertical lines through each point of measurement indicates the value of the standard deviation; frequency of the signal is 1000 Hz.

affect only brief sounds; for tone durations exceeding 20 to 30 msec no appreciable changes in frequency discrimination could be observed ([11, 12]; see also Fig. 9).

It should be noted that investigations of threshold intensities for sounds of different duration, carried out on patients with vascular focal lesions of the temporal region [13] and on patients with tumors localized in the region of the superior and middle parts of the temporal lobe (before and after removal of the tumors) [26a, 26b, 42], revealed the same finding, namely, that there is a rise in thresholds only for brief signals. These findings clarify the discrepancy between the electrophysiological and behavioral observations as to the role of the auditory cortex in frequency discrimination, which was mentioned in the opening paragraphs of this paper. This discrepancy arose because it was not realized that the electrophysiological data concerning frequency projection upon the auditory cortex [38, 43, 48, 80] should be related only to sounds of brief duration (1 to 20 msec) since this is the time in which the evoked cortical response develops [27, 28, 82]. On the other hand, the behavioral investigations used relatively long tones (1 sec and over)

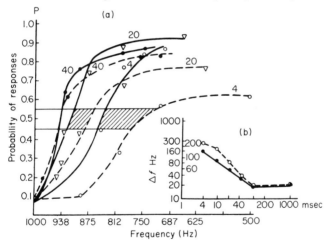

FIG. 9. Frequency discrimination before and after ablation of the temporal cortex in the dog. The extent of the lesion is the same as in Fig. 8. Left cortical regions AI, AII, Ep, and SS were removed. (a) Probability of correct responses to nonreinforced stimuli. Only the standard tone of 1000 Hz was reinforced. Continuous lines: control determinations; broken lines: determinations after cortical ablation. Duration of the sound signal in milliseconds is indicated for each curve. The shaded areas show the shift of response probability (for probability levels of 0.45-0.55) for signals of 4 and 20 msec in duration. (b) Difference limen for frequency (Δf in Hz) as a function of the duration of a 1000-Hz tone. Continuous line: control; broken line: determinations after the operation. In (a) and (b), statistically significant rise in threshold for frequency discrimination is observed only for sounds of brief duration (from 4 to 20 msec). After A. V. Baru [11, 12].

to explore hearing deficits after extensive bilateral ablations of the temporal region. Under such conditions, however, there is no substantial disturbance in frequency discrimination [14, 32, 57, 61]. How can we account for the basic fact that it is the detection and discrimination of brief sounds only which are impaired after lesions of the auditory cortex?

Analysis of single unit data at various levels of the auditory system suggests that transmission of information about the properties of brief sounds or of the initial time segment of any sound within the limits of 10 to 20 msec (i.e., within the time during which the effects of the lesion in the auditory cortex are detectable) is accomplished by the short-time constant neurons as well as by the initial burst discharge of the long-time constant neurons (the latter being observed during the action of sounds at suprathreshold intensities). As has been discussed, this flow of information must converge on neurons whose initial response develops during the first 10 to 20 msec after the onset of the sound signal. A destruction of these cortical neurons upon which there is a convergent projection from the short-time constant neurons as well as from those long-time constant neurons which have a short latent period, at supra-threshold intensities, may be regarded as one of the factors which causes impairment in the discrimination of brief sounds. If we assume that the short-time constant neurons are directly or indirectly connected predomi-nantly with the internal hair cells, then there exists presumably a system with a short-time constant which is capable of transmitting information from the receptor elements up to the cortical fields.

However, the cortical neurons which have the above-discussed convergent projection produce not only an initial response but also a late, delayed response. There are also other neurons which manifest delayed reactions whose duration does not depend on the duration of the stimulus [83, 84]; such reactions may be regarded as manifestations of memory. It may be assumed that short-time memory is of particular importance for the detection and discrimination of short sounds since their duration is much shorter than the time required for the development of the process of discrimination [7, 23]. Thus, the finding that in lesions of the auditory cortex the detection of brief sounds only is impaired is presumably accounted for by the destruction of neurons which act in transmission and processing of information within short segments of time and are also involved in the phenomena of short-time memory.

The discrimination of long-lasting sounds, which is dependent on activity of the long-time constant neurons, is not affected by lesions of the auditory cortex. It is clear that this activity is organized in a different way and involves other central groups. Precisely what these structures are remains obscure. Their location must, apparently, be looked for beyond the boundaries of the classical auditory region, possibly, in the limbic system. Some facts suggesting differences in the chemical susceptibility of the processes which are involved in detection of short- and long-lasting sounds deserve a comment. Thus, after an injection of caffein, one observes a statistically significant decline in thresholds for noise pulses with a duration of less than 16 msec. After an injection of phenamine, the thresholds for sounds with a duration of less than 10 msec do not show any change, but a decline in thresholds occurs for sounds with a duration from 10 to 1000 msec [10].

Thus, the detection of sounds of different duration is based evidently on processes which differ not only in the locus where they occur, but also in their biochemical organization.

The final problem of importance to be raised when studying the functions of the auditory system with sounds of different duration is the question of a change in the pitch of the sound. Thus, when the duration of a sound pulse of a given frequency decreases, there takes place, along with a regular increase of the differential frequency thresholds [51, 75] (see Fig. 9), a change in the pitch quality of the signal. According to Doughty and Garner [19], a short tonal pulse having a definite pitch turns into a click; such a click loses its pitch coloration when the signal is on the average 2 to 4 msec in duration (within the range of frequencies from 1000 to 8000 Hz). From the formal point of view of spectral analysis of the sound, both phenomena, i.e., the loss of the pitch quality and the increase in the differential frequency thresholds, are connected with the extension of the band of the signal spectrum when the duration of the signal decreases (see discussion in references 34 and 75).

The broadband pulses of short duration devoid of a clear musical pitch quality possess nonchromatic or timbre qualities which determine the frequency discrimination of such short sounds to a high degree. For frequency discrimination of such short sounds, the well-known problem of components of a tonal perception arises. The frequency-dependent quality of the auditory sensation was classified by many authors (see Teplov's review [79]) into two main groups of components: chromatic pitch components, connected with identification and reproduction of musical intervals, and nonchromatic components (timbre, brightness, volume) (see review of Stevens and Davis [76]) which are not directly connected with the musical scale. In the frequency discrimination of short-sound pulses, the nonchromatic components seem to dominate. In the frequency discrimination of long-lasting sounds the chromatic components evidently prevails.

Thus, it may be presumed that the mechanism for frequency discrimination of short sounds, which becomes defective as a result of lesions of the cortical auditory area, is connected with the nonchromatic components determining the discrimination. The chromatic ("musical") pitch components, which require sounds of longer duration, are not disturbed when the auditory cortical projection region is damaged. Of great interest for this problem are data relating to the differences in localization of central lesions which cause a disturbance of musical perception and the typical lesions of the temporal areas

causing sensory aphasia as well as deficits in the perception of brief sounds
[42]. Highly illustrative is a case of severe sensory aphasia recently described;
it relates to a person (a prominent composer) who suffered from a massive
lesion of the temporal region but preserved all his musical abilities [54]. The
locus of lesions causing disorders of musical perception is controversial. This
problem would require a special presentation which is beyond the scope of
the present article.

The data presented and the conclusions drawn from them support the point
of view that there exist in the auditory system two different mechanisms
which work, respectively, under a short- and a long-time constant regime. One
could presume that the first of these mechanisms operates predominantly in
nonexpressive sound perception including nonexpressive speech, and the second in music and expressive speech perception. Such a presumption is, at the
present time, certainly not sufficiently substantiated. However, there are some
reasons to advance it as a working hypothesis, a hypothesis which perhaps has
some speculative features.

Conclusion

It is still impossible to formulate a general theory of hearing, i.e., a theory
of the mechanisms which are responsible for the perception and utilization by
the organism of the entire domain of sounds.

However, even with the existing knowledge certain concepts concerning
some of the mechanisms can be developed.

The experimental facts and their evaluation presented in this article make it
evident that there are in the auditory system two mechanisms, which differ in
a number of attributes. They were designated as mechanisms which work,
respectively, under conditions of a short- and a long-time constant regime. It
seems possible to regard each part of the auditory system as consisting of
elements which are, in the main, functionally connected with one or the other
of these two mechanisms.

Whereas the basilar membrane as a whole possesses characteristics of a
frequency analyzer with a short-time constant (short-term analyzer, in the
terminology of Von Békésy [16]), it is already possible to differentiate the
element according to their time constants in the organ of Corti. This is
suggested by the work of Neubert [62] who has shown that the internal hair
cells, unlike the external ones, are mechanically adjusted to transient phenomena. If these data are correct, then the different properties of the internal and
external hair cells must involve also mechanical time constants.

Innervation of the internal hair cells by the radial fibers is characterized by
a connection of one nerve fiber with one to three hair cells, i.e., by a very
small receptive field (of the order of 10 to 30 μ). A small surface of the

receptive field in the presence of the supposed connections between the internal hair cells, the rapidly summating short-time constant neurons of the cochlear nuclei, as well as similar neurons in the inferior colliculus, would contribute to the work of the system under conditions of a short-time constant regime. On the other hand, the external hair cells with their large receptive fields and their connection with the slowly summating, tonic long-time constant neurons would favor the work of the system under conditions of a long-time constant regime.

The presented material shows that the properties of a short-time constant mechanism are demonstrable in all parts of the auditory system; this mechanism is revealed by the existence of short-time constant neurons in the brain-stem divisions of the auditory system and by the existence of certain neural groups in the auditory cortical fields. Thus, the properties of a short-time constant mechanism may be encountered with a varying probability in all divisions of the auditory system beginning, apparently, with the cochlea and ending with the auditory area of the cortex.

A remarkable property of the short-time constant mechanism is the very short time which it requires for transmission of information about the attributes of the sound from the periphery to the cortical auditory area, despite the existence of a multisynaptic chain and the great opportunities for convergence on the various synaptic structures at any level. The short-time constant mechanism must be regarded as a mechanism which is concerned with discrimination of the spectral properties of sounds within short segments of time and which measures time intervals between transients. This mechanism is impaired by lesions of the primary auditory cortex. It may be assumed that frequency discrimination in the short-time domain achieved by this mechanism is not connected with chromatic pitch sensation.

The long-time constant mechanism presumably secures a different and more precise discrimination of the spectral properties of sounds; it is likely to be more closely concerned with the sensation of the chromatic pitch, with musical perception, as well as with the emotional side of sound perception in general.

The character of the relation of the long-time constant mechanism with the cortical divisions is at present not clear; this mechanism manifests no disturbances as a result of extirpation of the auditory area, at least not under the conditions of our investigations.

REFERENCES

1. Altman, J. A. Responses of the inferior colliculus neurons of the cat to changes in time intervals between binaural presented stimuli. *Biophysics (USSR)* **11**, 488-497 (1966) (in Russian).

2. Altman, J. A. The alternated responses of neurons in the inferior colliculus. *J. Higher Nervous Activity (USSR)* **16**, 531-533 (1966) (in Russian).

3. Altman, J. A. Are there neurons detecting direction of sound source motion? *Exp. Neurol.* **22**, 13-25 (1968).

4. Altman, J. A. This volume, Chap. 13.

5. Altman, J. A., and Maruseva, A. M. Evoked potentials of the auditory system. *J. Higher Nervous Acitivty (USSR)* **15**, 539-549 (1965) (in Russian).

6. Altman, J. A., Radionova, E. A., and Ratnikova, G. I. Electrophysiological investigation of the cochlear nucleus in the cat. *Sechenov Physiol. J. USSR* **49**, 1163-1172 (1963) (in Russian).

7. Avakian, R. V., Vardapetian, G. A., and Gersuni, G. V. Effect of acoustic signal duration on the latency of a voluntary motor response. *J. Higher Nervous Activity (USSR)* **16**, 1037-1045 (1966) (in Russian).

8. Baru, A. V. Effects of lesions in the auditory cortex on detection of sound stimulus of different duration. *Abstr. 10th All-Union Conf. Physiologists, USSR, 1964*, Vol. 2, Pt. 2, pp. 79-80 (in Russian).

9. Baru, A. V. On the role of the temporal cortex in the detection of sounds of different duration in the dog. *J. Higher Nervous Activity (USSR)* **16**, 655-666 (1966) (in Russian).

10. Baru, A. V. Peculiarities in the detection of acoustic signals of different duration under the action of some drugs. *J. Higher Nervous Activity (USSR)* **17**, 107-115 (1967) (in Russian).

11. Baru, A. V. Frequency differential limens as a function of tonal signal duration after ablation of the auditory cortex in animals (dogs). *In* "Problems of Physiological Acoustics" (G. V. Gersuni, ed.), Vol. 6: Mechanisms of Hearing, pp. 121-135. Nauka, Leningrad, 1967 (in Russian).

12. Baru, A. V. This volume, Chapter 15.

13. Baru, A. V., Gersuni, G. V., and Tonkonogii, I. M. Measurement at absolute auditory thresholds of sound stimulus of different duration in temporal-lobe lesions. *J. Neuropathol. Psychiatry (USSR)* **64**, 481-485 (1964) (in Russian).

14. Belenkov, N. J. Conditioned reflex and subcortical structures. Medicae Press, Moscow, 1965 (in Russian).

15. Von Békésy, G. Experimental model of the cochlea with and without nerve supply. *In* "Neural Mechanisms of the Auditory and Vestibular Systems" (G. L. Rasmussen and W. F. Windle, eds.), pp. 181-200. Thomas, Springfield, Illinois, 1960.

16. Von Békésy, G. Hearing theories and complex sounds. *J. Acoust. Soc. Amer.* **35**, 588-601 (1963).

17. Cajal, S. R. "Histologie du Système Nerveux de l'Homme et des Vertébrés." A. Maloine, Paris, 1909.

18. Davis, H. Peripheral coding of auditory information. *In* "Sensory Communication" (W. A. Rosenblith, ed.), p. 119. M.I.T. Press, Cambridge, Massachusetts, 1961.

19. Doughty, J. M., and Garner, W. R. Pitch characteristics of short tones. *J. Exp. Psychol.* **37**, 351-365 (1947).

20. Evans, E. F., Ross, H. F., and Whitfield, I. C. The spatial distribution of unit characteristic frequency in the primary auditory cortex of the cat. *J. Physiol. (London)* **179**, 238-247 (1965).

21. Furman, G. G., and Frishkopf, L. S. Model of neural inhibition in the mammalian cochlea. *J. Acoust. Soc. Amer.* **36**, 2194-2201 (1964).

22. Gasanov, U. G. Threshold of evoked potentials of the auditory cortex in wakeful cats for signals of different duration. *In* "Problems of Physiological Acoustics" (G. V. Gersuni, ed.), Vol. 6: Mechanisms of Hearing, pp. 101-107. Nauka, Leningrad, 1967 (in Russian).

23. Gersuni, G. V. Evoked potentials and discrimination of external signals. *J. Higher Nervous Activity (USSR)* **13**, 882-890 (1963) (in Russian).

24a. Gersuni, G. V. Organization of afferent inflow and the process of discrimination of signals of various duration. *J. Higher Nervous Activity (USSR)* **15**, 260-273 (1965) (in Russian).

24b. Gersuni, G. V. Organization of afferent flow and the process of external signal discrimination. *Neuropsychologia* **3**, 95-109 (1965).

25. Gersuni, G. V., Altman, J. A., Maruseva, A. M., Radionova, E. A., Ratnikova, G. I., and Vartanian, I. A. This volume, Chap. 16.

26a. Gersuni, G. V., Baru, A. V., and Karaseva, T. A. On the role of the auditory cortical projection zone in discriminating acoustic signals. *J. Higher Nervous Activity (USSR)* **17**, 932-946 (1967) (in Russian).

26b. Gersuni, G. V., Baru, A. V., Karaseva, T. A., and Tonkonogii, I. M. This volume, Chap. 10.

27. Gersuni, G. V., Gasanov, U. G., Zaboeva, N. V., and Lebedinsky, M. M. Evoked potentials of the auditory cortex and the time characteristics of the sound stimuli. *Biophysics (USSR)* **9**, 597-606 (1964) (in Russian).

28. Gersuni, G. V., Shevelev, I. A., and Likhnitsky, A. M. Dependence of the primary response of the auditory cortical area in alert cats on temporal parameters of the signal. *J. Higher Nervous Activity (USSR)* **14**, 489-497 (1964) (in Russian).

29. Gersuni, G. V., and Zaboeva, N. V. Evaluation of the functional significance of electrical responses to the auditory system. *Sechenov Physiol. J. USSR* **48**, 1178-1186 (1962) (in Russian).

30. Goldstein, M. H., and Kiang, N. Y-S. Synchrony of neural activity in electric responses evoked by transient acoustic stimuli. *J. Acoust. Soc. Amer.* **30**, 107-114 (1958).

31. Greenwood, D. D., and Maruyama, N. Excitatory and inhibitory response areas of auditory neurons in the cochlear nucleus. *J. Neurophysiol.* **28**, 863-890 (1965).

32. Hananashwili, M. M. The role of auditory cortex in sound discrimination in dogs. *Abstr. 10th All-Union Conf. Physiologists, USSR, 1964*, Vol. 2, pp. 371-372 (in Russian).

33. Hananashwili, M. M. Discrimination of acoustic stimuli with different rise-time. *J. Higher Nervous Activity (USSR)* **15**, 788-795 (1965) (in Russian).

34. Harkevich, A. A. "The Spectra and Analysis." State Press, Moscow, 1962 (in Russian).

35. Harrison, J. M., and Warr, W. B. A study of the cochlear nuclei and ascending auditory pathways of the medulla. *J. Comp. Neurol.* **119**, 341-380 (1962).

36. Hartline, H. K., Wagner, H. G., and Ratliff, F. Inhibition in the eye of limulus. *J. Gen. Physiol.* **39**, 651-673 (1956).

37. Hilali, S., and Whitfield, I. C. Responses of the trapezoid body to acoustic stimulation with pure tones. *J. Physiol. (London)* **122**, 158-171 (1953).

38. Hind, J. E. An electrophysiological determination of tonotopic organization in auditory cortex of cat. *J. Neurophysiol.* **16**, 475-489 (1953).

39. Hind, J. E. Unit activity in the auditory cortex. *In* "Neural Mechanisms of the Auditory and Vestibular Systems" (G. L. Rasmussen and W. F. Windle, eds.), pp. 201-210. Thomas, Springfield, Illinois, 1960.

40. Hind, J. E., Goldberg, J. M., Greenwood, D. D., and Rose, J. E. Some discharge characteristics of single neurons in the inferior colliculus of the cat. II. Timing of discharges and observation on binaural stimulation. *J. Neurophysiol.* **26**, 321-341 (1963).

41. Karaseva, T. A. Specificities of short sound signal estimate in cases of local injuries of the temporal lobe of the brain. *In* "Problems of Physiological Acoustics" (G. V.

Gersuni, ed.), Vol. 6: Mechanisms of Hearing, pp. 135-146. Nauka, Leningrad, 1967 (in Russian).

42. Karaseva, T. A. "Testing of Hearing in Temporal-Lobe Damage." Dissertation, The Burdenko Neurosurgical Institute, Moscow, 1967 (in Russian).

43. Katchuro, I. I. Frequency localization within the auditory cortex of the cat. *Seche-nov Physiol. J. USSR* **49**, 659-665 (1963) (in Russian).

44. Katsuki, Y. Comparative neurophysiology of hearing. *Physiol. Rev.* **45**, 380-423 (1965).

45. Katsuki, Y., Sumi, T., Uchiyama, H., and Watanabe, T. Electric responses of auditory neurons in cat to sound stimulation. *J. Neurophysiol.* **21**, 569-588 (1958).

46. Katsuki, Y., Watanabe, T., and Maruyama, N. Activity of auditory neurons in upper levels of brain of cat. *J. Neurophysiol.* **22**, 343-359 (1959).

47. Kiang, N. Y-S. "Discharge Patterns of Single Fibers in the Cats Auditory Nerve. M.I.T. Press, Cambridge, Massachusetts, 1965.

48. Kiang, N. Y-S., and Goldstein, M. H. Tonotopic organization of the cat auditory cortex for some complex stimuli. *J. Acoust. Soc. Amer.* **31**, 786-790 (1959).

49. Kiang, N. Y-S., Pfeiffer, R. R., Warr, W. B., and Backus, A. S. N. Stimulus coding in the cochlear nucleus. *Ann. Otol. Rhinol. Laryngol.* **74**, 463-479 (1965).

50. Licklider, I. C. R. A duplex theory of pitch perception. *Experientia* **7**, 128-134 (1951).

51. Liang, Chic-an, and Chistovich, L. A. Frequency difference limens as a function of tonal duration. *Sov. Acoust. J.* **6**, 81-86 (1960) (in Russian).

52. Lorente de Nò, R. Anatomy of the eighth nerve. General plan of structure of the primary cochlear nuclei. *Laryngoscope* **43**, 327-350 (1933).

53. Lubinsky, I. A., and Posin, N. V. The modelling of information processing in the auditory system of frequency and intensity data. *In* "Problems of Physiological Acoustics" (G. V. Gersuni, ed.), Vol. 6: Mechanisms of Hearing, pp. 209-221. Nauka, Leningrad, 1967 (in Russian).

54. Luria, A. R., Tsvetkova, L. S., and Futer, D. S. Aphasia in a composer *J. Neurological. Sci.* **2**, 288-292 (1965).

55. Maruseva, A. M., Gersuni, G. V., Popov, A. V., and Radionova, E. A. Synaptic transformation of the afferent flow in the auditory system. *In* "Synaptic Processes" (P. G. Kostyuk, ed.), pp. 258-271. Naukova, Dumka, Kiev, 1968.

56. Maruseva, A. M. On the temporal characteristics of the auditory neurons in the inferior colliculus of rat with different types of responses to sound stimuli. *In* "Problems of Physiological Acoustics" (G. V. Gersuni, ed.), Vol. 6: Mechanisms of Hearing, pp. 50-62. Nauka, Leningrad, 1967 (in Russian).

56a. Maruseva, A. M. This volume, Chap. 11.

57. Mering, T. A. A study of the coupling function of the acoustic analyser during the formation of conditioned motor reflexes. *J. Higher Nervous Activity (USSR)* **10**, 747-755 (1960) (in Russian).

58. Morest, D. K. The laminar structure of the inferior colliculus of the cat. *Anat. Rec.* **148**, 314 (1964).

59. Morest, D. K. The laminar structure of the medial geniculate body of the cat. *J. Anat.* **39**, 143-160 (1965).

60. Moushegian, G. Rupert, A., and Galambos, R. Microelectrode study of ventral cochlear neculeus of the cat. *J. Neurophysiol.* **25**, 515-529 (1962).

61. Neff, W. D. Neural mechanisms of auditory discrimination. *In* "Sensory Communication" (W. A. Rosenblith, ed.), pp. 259-278. M. I. T. Press, Cambridge, Massachusetts, 1961.

62. Neubert, K. Innere Haarzellen des Cortischen Organs und Schallanalyse. *Naturwissenschaften* **47**, 526-527 (1960).

63. Oonishi, S., and Katsuki, Y. Functional organization and integrative mechanism of the auditory cortex of the cat. *Jap. J. Physiol.* **15**, 342-365 (1965).
64. Popov, A. V. Characteristics of activity of the central neurons in the auditory system of the locust. *In* "Problems of Physiological Acoustics" (G. V. Gersuni, ed.), Vol. 6: Mechanisms of Hearing, pp. 108-121. Nauka, Leningrad, 1967 (in Russian).
65. Popov, A. V. This volume, Chap. 17.
66. Radionova, E. A. Correlation of some characteristics of the auditory system neurons in their reaction to sound stimuli. *Biophysics (USSR)* **11**, 478-487 (1966) (in Russian).
67. Radionova, E. A. On the significance of time characteristics of the cochlear nucleus neurons. *In* "Problems of Physiological Acoustics" (G. V. Gersuni, ed.), Vol. 6: Mechanisms of Hearing, pp. 32-49. Nauka, Leningrad, 1967 (in Russian).
67a. Radionova, E. A. Inhibitory phenomena in impulse activity of the neurons in the cochlear nucleus of cats. *J. Higher Nervous Activity (USSR)* **18**, 133-136 (1968) (in Russian).
68. Radionova, E. A. This volume, Chap. 9.
69. Ratnikova, G. I. On the structure of the cochlear nuclei in the cat. *In* "Problems of Physiological Acoustics" (G. V. Gersuni, ed.), Vol. 6: Mechanisms of Hearing, pp. 182-195. Nauka, Leningrad, 1967 (in Russian).
70. Rose, J. E. Organization of frequency sensitive neurons in the cochlear nuclear complex of the cat. *In* "Neural Mechanisms of the Auditory and Vestibular Systems" (G. L. Rasmussen and W. F. Windle, eds.), pp. 116-136. Thomas, Springfield, Illinois, 1960.
71. Rose, J. E., Galambos, R., and Hughes, J. R. Microelectrode studies of the cochlear nuclei of the cat. *Bull. Johns Hopkins Hosp.* **104**, 211-251 (1959).
72. Rose, J. E., Greenwood, D. D., Goldberg, J. M., and Hind, J. E. Some discharge characteristics of single neurons in the inferior colliculus of the cat. I. Tonotopical organization, relation of spike counts to tone intensity and firing patterns of single elements. *J. Neurophysiol.* **26**, 294-320 (1963).
73. Rose, J. E., Gross, N. B., Geisler, C. D., and Hind, J. E. Some neural mechanisms in the inferior colliculus of the cat which may be relevant to localization of a sound source. *J. Neurophysiol.* **29**, 288-314 (1966).
74. Sando, I. The anatomical interrelationships of the cochlear nerve fibers. *Acta Oto-La-ryngol.* **59**, 417-436 (1965).
75. Sekey, A. Short-time auditory frequency discrimination. *J. Acoust. Soc. Amer.* **35**, 682-690 (1963).
76. Stevens, S. S., and Davis, H. "Hearing, Its Psychology and Physiology." Wiley, New York, 1938.
77. Stotler, W. A. The mode of termination of axons on the cells of the acoustic relay nuclei of the medulla. *Anat. Rec.* **103**, 585 (1949).
78. Suga, N. Functional properties of auditory neurons in the cortex of echo-locating bats. *J. Physiol. (London)* **181**, 671-700 (1965).
79. Teplov, B. M. "Psychology of muscial abilities." Pedagogical Academy Press, Moscow, 1947 (in Russian).
80. Tunturi, A. R. Physiological determination of the arrangement of the afferent connections to the middle ectosylvian auditory area in the dog. *Amer. J. Physiol.* **162**, 489-502 (1950).
81. Tunturi, A. R. Anatomy and physiology of the auditory cortex. *In* "Neural Mechanisms of the Auditory and Vestibular Systems" (G. L. Rasmussen and W. F. Windle, eds.), pp. 181-200. Thomas, Springfield, Illinois, 1960.
82. Vardapetian, G. A. Electrophysiological study of temporal summation in different

levels of the auditory system of cats. *J. Higher Nervous Activity (USSR)* **16**, 470-479 (1966) (in Russian).

83. Vardapetian, G. A. Characteristics of single unit responses in the auditory cortex of cat. *In* "Problems of Physiological Acoustics" (G. V. Gersuni, ed.), Vol. 6: Mechanisms of Hearing, pp. 74-90. Nauka, Leningrad, 1967 (in Russian).
84. Vardapetian, G. A. This volume, Chapter 14.
85. Vartanian, I. A. Quantitative characteristics of temporal summation in inferior colliculus and lateral lemniscus of the rat brain. *J. Higher Nervous Activity (USSR)* **16**, 103-111 (1966) (in Russian).
86. Vartanian, I. A. This volume, Chap. 12.
87. Vartanian, I. A., and Ratnikova, G. I. Frequency localization and temporal summation in the auditory centres of the midbrain. *In* "Problems of Physiological Acoustics" (G. V. Gersuni, ed.), Vol. 6: Mechanisms of Hearing, pp. 62-74. Nauka, Leningrad, 1967 (in Russian).
88. Wall, P. D. Repetitive discharge of neurons. *J. Neurophysiol.* **22**, 305-320 (1959).
89. Whitfield, I. C., and Evans, E. F. Responses of auditory cortical neurons to stimuli of changing frequency. *J. Neurophysiol.* **28**, 655-672 (1965).
90. Zaboeva, N. V. The responses of cochlear nerve to acoustic signals with different rise-time. *Sechenov Physiol. J. USSR* **52**, 346-354 (1966) (in Russian).
91. Zaboeva, N. V. Temporal summation in the auditory cortex for stimulation with different frequencies and white noise. *In* "Problems of Physiological Acoustics" (G. V. Gersuni, ed.), Vol. 6: Mechanisms of Hearing, pp. 90-101. Nauka, Leningrad, 1967 (in Russian).
92. Zaboeva, N. V. Primary responses of the auditory cortex to acoustic signals of various rise-time. *Sechenov Physiol. J. USSR* **53**, 752-760 (1967) (in Russian).
93. Zwicker, E. Temporal effects in simultaneous masking and loudness. *J. Acoust. Soc. Amer.* **38**, 132-141 (1965).

7
Cortical Feedback Mechanism in the Auditory System of the Cat

Yasuji Katsuki

Much information has been accumulated to date on the neural mechanism of sensations from the recording of single neuronal responses to various stimuli. From such information, the detailed neural mechanism has been revealed particularly in the ascending system of higher animals. Actually, the concept of the control of the ascending information in the sensory tracts only recently began to attract the attention of neurophysiologists, although many years ago such a control system was already thought to exist [5, 6]. This idea grew out of the knowledge that control mechanisms were found in the lower animals, like crustacea and mollusca, and even in the sensory end organs of higher animals, two kinds of synapses were found by electron microscopy studies.

In the auditory system of the cat, a peripheral control mechanism was first revealed by histological as well as electron microscopy study, and then by electrophysiological technique. The efferent system originally described by Rasmussen [15, 16] was found to produce the inhibitory effect on the hair cell activities in the cochlea. Its functional characteristic, as a negative feedback mechanism, was demonstrated electrophysiologically by Galambos [4], Desmedt and Monaco [2], and Fex [3]. In contrast to this, the control system at the upper level of the brain was described only histologically and has not yet been functionally identified with certainty.

Otani and Hiura [14] reported recently that the cortical auditory area of the cat has several efferent fiber tracts projecting from the auditory cortex. These tracts connect with the ipsilateral medial geniculate body, the bilateral inferior colliculi, adjacent gray matter, and the ipsilateral dorsal nucleus of the lateral lemniscus. They have somewhat tonotopic localization. Desmedt and Mechelse [1] showed that a lesion near the pseudosylvian fissure in the cat caused degeneration to occur mainly in a region situated between the medial geniculate nucleus and the medial lemniscus. The electrical stimulation of this region suppressed the response of the cochlear nucleus to sound.

Our aim in the present study was to understand how stimulation of the auditory cortex might influence the unit responses of the medial geniculate body and inferior colliculus to sound stimulation through efferent systems.

Method

More than 20 adult cats were lightly anesthetized with Nembutal (30 mg/kg) and maintained thereafter with Flaxedil or with a gasous mixture of 2% Fluothane in oxygen, when necessary. The experimental animal was fixed on the stereotaxic instrument and the skull was trephined in several places to allow insertion of the recording capillary microelectrode and placement of the stimulating bipolar electrodes on the surface of the auditory cortex. As a rule, the right ear was used for sound stimulation, and the recording of unitary responses was taken from the left medial geniculate body. The auditory cortex was stimulated electrically at the left side. In some animals, the recording of responses was performed from the inferior colliculus, and the right auditory cortex was also stimulated electrically when it was necessary.

Routine glass capillary microelectrodes filled with 3 M KCl solution and with an ohmic resistance of between 10 to 50 MΩ were used. These electrodes were inserted vertically into the left medial geniculate body from the surface of the cortex, located at Fr. (frontal) 4.3-4.5 mm, left L. (lateral) 8.0 mm (sterotaxic planes of Jasper and Ajmone Marsan, [7]). Click and tone-burst stimuli were delivered through a closed sound system to the external ear. For cortical stimulation, single or brief bursts (200-700/sec) of electric pulses were applied on the auditory cortex through a pair of platinum wire 1 mm apart, insulated except at the tips. The electrical stimulus, a square pulse of 0.5 msec duration and 3-8 V, was delivered through an isolation unit. The number of pulses in a volley was determined by changing the frequency of the pulse generator, but the duration of a volley was fixed by a gate pulse of constant duration (10 msec).

These electrical stimuli were applied to the anterior and middle ectosylvian gyrus in the primary (AI), the secondary (AII) auditory area, and Ep. By the use of a distributor, stimuli to the various parts of the cortex were delivered systematically one after another through each pair of electrodes. The time relation between electrical stimulation on the auditory cortex and tonal stimulus ranged from a few milliseconds to over 100 msec. The position of the tip of the recording electrode in most animals was examined by a histological staining method by passing a small electric current through the electrode after the experiments. It was thus shown that the recordings had been performed from the pars principalis of the medial geniculate body (m.g.b.).

Results

Recordings were taken from more than 300 units extracellularly, mainly from m.g.b. and partly from the inferior colliculus (i.c.).

The auditory response of approximately 9% of that obtained from m.g.b. studied by combined cortical and ear stimulation was either inhibited or facilitated by preceding electrical stimulation on the surface of the auditory cortex; 8% of them responded to the cortical stimulation alone. Some of these neurons responded to sound stimuli alone, but without modification of the response pattern to sound stimuli by a preceding cortical stimulation.

Those neurons modified were either inhibited or facilitated, and twice as many were inhibited as were facilitated. However, many neurons, almost two-thirds of them, showed no modification. They responded to sound stimulation and no change was induced by electrical stimulation. In most of those neurons studied, a low, irregular spontaneous discharge was seen. Particular attention was not given to this subject in this chapter.

Modification of Auditory Response

INHIBITION

As shown in Fig. 1, by repetitive shocks (1 to 7 pulses) on AI, inhibitory effects were produced in 14 m.g.b. units. Electrical stimulation of AI inhibited the responses to both clicks (Fig. 1) and tone bursts. The left column is the control record where the unitary responses to clicks are observed with a fairly high firing probability. In the right column, spike responses to clicks, taken from a m.g.b. unit, are inhibited by the preceding conditioning stimulus at AI, although a small evoked potential can still be seen. The evoked potential arises from surrounding units in response to cortical stimulation, since the click stimulus occurs after the appearance of the evoked potential. Such an inhibitory effect depended upon the conditioning stimulus parameters. An increase in stimulus intensity and/or number of electrical pulses in the burst applied to the cortex resulted in an increase in the duration and intensity of the inhibitory effect as shown in Fig. 2.

Regarding the relationship between the threshold for a click and the

L A I

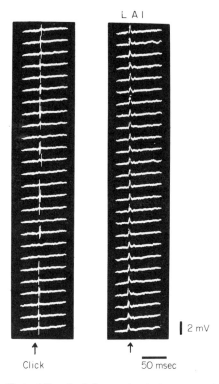

2 mV

↑
Click

↑

50 msec

FIG. 1. Inhibitory effect of five-shock burst stimulation (at 500/sec) at left AI on unit responses to clicks in the medial geniculate body. Left column: control record of single neuron responses to clicks. Right column: single neuron responses to click are inhibited by preceding electrical stimulation at AI, but positive small evoked potentials remain about 10 msec after electrical artifacts. The large positive (upward) deflections on each trace are electrical artifacts from the five stimuli, which preceded the click by 10 msec.

number of stimulating pulses, an increase in the number of pulses elevated the threshold for click. By changing the time interval between conditioning electrical pulses and sound stimulus, the latency and duration of inhibition were determined. In one example, the earliest onset of inhibition after the last conditioning shock was 8.3 msec, the latest 31.8 msec. The duration of the inhibition ranged between 30 and 200 msec.

FACILITATION

Facilitatory effects were observed in six m.g.b. units. Such facilitatory effects were elicited by electrical stimulation at the secondary auditory area (AII). Figure 3 gives an example of facilitation. The tone burst is indicated at the bottom of each column. The control record in the left column shows sporadic

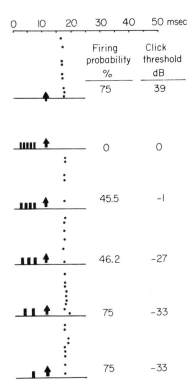

FIG. 2. The dotted pattern of the responses to clicks and its inhibitory effect by electrical stimulation at AI. Arrow indicates the presentation of a click. Vertical bars show the number of stimulating pulses. The first record with no vertical bars is the control condition with no cortical stimulation.

spike responses to tone bursts (at 900 Hz, -30 dB); the spike latencies are somewhat variable. Electrical conditioning stimulation at AII, however, facilitated clearly the responses by decreasing and stabilizing their latencies as shown in the right column.

The relationship between the threshold of the response and the number of stimulating pulses could be measured, but the results are not shown in this chapter. The latency of the facilitated spikes was from 10 to 37.5 msec, whereas the duration of the facilitation was not determined systematically [20].

No Modification of Auditory Response

Almost 80% of neurons in response to sound stimulation did not show any response to electrical stimulation on the cortex.

L. A II

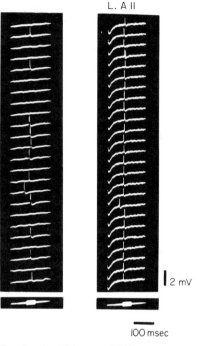

2 mV

100 msec

Tone burst   900 cps   −30 dB

FIG. 3. Facilitative effect of five-shock stimulation at AII on single unit responses of the medial geniculate body to tone bursts. Left column: control record of single unit responses to 900 Hz tone burst at −30 dB. Right column: unit responses to tone bursts are facilitated by electrical stimulation at AII. A stimulus artifact is present at the beginning of each sweep.

In 13 cases, responses were elicited both by cortical and by ear stimulation. By cortical stimulation, single spikes were elicited, regardless of the number of stimulating pulses. There were no modifications in responses in either an inhibitory or a facilitatory mode by both stimulation.

When the time delay between the cortical and the sound stimulus was very short, the initial response to cortical or sound stimulation sometimes disturbed the response to the second stimulus. This effect seemed not to be inhibitory (synaptic), but merely the refractory one.

Five neurons responded only to cortical stimulation. The latency of response to a single shock ranged from 3 to 30 msec. Judging from those latencies, some pathways were thought to be at least monosynaptic and others were thought to involve more than two synapses.

Stim. electrode placement

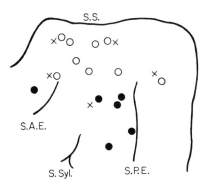

FIG. 4. Schematic presentation of stimulating electrode placement on auditory cortex of left hemisphere in cat. Filled circles show the facilitative effect and open circles the inhibitory effect to the medial geniculate neurons. Crosses denote the effective sites for spike responses in the m.g.b. s.s., suprasylvian sulcus; S. A. E., anterior ectosylvian sulcus; S. Syl., pseudosylvian sulcus; and S. P. E., posterior ectosylvian sulcus.

Sites of Cortical Electrical Stimulation

Figure 4 schematically diagrams the placement site of cortical stimulating electrodes for evoking the inhibitory and facilitatory effects in the m.g.b. Open circles indicate the sites producing inhibitory effects; filled ones represent facilitatory effects. Crosses denote the points where responses occurred but without either inhibition or facilitation. The general tendency was for the stimulation at AI to produce the effects to inhibit sound responses in the m.g.b., whereas stimulation at AII appeared to be facilitatory. However, there was no mutual interaction between AI and AII, namely, only the stimulation at AI or AII was effective to units in the m.g.b., and both were never simultaneously effective.

Effects caused by cortical stimulation upon slowly evoked potentials by sound stimulation were studied. Slowly evoked potentials were recorded by the use of a glass microelectrode in the m.g.b. The evoked potentials were more clearly observed by a C.A.T. computer average. Although it was very difficult to observe the effect of cortical stimulation on the potential evoked by a sound stimulation in each single trace, by averaging the responses, the inhibition by the conditioning cortical stimulation could be demonstrated. This small inhibitory result may suggest that the number of efferent fibers terminating in the m.g.b. is not very great.

Influences of the Efferent Systems on the Response Areas of Medial Geniculate Neurons

The inhibitory effects of cortical stimulation on the response area of the m.g.b. neuron were studied in detail.

It was not easy to complete both the response area and the inhibited area of the same neuron. Many units were lost during the course of complete experiments.

Two cases are shown in Fig. 5. Filled circles and lines show the response areas without cortical stimulation of m.g.b. neurons which have the characteristic frequencies of 1.2 and 3.5 kHz, respectively. The acoustic responses of both neurons were inhibited by cortical stimulation. The filled circle in the right inset indicates the site of electrical stimulation at AII, where no inhibitory effect was observed. Open circles and filled and open triangles show the change (inhibition) of response areas and the site of electrical stimulation of the anterior, middle, and posterior (Ep) ectosylvian gyri, respectively, in the inset.

In the case of a neuron with 3.5 kHz characteristic frequency, parallel threshold elevation was seen by conditional cortical stimulation. A remarkable thing was the different elevation of threshold at the characteristic frequency of the neuron by cortical stimulation at different cortical regions. When

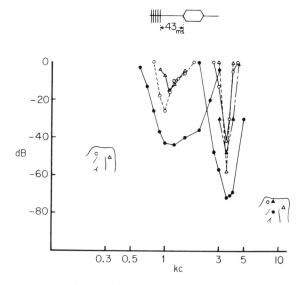

FIG. 5. Response areas of two inhibited units and their changes by cortical stimulation as indicated in the inset. See text for explanation.

electrical stimulation was applied at the anterior ectosylvian gyrus (open circle in the right inset), the most prominent inhibitory effect occurred.

This result suggests that there might be some relation between the tonotopic localization of the auditory cortex and the characteristic frequency of the m.g.b. neuron.

In another example, that of a neuron with a lower characteristic frequency, the inhibitory effect, not the parallel elevation of threshold, was different. Electrical stimulation at the anterior ectosylvian gyrus affected mainly the high-frequency side (open circle) while stimulation at the posterior ectosylvian gyrus elevated the threshold at the low-frequency side (open triangle).

Of course, the change of the time interval between conditioning and tonal stimuli, and also the number of electrical pulses, produced different threshold elevation in their response areas.

The facilitative effects produced by AII stimulation were also observed in several neurons. Unfortunately, the measurements of effects were not completed, as a result of the reasons described above.

Effects of Cortical Electrical Stimulation on the Inferior Colliculus (i.c.)

The neuron in the inferior colliculus was observed in response to cortical stimulation of both homo- and contralateral AI. The threshold for ipsilateral cortical stimulation was lower than that for contralateral stimulation. However, there was no appreciable difference in the latencies. The effects produced by cortical stimulation, either inhibition or facilitation of spike responses, were observed in 29.2% of the neurons (five inhibited, two facilitated) examined in the i.c. This value is about 1.7 times greater than the percentage of modified neurons in the m.g.b. The latency of both the inhibitory and the facilitative effects was longer than for corresponding effects in m.g.b. neurons, in the range of 30 to 40 msec.

Discussion

The centrifugal nerve fibers terminating within the receptor organs and controlling sensory afferent activity have been found in the crustacean stretch receptor [9] and in the vertebrate cochlea [3, 15, 16]. They were revealed to be inhibitory in their action. The control mechanisms of efferent gamma fibers of muscle spindles were also studied and found to be the control of the contraction of intrafusal muscle fibers. Control mechanisms at the intermediate nuclei along the ascending sensory pathways have also been studied by many authors and the corticofugal gating effect has been suggested. Whereas in the visual system, the efferent system at the upper levels has already been reported, similar studies have rarely been reported in the auditory system.

The present study has shown some modification of activity at the level of m.g.b. and i.c. by cortical stimulation. However, this effect was not very strong; only about 9% of the neurons studied in the m.g.b. showed either inhibition or facilitation. In order to reject the effect of anesthetics, the control experiment, was performed by immobilization with Flaxedil. No marked difference was observed in the small number of the m.g.b. neurons modified by cortical stimulation. Therefore, the weakness of the corticofugal effect is probably not due to the influence of the barbiturate anesthetic.

The corticofugal control influence was usually inhibitory. This was borne out in the present study also, where inhibitory influence was about twice as common as facilitation.

The anatomical findings by Otani and Hiura [14] agree well with the electrophysiological results. Namely, the AII area, which corresponds to the site of facilitation, has only sparse projections to the m.g.b.

The corticofugal inhibitory effect such as we have observed has been found widely, while descending facilitating effects are not so common. In the somatosensory system, some facilitative effects were found in the dorsal column nuclei of the cat. Suzuki and Taira [18] also reported that stimulation of the reticular formation augments postsynaptic potentials in the lateral geniculate body, and further that the single unit activity of the radiation fibers coming from the lateral geniculate body is both facilitated and inhibited by the stimulation of the reticular formation.

All of the neurons activated by auditory stimulation may be considered to be the classical m.g.b. neurons that transport the auditory information to the cortex. About 9% of them were inhibited or facilitated by the electrical stimulation at the cortex. The five neurons that responded to the electrical, but not auditory stimuli, may be internuncial neurons on the corticofugal pathway. The 13 neurons that responded independently to both electrical and auditory stimulation may well be the inhibitory internuncial neurons, activated by corticofugal impulses and also by axon collaterals from classical m.g.b. neurons. Morest [10-12] has shown histologically that those neurons have axon collaterals with many branches.

Inhibitory interneurons in the brain have been shown to produce repetitive discharges as observed in Renshaw cells of the spinal cord. In the l.g.b. neurons of the rat, similar observations were made [17].

In the present study, we could not directly identify either excitatory or inhibitory interneurons from our extracellular recordings, nor did we observe repetitive discharges from any neurons.

In Fig. 5, influences of the cortical efferent system on the response area of the m.g.b. neuron are illustrated. The threshold change of the response is associated with various stimulating parameters—the intensity, the number of stimulating pulses, the time interval between cortical and acoustic stimuli, and also the site of electrical stimulation at the auditory cortex AI and AII. To date, the possible integrative mechanism at the auditory cortex has already been clarified to a certain extent by Oonishi and Katsuki [13]. After the auditory information reaches its destination in the auditory cortex through the perceptual integration as reported [13], a feedback action via cortical efferent pathway might contribute in preventing the inadequate, and in facilitating the adequate, impulses to reach their final destination. On the other hand, the feedback control mechanism by olivocochlear bundle originating from the superior olive is merely reflexive in its action, and the mechanism is quite different from that of the cortical origin.

Otani and Hiura's anatomical findings [14] showed a topical relation between the region of cortical ablation and the degenerating terminals within the m.g.b. and the i.c. The anterior region of the auditory area projects to the anterior part of the m.g.b. and the posterior, dorsal, and ventral regions project to caudal, dorsolateral, and ventromedial parts of the m.g.b., respectively. Within the cortex, a tonotopic organization was found in the cat auditory cortex. Therefore, it is highly conceivable that each cortical efferent fiber has a frequency-specific effect, inhibitory as well as facilitative, to neurons at the lower level, and that such a cortical feedback control action may play an important role in the frequency-specific "gating" mechanism of the central auditory system. This system may be activated when, for example, a person wishes to discriminate one particular sound from among a variety of background sounds.

Cortical Effects upon Collicular Neurons

As described above, the possibility exists that the cortical efferent flow influences the auditory neurons below the m.g.b., such as the i.c. So our observation might be based upon the results of events peripheral to the m.g.b. This is excluded, however, by the fact that the neurons of the i.c. were activated by efferent fibers from both ipsi- and contralateral auditory cortices, and the latency of response to electrical stimulation was for the most part longer than that of the m.g.b., and, so far as has been examined, no distinct modification of activity in the m.g.b. was observed by contralateral cortical stimulation.

Acknowledgments

All experiments in this chapter were performed by Dr. Takeshi Watanabe and other members at the author's laboratory. The author expresses his indebtedness to Dr. A. Leonard Diamond for editing the manuscript.

REFERENCES

1. Desmedt, J. E., and Mechelse, K. Corticofugal projections from temporal lobe in cat and their possible role in acoustic discrimination. *J. Physiol. (London)* **147**, 17-18 (1959).
2. Desmedt, J. E., and Monaco, P. Mode of action of the efferent olivo-cochlear bundle on the inner ear. *Nature (London)* **192**, 1263-1265 (1961).
3. Fex, J. Auditory activity in centrifugal and centripetal cochlear fibers in cat: A study of a feedback system. *Acta Physiol. Scand.*, **55**, Suppl. 189 (1962).
4. Galambos, R. Suppression of auditory nerve activity by stimulation of efferent fibers to cochlea. *J. Neurophysiol.* **19**, 424-437 (1956).
5. Hagbarth, K. E., and Kerr, D. I. B. Central influences on spinal afferent conduction. *J. Neurophysiol.* **17**, 295-307 (1954).
6. Hernández-Peón, R., Scherrer, H., and Jouvet, M. Modification of electrical activity in cochlear nucleus during "attention" in unanesthetized cats. *Science* **123**, 331-332 (1956).
7. Jasper, H. H., and Ajmone-Marsan, C. "A Stereotaxic Atlas of the Diencephalon of the Cat." Nat. Res. Council, Canada, 1954.
8. Katsuki, Y., Watanabe, T., and Maruyama, N. Activity of auditory neurons in upper levels of brain of cat. *J. Neurophysiol.* **22**, 343-359 (1959).
9. Kuffler, S. W. Synaptic inhibitory mechanisms. Properties of dendrites and problems of excitation in isolated sensory nerve cells. *Exp. Cell Res. Suppl.* **5**, 493-519 (1958).
10. Morest, D. The probable significance of synaptic and dendritic patterns of the thalamic and midbrain auditory system. *Anat. Rec.* **148**, 390-391 (1964).
11. Morest, D. The neuronal architecture of the medial geniculate body of the cat. *J. Anat.* **98**, 611-630 (1965a).
12. Morest, D. The laminar structure of the medial geniculate body of the cat. *J. Anat.* **99**, 143-160 (1965b).
13. Oonishi, S., and Katsuki, Y. Functional organization and integrative mechanism on the auditory cortex of the cat. *Jap. J. Physiol.* **15**, 342-365 (1965).
14. Otani, K., and Hiura, H. Projection fibers from the auditory cortex of the cat. *Progr. Neurol. Psychiat.* **7**, 483-494 (1962) (in Japanese).
15. Rasmussen, G. L. The olivary peduncle and other fibers projections of the superior olivary complex. *J. Comp. Neurol.* **84**, 141-220 (1946).
16. Rasmussen, G. L. Descending or "feedback" connections of auditory system of the cat. *Amer. J. Physiol.* **183**, 653 (1955).
17. Sefton, A. J., and Burke, W. Reverberating inhibitory circuits in the lateral geniculate nucleus of the rat. *Nature (London)* **205**, 1325-1326 (1965).
18. Suzuki, H., and Taira, N. Effect of reticular stimulation upon synaptic transmission in cat's lateral geniculate body. *Jap. J. Physiol.* **11**, 641-655 (1961).
19. Watanabe, T. A single neuron activity in the secondary cortical auditory area in the cat. *Jap. J. Physiol.* **9**, 245-256 (1959).
20. Watanabe, T., Yanagisawa, K., Kanzaki, J., and Katsuki, Y. Cortical efferent flow influencing unit responses of medial geniculate body to sound stimulation. *Exp. Brain Res.* **2**, 302-317 (1966).
21. Winter, D. L. *N. Gracilis* of cat. Functional organization and corticofugal effects. *J. Neurophysiol.* **28**, 48-70 (1965).

8
Central Control of Single Unit Responses to Acoustic Stimuli

J. Bureš and O. Burešová

Stimulus-response relationships, quantitatively describing the transformation of physical stimuli into nerve impulses at the level of receptors, cannot be simply applied to higher sensory centers. The individual elements of complex neural nets are provided not only with the specific sensory inputs, but also with a number of other afferents controlling their excitability, spontaneous activity, and connectivity. The purpose of the present paper is to illustrate by several examples the significance of the above factors, and to discuss the potential behavioral implications.

All experiments were performed on unanesthetized, curarized rats, aged three months. Unit activity was led off with capillary microelectrodes filled with 3M-KC1 or with saturated sodium glutamate, and recorded on the screen of a CRO. Automatic plotting of poststimulation histograms was used to detect and evaluate the unit responses.

Spontaneous and Evoked Activity

Most central neurons are spontaneously active, their activity forming the referent background level for all unit responding. Since spontaneous activity is a statistical process (often approaching a Poisson distribution), signal transmission to the next link of the neural net can occur only when the difference ΔF between the mean background frequency F and the response firing rate F_R reaches a certain minimum probability. In most papers on neural coding at the single neuron level, the above probability (dependent variable) is studied in relation to the physical properties of the stimulus (independent variable), while spontaneous activity is considered constant. This is an evident oversimplification, however, since spontaneous activity may fluctuate over a wide range, and since the neural effects of the same physical stimulus may vary considerably with attention, habituation, conditioning, etc. We attempted, therefore, to approach this problem from another point of view, using a constant stimulus and manipulating the background firing rate as the independent variable [2]. Changes of spontaneous firing rate caused by anesthesia, cooling, arousal, etc., affect vast neuronal populations and may thus modify the sensory signal before it reaches the neuron under examination. To overcome this difficulty, spontaneous activity was changed only in the recorded unit using extracellular polarization or electrophoretic application of ions through the recording microelectrode.

In general, two classes of neurons can be recognized by using this technique in the inferior colliculus of rats (Fig. 1): (a) neurons in which, in spite of considerable changes of the background firing rate F, the stimulus-induced difference ΔF remains constant; such neurons can be termed additive, since

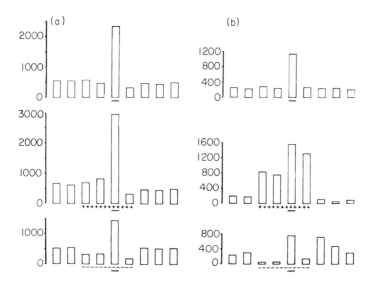

FIG. 1. Excitatory reactions of collicular units to the acoustic stimulus. The columns of the poststimulation histograms correspond to nine consecutive 1-sec intervals. Numbers of spikes accumulated in the individual intervals is given on the ordinate. Ten responses were added to obtain one poststimulation histogram. Above: control recording; middle and below: background activity changed by positive (+++) or negative (---) voltage applied to the microelectrode. (a) multiplicate, (b) additive reactions. Data are from Bureš and Burešová [2].

their output activity is the result of simple addition of the background
activity and of the response increment or decrement; (b) neurons in which the
difference ΔF varies with the background activity. In the most common type,
the response increases or decreases proportionally to the spontaneous activity
in a way such that the response-background ratio $\Delta F/F$ remains constant.
Such neurons may be termed multiplicative, since their output firing rate
corresponds to the background activity multiplied by a stimulus-specific constant. Examination of 128 neurons in colliculus indicated that both types are
equally frequent (Fig. 2).

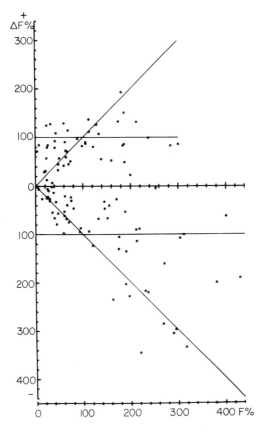

FIG. 2. A correlogram of the normalized data. Each point corresponds to a reaction
obtained with a given change of background frequency. Above: excitatory reactions (+
F); below: inhibitory reactions (− F) expressed in percentage of the corresponding control
reactions (F_0 = 100%). Abscissa: the variable background frequency (F) expressed in
percent of the corresponding control background (F_0 = 100%). For further explanations,
see text. Data are from Bureš and Burešová [2].

The additive units comply best with the conventional model of a nerve cell based on the electrophysiological properties of spinal motoneurons. Even in these cells, Granit *et al.* [8] have recently demonstrated deviations from additive responding when the spontaneous firing rate was changed by intracellular polarization beyond certain limits. Different membrane properties of individual cells may account for differences between additive and multiplicative neurons. But even if the nervous system were to consist of additive elements only, it is possible to conceive of them as organized into circuits with multiplicative properties which may suit some central functions better than linear additivity. Sequential linking of additive neurons into chains would cause unreliable transmission of threshold signals, since with increasing background activity, its standard deviation may rise to such an extent, that threshold reactions are lost in the noise. This is not the case with multiplicative neurons (or circuits), in which the signal-to-noise ratio remains constant. It can be expected, therefore, that multiplicative neurons are mainly encountered in neural structures ensuring highly reliable signal transmission. It must be stressed, however, that improvement of the S/N ratio can be also attained by other mechanisms [16].

Dominant Reactions

In another group of neurons, reactions to external stimuli appear only after their spontaneous activity has been changed by polarization and/or microelectrophoresis. Such "dominant"-type reactions to indifferent acoustic stimuli appear in about 50% of initially nonresponding neurons in colliculus inferior [2]. Increase and decrease of the spontaneous firing rate have the same activating effect (Fig. 3). Reactions of the dominant type may apparently play an important role in modifying the connectivity of neuronal nets by gating the flux of nerve impulses into new channels. On the contrary, there are many neurons, the receptive field of which is not appreciably changed by polarization. Reactions closely resembling the dominant type were described in stimulated cortical neurons by Spehlmann and Kapp [14] and by Voronin [15]. Dominant reactions might be caused by excitability shifts which change subthreshold stimuli into suprathreshold ones and thus increase the responsiveness of the given neurons to a wide variety of stimuli.

Unit Conditioning

While dominant reactions are rather nonspecific, more selective plastic processes underly the formation of conditioned reflexes. An attempt was made, therefore, to approach this type of plasticity by reinforcing indifferent

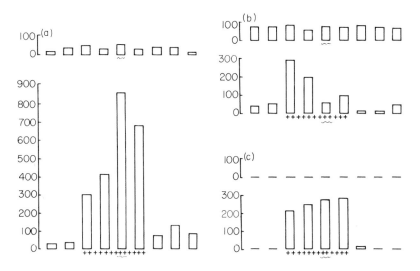

FIG. 3. Examples of three collicular units which did not react to the acoustic stimulus under control conditions (above). During polarization (below, +++) the acoustic stimulus remained ineffective (c) or began to evoke excitatory (a) or inhibitory (b) reactions. Data are from Bureš and Burešová [2].

acoustic stimuli (CS) by direct polarization of the recorded neurons (UCS). More than 100 units in the cortex, hippocampus, nonspecific thalamus, and reticular formation were examined in this way [34]. An acoustic signal (2000/sec) lasting for 3 sec was reinforced during the last second by polarization. Although in most cases (58%) the conditioned stimulus remained without effect in spite of up to a hundred reinforcements, in a few neurons (13%), the sound began to elicit a clear-cut reaction which could be extinguished by nonreinforcement (Fig. 4). In another 29% nerve cells conditioned acoustic reactions were observed only occasionally. Similar results were also recently obtained when using a tactile stimulus, such as a puff of air applied to the trigeminal region, as the CS [7].

The low incidence of positive reactions in the acoustically nonresponsive neurons may be due to the lack of acoustic inputs. In another series of experiments, therefore, an attempt was made to use the same technique in the inferior colliculus neurons which displayed marked reactions to acoustic stimuli before the conditioning started. Significant and reversible modification of the initial response was obtained in 78% of neurons (Fig. 5). It seems that modification of preformed reactions is much simpler than formation of new reactions in the nonresponsive neurons, and that it may constitute the first link of the plastic processes of learning.

There are other reasons why plasticity is so rarely observed in the initially nonresponsive neurons. Under normal conditions, learning involves large neuro-

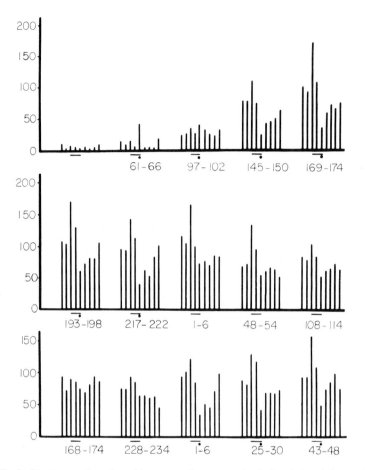

FIG. 4. Plastic reaction in a hippocampal neuron. Analyzing interval 1 sec. Sound stimulation indicated by the horizontal bar below columns 3-5, polarizing current by dot below the column 5. The first block of measurement constitutes a control set. Serial numbers of the integrated trials are given below the histograms. Number of spikes accumulated in the individual intervals is given on the ordinate. Polarization (outward current, 15 na, KCl electrode) evokes at first an excitatory, later an inhibitory reaction. An excitatory acoustic reaction develops after 150 reinforcements. It disappears after about 200 extinction trials but can be restored by reinforcement. Data are from Bureš and Burešová [4].

nal populations activated both by the CS and UCS. It is not surprising that excitation limited to the polarized neuron only is perhaps an inadequate UCS. On the other hand, it is indeed possible that only a fraction of neurons is capable of plastic change, while the remainder form rather rigid output or input circuits. The low incidence of plastic reactions in the above experiments

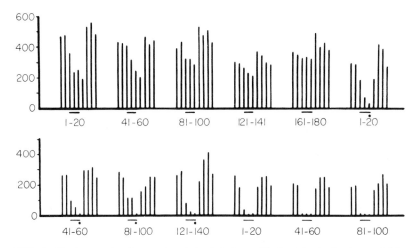

FIG. 5. Plastic reaction in a unit of the inferior colliculus. Analyzing interval 0.3 sec, massed training procedure. Other description as in Fig. 4. The inhibitory acoustic reaction was habituated first and only then reinforced by polarization (outward current, 20 na, sodium glutamate electrode), which immediately induced recovery. The acoustic inhibitory reaction was further increased by reinforcement and remained very intense even after the polarization was discontinued. Data are from Bureš and Burešová [4].

may then simply express the relative frequency of plastic and rigid neurons. Using paired stimulation of two afferent nerves as CS and UCS, respectively, Kandel and Tauc [11] found plasticity in only 17% of neurons in the isolated abdominal ganglion of Aplysia, which agrees very well with the approximately 15% of plastic neurons found in our experiments.

Multiplicative, dominant, and conditioned reactions are examples of mechanisms that may modify the response of a given neuron to a constant external stimulus. Unfortunately it is impossible to decide at present, whether the underlying processes must be sought in the synaptic contacts, in the membrane properties, or in the neural circuitry of the examined nerve cells. Similar changes of unit reactions occurring after elimination of remote tonic influences [1], during habituation [9, 13] and conditioning [5, 10, 12, 17] are probably due to complex interaction of large neuronal populations. Under these conditions, the primarily affected neurons cannot be distinguished by the present electrophysiological technique from those which are only passively involved because of their preformed connections with the primarily activated elements. In spite of the rather artificial conditions, direct stimulation of single neurons makes it possible to simplify the above problem by restricting the respective neural changes to the immediate connections of the examined nerve cell. We can therefore expect that this method will permit the physiologists to approach the problem of neural plasticity in a more analytic way.

REFERENCES

1. Bureš, J., and Burešová, O. The influence of cortical spreading depression on the evoked activity of reticular units. *Physiol. Bohemoslov.* 13, 584-593 (1964).
2. Bureš, J., and Burešová, O. Relationship between spontaneous and evoked unit activity in the inferior colliculus of rats. *J. Neurophysiol.* 28, 641-654 (1965).
3. Bureš, J., and Burešová, O. Plasticity at the single neuron level. *Proc. 23rd Int. Congr. Int. Union Physiological Sci., Tokyo, 1965*, Vol. IV, pp. 359-364.
4. Bureš, J., and Burešová, O. Plastic changes of unit activity based on reinforcing properties of extracellular stimulation of single neurons. *J. Neurophysiol.* 30, 98-113 (1967).
5. Burešová, O., and Bureš, J. Classical conditioning and reticular units. *Acta. Physiol.* 26, 53-57 (1965).
6. Burešova, O., Maruseva, A. M., Bureš, and Fifková, E. The influence of cortical spreading depression on unit activity in the colliculus inferior of the rat. *Physiol. Bohemoslov.* 13, 227-235 (1964).
7. Gerbrandt, L. K., Skrebitsky, V. G., Burešová, O., and Bureš, J. Plastic changes of unit activity induced by tactile stimuli followed by electrical stimulation of single hippocampal and reticular neurons. *Neuropsychologia* 6, 3-10 (1968).
8. Granit, R., Kernell, P., and Lamarre, Y. Synaptic stimulation superimposed on motoneurone firing in the "secondary range" to injected current. *J. Physiol. (London)* 187, 401-415 (1966).
9. Horn, G., and Hill, R. M. Habituation of the response to sensory stimuli of neurons in the brain stem of rabbits. *Nature (London)* 202, 296-298 (1964).
10. Kamikawa, K., McIlwain, J. T., and Adey, W. R. Response patterns of thalamic neurons during classical conditioning. *EEG clin. Neurophysiol.* 17, 485-496 (1964).
11. Kandel, E. R., and Tauc, L. Heterosynaptic facilitation in neurons of the abdominal ganglion of *Aplysia depilans. J. Physiol. (London)* 181, 1-27 (1965).
12. Shulgina, G. I. Examination of activity of cortical neurons during early stages of conditioning. *Sovrem. Probl. Elektrofiziol. Centr. Nerv. Sistemy (Moscow)* 296-308 (1967) (in Russian).
13. Sokolov, E. N. Inhibitory conditioned reflex at single unit level. *23rd Proc. Int. Congr. Int. Union Physiological Sci., Tokyo, 1965,* Vol. IV, pp. 340-343.
14. Spehlmann, R. S., and Kapp, H. Direct extracellular polarization of cortical neurons with multibarelled microelectrodes. *Arch. Ital. Biol.* 102, 74-94 (1964).
15. Voronin, L. L. Influence of extracellular polarization of single units of the sensorimotor cerebral cortex of the rabbit on their evoked activity. *Zh. Vyssh. Nerv. Deyatel. I. P. Pavlova* 16, 667-677 (1966).
16. Werner, G., and Mountcastle, V. B. The variability of central neural activity in a sensory system, and its implications for the central reflection of sensory events. *J. Neurophysiol.* 26, 958-977 (1963).
17. Yoshii, N., and Ogura, H. Studies on the unit discharge of brainstem reticular formation in the cat. I. Changes of reticular unit discharge following conditioning procedure. *Med. J. Osaka Univ.* 11, 1-17 (1960).

9
Two Types of Neurons in the Cat's Cochlear Nuclei and Their Role in Audition

E. A. Radionova

One of the important properties of the auditory system is its capacity to work in a wide time range, as a device for both quick performance and for accumulating information about a signal over a rather long period of time. This capacity of the auditory system makes its performance rather unique as compared with other known analyzing systems. The question of the means by which this capacity is achieved is of great interest.

This problem was investigated at the level of the cochlear complex which is the first central synaptic region of the auditory system. It was shown [11] that two widely diverse types of neurons exist which possess quite different time characteristics. In this chapter additional work is presented on these two types of neurons, and their functional significance is considered.

Material and Methods

More than 500 neurons were studied in the cat's cochlear complex. The cats were anesthetized with chloralose (30 mg/kg) and urethane (500 mg/kg) given intraperitoneally. The body temperature of the animals was maintained near 37.5°. After insertion of a tracheal cannula, the cochlea contralateral to the side of operation was destroyed and a part of the cerebellum was removed to expose the cochlear complex.

Tungsten microelectrodes with equivalent resistance of 10 to 30 MΩ, when measured at 1000 Hz, were used for recording. The spikes were displayed on the tube face of the oscilloscope in the conventional manner or reduced to a "dot" [20]. In addition, the spike activity was recorded on magnetic tape and the data were processed automatically to obtain poststimulus time (PST) histograms and latency distributions [19]. In order to secure a reliable separation of spikes from background activity, a threshold circuit [18, 19] was employed whenever indicated, so that the spike had to reach a preset amplitude before it was registered.

Sound signals were delivered through an electrostatic loudspeaker with a frequency bandwidth of 3 to 20 kHz; the loudspeaker was placed at a distance of 5 cm from the animal's ear. For work in the low-frequency range, a dynamic loudspeaker was used with a frequency bandwidth of 70 to 8000 Hz; this loudspeaker was placed in the midline at a distance from both ears of 30 cm.

In order to obtain larger samples for statistical evaluations of different response characteristics (such as threshold, latency, number of spikes, etc.) each stimulus was presented 10 to 20 times (sometimes 30 to 40 times). The repetition rate of the signals was 0.5 to 0.7 Hz.

The electrode tip was located by the method described by Fox and Eichman [1]. In some experiments, the locus of a unit was known only approximately from the depth of the electrode insertion.

Other aspects of the methods used have been described in more detail previously [10-14].

Results

The experimental data indicate that some discharge characteristics observed under conditions of threshold stimulation were highly correlated with each other. Thus, the following functions were found to be interrelated: pattern of spike discharges near threshold, dependence of latent period (LP) and its dispersion (σ_{LP}) on signal intensity (I), [LP(I), $\sigma_{LP}(I)$], dependence of threshold* (I_o) on duration (t) and risetime (t^1) of the signal [($I_o(t)$, $I_o(t^1)$], probability (p) of spike discharge depending on signal intensity [$p(I)$]. Since these functions are correlated, two diverse types of neurons possessing widely different properties at threshold could be distinguished.

It should be mentioned that in this chapter the term "neuron type" is used to characterize the properties of the neuron as they appear in response to the best (characteristic) frequency. Since with a frequency change the characteristics of a neuron may change as well, it will be convenient to speak in such cases about "reaction type," rather than "neuron type."

---

* Threshold was defined as that sound intensity at which a neuron responds (with at least one spike) with a probability of 0.5.

THE TEMPORAL PATTERN

The pattern of spike discharges is one of the most obvious characteristics which permits a distinction between the two types of neurons (Fig. 1). The first type is characterized by a tonic discharge pattern, which coincides in time with the duration of the signal over a wide intensity range including near-threshold intensities. For instance, neuron 532 (Fig. 1) with a threshold at −8 dB discharged tonically at an intensity level as low as −7 dB. The second type of neuron always has a phasic discharge pattern ("on" or "on-off") near threshold; sometimes this type of neuron retains the phasic discharge pattern over a wide intensity range up to the level of 90 dB (neuron 222 in Fig. 1), but more often, neurons of this type display tonic discharge patterns at high-intensity levels [(11); see also Fig. 4(II)].

Thus, the separation of neurons into two types according to their discharge patterns is based on differences between these patterns near threshold. It may be mentioned that a proper classification is easily made despite the great variety of patterns which were observed at high-intensity levels in complete agreement with other workers [5, 7, 13, 16].

THE LATENT PERIOD

The latent period (LP) and its variations with stimulus intensity make it possible to separate these two groups of neurons on the basis of the latency criterion and thus to recognize a "long-latency" and a "short-latency" group [Fig. 2(a)]. At sufficiently high intensity levels, the latent periods of the neurons of both groups are nearly the same; usually, the shortest latent period is 2 to 4 msec. The difference between two neuron types becomes apparent as the stimulus intensity decreases and approaches threshold. Under such conditions, the latent period increases greatly [Fig. 2(aI)], usually by several dozens of milliseconds, for neurons with tonic discharge patterns. For neurons with phasic discharge patterns, the latent period changes only slightly (only by several milliseconds) under the same stimulus conditions [Fig. 2(a,II)].

THE DISPERSION OF LATENT PERIOD VALUES

σ_{LP} changes in step with the mean latent period itself. At high-intensity levels, σ_{LP} is usually small (sometimes as small as a fraction of a millisecond) for both groups of neurons; however, at threshold intensity, its value rises to several dozens of milliseconds for the long-latency neurons, but to not more than several milliseconds for the short-latency units (Fig. 3). Figure 4 gives another example of latent period distributions for neurons of the long- and

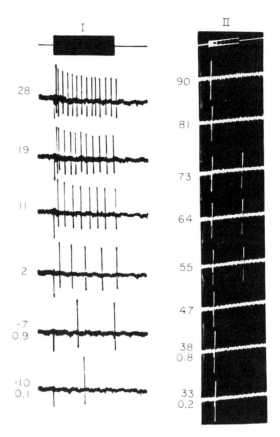

FIG. 1. Two types of discharge patterns seen for the units in cochlear complex in response to best frequency tones. Left (I): neuron 532, sound signal of 7.9 kHz; duration, 110 msec; location, anteroventral cochlear nucleus. Right (II): neuron 222, sound signal of 5 kHz; duration, 140 msec; location, not determined. Numbers to the left of each record indicate sound intensities in decibels SPL and probability (p) of firing if $p < 1$. Stimulus signals are shown in the uppermost traces; the first downward deflection in each unit record is the stimulus artifact which marks the onset of the stimulus.

short-latency type. Thus, the discharges of short-latency units are, in contrast to the long-latency elements, extremely precise and stable in indicating the stimulus onset.

TEMPORAL SUMMATION

The long- and short-latency neurons differ in their temporal summation capacity. For the long-latency neurons there is a lowering of threshold with increase of sound duration, and in this way the neuron can accumulate

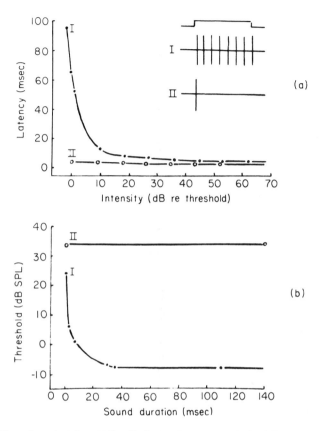

FIG. 2. Time characteristics of the discharges in response to best frequency tones for the two types of neurons. Curve I represents neuron 532; curve II, represents neuron 222 (see Fig. 1). (a) graphs the signal intensity against the latent period of the spike. Signal duration is about 100 msec. (b) graphs the sound duration against threshold value for the response. Inset: discharge patterns of the two neurons.

information concerning the signal in time. Practically no temporal summation occurs for short-latency neurons [Fig. 2(b)]. The lowering of thresholds correlates closely with the latency values at threshold (LP_o); the correlation coefficient is as high as 0.91 between the LP_o and the threshold shift when stimulus duration is increased from 1 to 100 msec.

REACTION TO VARIATIONS IN RISETIME OF THE STIMULUS

This reaction is also different for the long- and short-latency units. As the risetime (t^1) of the signal amplitude increases from zero to its maximal

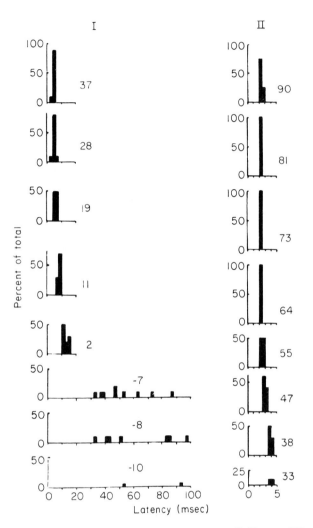

FIG. 3. Latency distributions in the two neuron types. (I) Neuron 532; (II) neuron 222 (see Figs. 1 and 2). Abscissa: classes of latency values. Ordinate: percentage of events in each class. Number near each histogram indicates the sound intensity in dB SPL. Sound signals were best frequency tones of about 100-msec duration. Note that the width of a class in (I) is four times larger than in (II).

value,* the long-latency neurons do not change their threshold, whereas for the short-latency neurons the threshold increases sharply even with a small increase of t^1 (Fig. 5). The difference between the long- and short-latency neurons seems to be similar in this respect to the difference in accommodation capacity established for motoneurons of different types [17].

* The value of t^1 was varied from zero to 110 msec, the amplitude changing as a linear function of time.

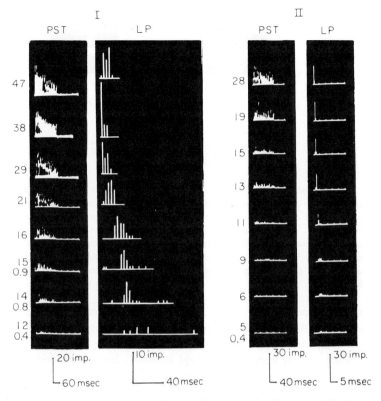

FIG. 4. Poststimulus histograms (PST) and latency distributions (LP) for the two neuron types in response to best frequency tones. (I) Neuron 253: sound signal of 3.1 kHz; duration, 180 msec; location, presumably in the dorsal cochlear nucleus. (II) Neuron 289: sound signal of 9 kHz; duration, 120 msec; location, anteroventral cochlear nucleus. Numbers to the left of histograms indicate sound intensity in dB SPL and probability (p) of firing if $p < 1$. Each histogram is based on a sample consisting of responses to 25 presentations of the signal.

THE DISTRIBUTION OF THRESHOLD VALUES

This distribution is different for long- and short-latency units as well. The probability function $[p(I)]$, which is an integral expression of such a distribution and indicates the reliability of signal detection by the neuron, has a different slope for the long- and short-latency units (Fig. 6). When the steepness of this function is measured by the intensity range (S) over which the response probability of the neuron changes from $p = 0.25$ to $p = 0.75$, S is less than 2 dB for the majority of long-latency units, whereas it is usually about 3 to 4 dB for the short-latency units. Thus, the threshold values fluctuate over a narrower intensity range for the long-latency units than they do for the short-latency neurons.

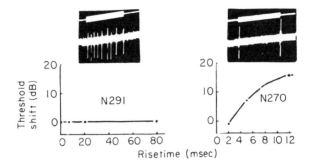

FIG. 5. Thresholds for the two neuron types as a function of the risetime of the signal. Left: neuron 291 (see also Fig. 8); sound signals were best frequency tones of 12 kHz; duration, 210 msec; location, presumably in the posteroventral cochlear nucleus. Right: neuron 270; sound signals were best frequency tones of 7 kHz; duration, 210 msec; location, presumably in the posteroventral cochlear nucleus. Abscissa: risetime of the signal. Ordinate: threshold shift as compared with the threshold value for risetime t^1 = 0. Records show the discharge patterns of the two units at an intensity about 15 dB above threshold.

Interdependence between all the characteristics discussed is high. If one of them is known, it is possible to predict, at least in a general way, the others. Thus, the long-latency-type neurons are characterized by a long latent period (of the order of 100 msec) at threshold intensity, large dispersion of latency values near threshold, a marked dependence of thresholds on signal duration, insensitivity to the risetime of the signal, a steep probability function $p(I)$, and a tonic discharge pattern at near-threshold intensities. In contrast, the short-latency-type neurons are characterized by a short latent period (no more than 10 msec) at threshold intensity, small dispersion of latency values near threshold, slight dependence of thresholds on sound duration, marked dependence of thresholds on the stimulus risetime, a more sloping probability function $p(I)$, and a phasic discharge pattern at near-threshold intensity. Among the examined neurons of the cochlear complex, about 60% were long-latency neurons, about 20% were of the short-latency type, and about 20% of the neurons had intermediate properties.

Having established the two neuron types, it is of interest to consider to what extent the reaction type depends on such stimulus parameters as its intensity, duration, and frequency.

THE SIGNIFICANCE OF SOUND INTENSITY

With the stimuli at various intensities of the best frequency tone, the significance of sound intensity was examined. The tones had a rectangular envelope and were about 100 msec in duration. At sufficiently high intensity

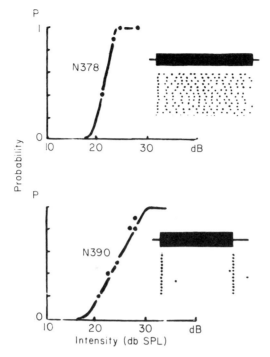

FIG. 6. Two types of probability functions in response to best frequency signals. Abscissa: sound intensity in dB SPL. Ordinate: probability of spike occurrence. Insets: discharge patterns at relatively high-intensity level recorded with the "dot" method (20). Upper figure represents neuron 378, sound signal of 5.23 kHz; duration, 185 msec; location, posteroventral cochlear nucleus. Lower figure represents neuron 390, sound signal of 14.5 kHz; duration, 120 msec; location, not determined. Stimulus onset is not recorded by the dots.

levels the discharge pattern, the latent period, and its dispersion are not necessarily different for the neurons of the long- and the short-latency types (Figs. 2-4; see also Radionova [11 and 12]). However, these characteristics differ greatly at near-threshold intensities (Figs. 1-4, and 7). Therefore, for these characteristics the differences between the two neuron types are most pronounced at near-threshold intensities. The other functions $[I_o(t), I_o(t^1)$, and $p(I)]$ are also characteristic for the neuron type only under threshold conditions of stimulation.

THE SIGNIFICANCE OF SIGNAL DURATION

The significance of signal duration was examined for the best frequency tone with a rectangular envelope at near-threshold intensity. For a stimulus of short duration (1 msec), the latent period and its dispersion, the discharge pattern and the steepness of the probability function do not differ essentially in neurons of the long- and short-latency types [(IA) and (IIA) in Fig. 7]. However, for signals of sufficient duration [(IB) and (IIB) in Fig. 7] the differences between these characteristics become well pronounced. Therefore, the differences between the two neuron types are most pronounced when the stimulus is of sufficient duration. Other functions [$I_o(t)$ and $I_o(t^1)$] are characteristic for the neuron type only when the signals are sufficiently long.

THE SIGNIFICANCE OF SOUND FREQUENCY

For the reaction type of a neuron, stimulus frequency is sometimes critical. The two neuron types were established in responses to the best (characteristic or optimal) frequency. However, for the long-latency neurons all the characteristics can change with a change in stimulus frequency so that a neuron that is a long-latency neuron for the best frequency may display all the characteristics of a short-latency neuron for another frequency. Thus, its latent period at threshold becomes short (Fig. 8), the latent period dispersion values decrease greatly (Fig. 9), its capacity for temporal summation practically disappears (Fig. 8), its threshold becomes critically dependent on the risetime of the signal (Fig. 9), the discharge pattern becomes phasic (at least for near-threshold intensities) (Figs. 8, 9), and the probability function becomes less steep [Fig. 10(I)]. What factors may determine such a change of all the reaction-type characteristics has thus far not been determined. It may be mentioned, however, that with different neurons this change can take place at various distances from the best frequency of the neuron.

It should be pointed out that a change in the properties of the long-latency neurons, with a change in signal frequency, does not occur in every case. A great many neurons of the long-latency type remain true to type over the whole frequency range to which they respond; the long-latency-type characteristics, however, are less pronounced for frequencies other than the best frequency.

Essentially, the short-latency neurons retain their properties when the best frequency is substituted by another one; however, their probability functions become steeper [Fig. 10(II)].

It can therefore be concluded that the differences between the two neuron types are most prominent for the optimal sector of the spectrum of the sound signals which activate the neuron.

The changes in time characteristics for the long-latency neurons taking place with a change in signal frequency are of great importance for the frequency analysis in the auditory system. Since the temporal summation is well pronounced for the best frequency of the signal, and slightly (if at all) for frequencies which are marginal in the response area, the increase of sound duration causes a sharpening of the tuning curve of the neuron by lowering

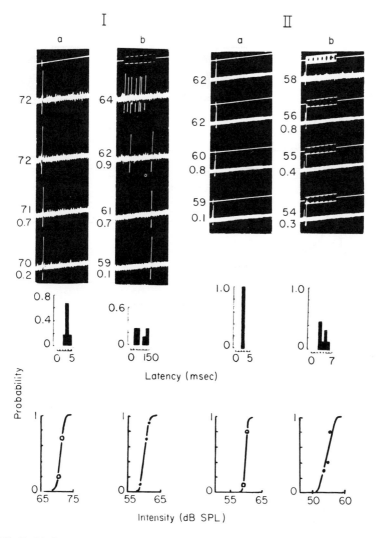

FIG. 7. Discharge characteristics for the two types of neurons (I, II) in response to best frequency tones at threshold. a: Sound duration, 1 msec; b: sound duration, 140 msec. Numbers to the left of each record represent sound intensity (dB SPL) and probability (*p*) of firing if $p < 1$. In the records for (II), the first small upward deflection is the stimulus artifact which indicates stimulus onset. Upper graphs represent latency distributions at sound intensities when the probability of firing (*p*) was 0.7 (I) and 0.8 (II), respectively. Abscissa: classes of latency values (msec). Ordinate: probability of spike occurrence. Lower graphs indicate probability curves. Abscissa: sound intensity (dB SPL). Ordinate: probability of spike occurrence. The record and the graphs in each vertical column refer to the same data. (I) Neuron 252, sound signal of 2.75 kHz. (II) Neuron 251, sound signal of 2.5 kHz. Both neurons were presumably located in the posteroventral cochlear nucleus.

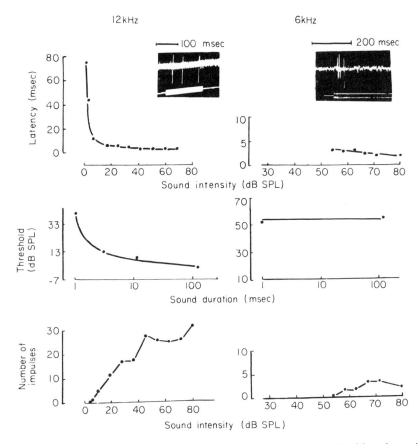

FIG. 8. Changes in response characteristics of a long-latency-type unit with a change in sound frequency from the optimal of 12 kHz to a nonoptimal of 6 kHz; neuron 291 (see also Fig. 5). Graphs in each vertical column designate latency (msec) as a function of sound intensity (dB SPL), stimulus duration of 120 msec; threshold (dB SPL) as a function of sound duration (msec); number of impulses in a response as a function of stimulus intensity (dB SPL), stimulus duration of 120 msec. Insets: records of the discharges for the two different sound frequencies of 12 and 6 kHz at intensities of about 5 dB above threshold level. In the response to 6 kHz, the relevant spike discharge is preceded by an evoked response.

the thresholds for the near-optimal frequency band (Fig. 11). On the other hand, since the threshold dependence on the risetime of the signal is quite different for the optimal and nonoptimal frequencies (Fig. 9), the increase of the signal risetime is effective in sharpening the tuning curve by causing a rise in thresholds for nonoptimal frequencies (Fig. 12). Thus, the capacity of

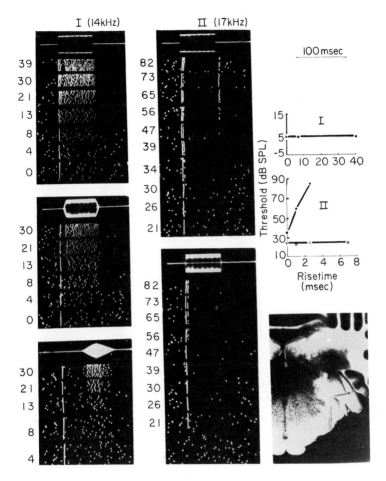

FIG. 9. Changes in characteristics of a long-latency unit responding to sound signals with different risetime as the sound frequency is changed from the optimal frequency of 14.0 kHz (I) to a nonoptimal of 17.0 kHz (II). Risetime in the records for the 14.0 kHz signals is zero, 7, and 40 msec, respectively; in the records for the 17.0 kHz signals, zero and 1 msec. Numbers to the left of the records: sound intensity (dB SPL). The first vertical string of dots in each block of records represents time marks which occur at the beginning of the stimulus in the left and right upper records, 2 msec before stimulus onset in the right (II) lower record, 6 msec before stimulus onset in the left (I) middle record, and 40 msec before stimulus onset for the left (I) lower record. The lowermost part of right (II) lower record shows the spontaneous activity of the neuron. Graphs plot the stimulus risetime against the threshold intensity (dB SPL) for the neural response. Dots indicate the discharge threshold; circles indicate the threshold for inhibition of spontaneous activity. Bottom right: arrow indicates the electrode location in a frontal section through the cochlear complex. Neuron 344: location, dorsal cochlear nucleus.

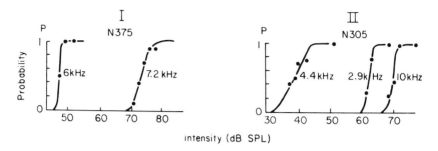

FIG. 10. Change in the steepness of the probability functions in neurons of two types (I, II) with a change of the sound frequency from the optimal frequency (best) to a nonoptimal one. (I) A long-latency unit (neuron 375); (II) a short-latency unit (neuron 305; for further information, see Fig. 11). The curves on the left in (I) and (II) are for signals at the optimal frequencies; the others are for signals at nonoptimal frequencies. Abscissa: sound intensity (dB SPL). Ordinate: probability of firing. Sound duration, about 100 msec. Both neurons were located in the posteroventral cochlear nucleus.

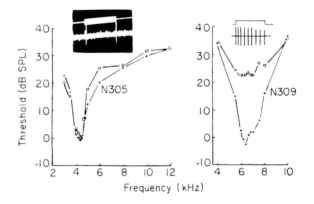

FIG. 11. Threshold tuning curves for a long-latency unit (right, neuron 309) and a short-latency neuron (left, neuron 305) obtained for signals of different duration: 90 msec (filled circles); 1 msec (circles). Abscissa: sound frequency in kilohertz. Ordinate: threshold intensity (dB SPL). Insets: discharge patterns in response to the best frequency sounds of 90-msec duration. Location of neuron 305: posteroventral cochlear nucleus (see also Fig. 10); location of neuron 309: not determined.

long-latency neurons to change their characteristics as the frequency is changed provides two mechanisms for sharpening which could be acting in the frequency analysis performed by neurons (Figs. 11, 12). It is clear that the auditory system could utilize both these mechanisms under natural conditions since sounds heard by man and animals vary greatly both in their duration and in steepness of the envelope.

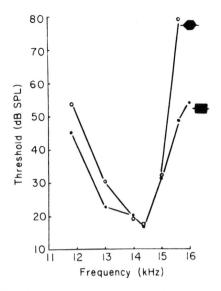

FIG. 12. Threshold tuning curves for a long-latency-type neuron obtained with signals of different risetime. Filled circles: signal risetime of 0; circles: signal risetime of 30 msec. The envelopes of the signal are shown to the right of the curves. Sound duration: 85 msec. Abscissa: sound frequency in kHz. Ordinate: threshold intensity (dB SPL). Neuron 581, location, anteroventral cochlear nucleus.

Discussion

Classification of the units of the cochlear complex into two widely diverse groups was made on the basis of a number of characteristics which are apparent when the stimulus intensity is near threshold. This classification does not encompass the large variety of discharge patterns which can be seen at sufficiently high-intensity levels [5, 7, 13, 16]. However, the proposed classification does not conflict with that of other authors [7], which is based on neuron discharge patterns. A neuron with any discharge pattern at a high-intensity level can be classified as belonging to a long- or short-latency group (or to an intermediate group) when its threshold characteristics are determined.

On the basis of the data obtained, some suggestions can be made concerning the functional significance of the two neuron types.

The long-latency-type neurons which react to a signal with a tonic discharge are capable of reflecting such properties of the signal as its intensity, duration, and character of the envelope even at near-threshold intensities. They are thus capable of measuring these parameters more or less precisely. Signal intensity is reflected in the discharge rate [Figs. 1(I), 7(IB), 8, and 9(I)], signal duration in the duration of the discharge train [Fig. 7(IB)], and the risetime of the envelope in the latent period value and its dispersion, as well as in the temporal pattern of the discharges (Fig. 9). All these properties obviously arise as a consequence of the capacity of such neurons for temporal summation and temporal accumulation of information concerning the signal. In addition, lack of dependence of the threshold on the signal risetime (Fig. 5) and reliable detection of the signal which results from the steep probability function in these neurons (Fig. 6) suggests that the long-latency neurons are well capable of detecting weak signals of sufficient duration.

The short-latency-type neurons, unlike those of long latency, are practically incapable of accumulating in time any information concerning the signal and of measuring its parameters at near-threshold intensities [Figs. 1(II), 2, and 7(IIB)]. Their capacity for detecting weak signals of sufficient duration is also small as compared with that of the long-latency neurons. (1) The threshold values of the short-latency neurons are distributed over a higher intensity range (by about 20 dB) than is the case for the long-latency elements. (2) Their threshold rises with an increase in the risetime of the signal (Fig. 5). (3) Their probability function is less steep than that of the long-latency units (Fig. 6). However, unlike those of long latency, the short-latency neurons are capable of indicating the onset of the signal with great precision, since their latent period is short and the dispersion around this value is small even at threshold intensities (Figs. 1-4, and 7). Thus, these neurons secure a reliable detection of the signal over the time scale [10]. Besides, there is some evidence which suggests that these neurons are properly adjusted for the detection of brief signals. Thus, first, when brief sounds are presented, their thresholds are close to thresholds of long-latency neurons (Fig. 2), and in some cases they are even considerably lower [12]. Second, for brief signals the probability function of these neurons becomes steep (Fig. 7), and is steeper as a rule than the probability function for the long-latency neurons. This implies that the reliability of brief signal detection is higher for the short-latency units than for the long-latency neurons. Finally, as was already mentioned (Fig. 11), short-latency units may have rather sharp tuning curves even for brief sounds.

Thus, each of the two groups of neurons possesses advantages over the other as regards some aspects in the sound analysis. It is clear that these two groups, in combination with a large group of neurons that have intermediate properties, may be utilized by the auditory system in sound detection, accumulation of information concerning signals, and in measuring signal properties. In particular, the organization modes of neuron activity described above may be thought of as designed, on the one hand, for sufficiently quick response to sound signals and, on the other hand, for accumulation of information about a signal over a long period of time. The difference between the two neuron types is most pronounced for tones of best frequency at threshold intensity and sufficiently long duration. This suggests that the differentiation of these two neuron groups is connected with the need to detect signals and accumulate information contained in the optimal segment of the sound spectrum to which a neuron is most sensitive.

It should be noted that development of the two neuron groups described seems to be an essential feature of the auditory system since two such groups can also be distinguished in the inferior colliculus of the cat and rat [4, 8] and in the auditory system of insects [9]. The meaning of such an organization is considered elsewhere in more detail [3].

When considering the mechanisms of the neuron that may be responsible for one or the other reaction type, the diagram in Fig. 13 may be helpful.

Since a neuron is a system with a definite time constant, the depolarization process caused by a stimulus can be expected to grow according to the curves 1, 2, 3, or n in Fig. 13. The shape of the curve will be determined by the stimulus intensity and time constant of the process. The scheme of Fig. 13 shows that the latent period of the spike measured by intercepts 0A, 0B, 0C, and 0D increases with a drop in stimulus intensity from n to 3, 2, and 1; on the other hand, with the increase of stimulus duration from 0A to 0B, 0C, and 0D the threshold intensity of the stimulus will decrease from n to 3, 2, and 1, respectively. Thus, the latency curve as a function of stimulus intensity [LP(I)] will coincide with the threshold curve as a function of stimulus duration [$I_0 (t)$]. This is actually the case for the units in the cochlear nuclei after the conduction time of the impulse from the cochlea is taken into account [11]. Thus, the scheme shown in Fig. 13 readily accounts for correlation between the functions LP(I) and $I_0(t)$. By introducing into this

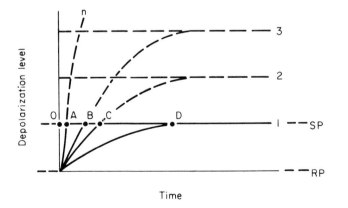

FIG. 13. Scheme of a depolarization process in a neuron at different stimulus intensities (1, 2, 3, n). Abscissa: time after the stimulus onset. Ordinate: amount of depolarization. RP, resting potential; SP, critical depolarization level necessary for generating a spike. The intensity 1 corresponds to rheobase.

scheme a noise in the form of RP or SP fluctuations (Fig. 13) according to a Gaussian distribution, interrelation of these characteristics with functions $\sigma_{LP}(I)$ and $p(I)$ becomes understandable as well. Correlation with other characteristics $[I_o \ (t^1)$ and the discharge pattern] is more difficult to understand, since further assumptions concerning accommodation and other neuronal properties would have to be made (for example, an assumption could be made that the greater the time constant of the process shown in Fig. 13, the greater the time constant of the accommodation process).

Thus, in accordance with Frank and Fuortes [2] and Katz [6], the general scheme shown in Fig. 13 describes processes that must essentially determine a number of properties of the neurons described in this chapter. Physical realization of such a scheme is theoretically possible in various structures such as neuronal membrane, neuron as a whole, or as a group of interconnected neurons. Hence, elementary properties of the neuron or properties of a system of interconnected neurons may be responsible for one or the other reaction type, which ultimately depends on the speed of the depolarization process, i.e., on the steepness of the curves 1, 2, 3, and n in Fig. 13.

It appears that simultaneous realization of the following conditions is essential for a long-latency-type reaction: (a) a sufficiently long time constant and slow accommodation rate of the active region of the neuronal membrane [11]; (b) a lack or a low level of inhibitory input activity; and (c) a sufficiently high time dispersion of impulses at neuron inputs. When all these requirements are simultaneously realized, the latent period at threshold may shift sufficiently to secure the capacity for temporal summation, a threshold stability despite changes in signal risetime, and reliable sound detection over a given intensity range [steep slope of the function $p(I)$]. The long-latency reaction type may be visualized as occurring for signals of optimal frequency (when inhibitory effects upon a given neuron produced by other neurons are relatively slight), the active synaptic endings having a location on well-ramified dendrites (where the most favorable conditions for summation of time-dispersed impulses may be expected).

For the short-latency-type reaction, the realization of at least one of the following factors is probably essential: (a) a low time constant and a high accommodation rate of the active membrane region; (b) a sufficiently high level of activity of inhibitory inputs (13); and (c) a low impulse dispersion at neuron inputs. The realization of any one of these requirements causes the latency shift at threshold to become limited, hence all other characteristics of the short-latency reaction type are realized as well. Thus, the short-latency reaction type may be realized either with signals of nonoptimal frequency (when inhibitory effects upon a given neuron are comparatively strong), or when synaptic endings are located in a region with low capacity for temporal and spatial summation (somas of small neurons, short, slightly ramified dendrites), or when there is a small number of slightly ramified afferent endings on a given neuron (e.g., end bulbs of Held) and thus time dispersion of arriving impulses seems to be insignificant.

The data concerning location of neurons with different reaction types are in agreement with such considerations. Thus, short-latency units were found to be located in the dorsal cochlear nucleus which possesses a great number of small neurons [15] and displays well pronounced inhibitory phenomena [5] as well as in the regions of the posteroventral and anteroventral cochlear nuclei adjacent to the interstitial nucleus, where there are synaptic endings in the form of Held bulbs or their modifications. Long-latency units were common in all divisions of the cochlear complex. These data are in agreement with results obtained by others [7].

Thus, the occurrence of the two reaction types in the cochlear complex may be thought of as being realized both by the elementary properties of the neurons and by their functional, morphological, and spatial organization.

Summary

1. Two widely diverse reaction types of the cochlear nuclei units are described. The long-latency type is characterized by (a) a long latent period (about 100 msec) and large dispersion of the latent period values near threshold; (b) a marked capacity for temporal summation; (c) independence of threshold on the risetime of the signal; (d) a steep slope of the probability function; and (e) a tonic discharge pattern. The short-latency type is characterized by (a) a short latent period (not more than 10 msec) and a small dispersion of latent period values near threshold; (b) a small capacity for temporal summation; (c) a dependence of threshold on risetime of the signal; (d) an inclined slope of the probability function; and (e) a phasic discharge pattern at near-threshold intensities.

2. The characteristic features of both these reaction types are best pronounced when (a) the signal intensity is near threshold; (b) the signal duration is of the order of 100 msec; and (c) the frequency of the signal is optimal for the given neuron. The existence of the two reaction types is assumed to be an adaptation for (a) detection of weak signals; (b) temporal accumulation of information about it; and (c) extraction of information contained in the optimal part of the sound spectrum.

3. The following neurophysiological mechanisms are considered as securing the occurrence of one or the other reaction type: (a) capacity of a given neuron to summate, and (b) inhibitory interactions between neurons. The interplay between these two factors is assumed to arise as a consequence of the properties of the neurons and through their functional, morphological, and spatial organization.

Acknowledgments

Special thanks are due to G. I. Ratnikova for histological assistance and S. S. Kochubey for technical assistance throughout the work.

REFERENCES

1. Fox, C. A., and Eichman, J. A rapid method for locating intracerebral electrodes. *Stain Technol.* **34**, 39-42 (1959).
2. Frank, K., and Fuortes, M. G. F. Stimulation of spinal motoneurons with intracellular electrodes. *J. Physiol.* **143**, 451-470 (1956).
3. Gersuni, G. V. On the mechanisms of hearing (in connection with studies of time and time-frequency characteristics of the auditory system). *In* Mechanisms of Hearing. "Problems of Physiological Acoustics" (G. V. Gersuni, ed.), Vol. 6: Mechanisms of Hearing, pp. 3-32. Nauka, Leningrad, 1967 (in Russian).
4. Gersuni, G. V., Altman, J. A., Maruseva, A. M., Radionova, E. A., Ratnikova, G. I., and Vartanian, I. A. This volume, Chap. 10.
5. Greenwood, D. D., and Maruyama, N. Excitatory and inhibitory response areas of auditory neurons in the cochlear nucleus. *J. Neurophysiol.* **28**, 863-892 (1965).
6. Katz, B. "Electric Excitation of Nerve." Oxford University Press, London, 1939.
7. Kiang, N. Y.-S., Pfeiffer, R. R., Warr, W. B., and Backus, A. S. N. Stimulus coding in the cochlear nucleus. Ann. Otol. Rhinol. Laryngol. **74**, 463-479 (1965).
8. Maruseva, A. M. On the time characteristics of neurons of different types in the inferior colliculus of the rat. *In* "Problems of Physiological Acoustics" (G. V. Gersuni, ed.), Vol. 6: Mechanisms of Hearing, pp. 50-62. Nauka, Leningrad, 1967, (in Russian).
9. Popov, A. V. Characteristics of activity of the central neurons in the auditory system of the locust. *In* ."Problems of Physiological Acoustics" (G. V. Gersuni, ed.) Vol. 6: Mechanisms of Hearing, p. 108-121 Nauka, Leningrad, 1967 (in Russian).
10. Radionova, E. A. Detection of the useful signal from noise in the neuronal impulse activity of the cochlear nucleus of cats. *J. Higher Nervous Activity (USSR)* **15**, 481-490 (1965) (in Russian).
11. Radionova, E. A. Correlation between some characteristics in the response of the auditory system neurons to sound stimuli. *Biophysics (USSR)* **11**, 478-487 (1966) (in Russian).
12. Radionova, E. A. On the significance of time characteristics of the response of the cochlear nucleus neurons. *In* "Problems of Physiological Acoustics," (G. V. Gersuni, ed.), Vol. 6: Mechanisms of Hearing, pp. 32-50. Nauka, Leningrad, 1967, (in Russian).
13. Radionova, E. A. Inhibitory phenomena of the neuronal impulse activity in the cat cochlear nucleus. *J. Higher Nervous Activity (USSR)* **18**, 133-136 (1968) (in Russian).
14. Radionova, E. A. Threshold values distribution of two types of neurons in the auditory system. *Biophysics (USSR)* **13**, 124-133 (1968) (in Russian).
15. Ratnikova, G. I. On the structure of cochlear nucleus in the cat. *In* "Problems of Physiological Acoustics" (G. V. Gersuni, ed.), Vol. 6: Mechanisms of Hearing, pp. 182-195. Nauka, Leningrad, 1967 (in Russian).

16. Rose, J. E., Galambos, R., and Hughes, J. R. Microelectrode studies of the cochlear nuclei of the cat. *Bull. Johns Hopkins Hosp.* **104**, 211-251 (1959).
17. Sasaki, K., and Otani, T. Accommodation in spinal motoneurons of the cat. *Jap. J. Physiol.* **11**, 443-456 (1961).
18. Vaitulevich, S. F. Method of improved oscillographic records of impulse unit activity. *J. Higher Nervous Activity (USSR)* **16**, 942-943 (1966) (in Russian).
19. Vaitulevich, S. F., and Likhnitsky, A. M. Use of impulse analyser AI-100 for temporal analysis of impulse activity. *J. Higher Nervous Activity (USSR)* **16**, 747-752 (1966) (in Russian).
20. Wall, P. D. Repetitive discharge of neurons. *J. Neurophysiol.* **22**, 305-320 (1959).

10

Functional Classification of Neurons in the Inferior Colliculus of the Cat according to Their Temporal Characteristics

G. V. Gersuni, J. A. Altman, A. M. Maruseva, E. A. Radionova, G. I. Ratnikova, and I. A. Vartanian

Studies of responses in various regions of the auditory system, carried out in recent years in our laboratory, have demonstrated that in each region one can distinguish several types of neurons according to their temporal characteristics [2-4, 7, 8, 10-12].

The analysis of the different response types is, we believe, essential for understanding the character of transmission and of information processing in the central synaptic regions of the auditory system. Classification of the responses of the auditory neurons into several distinct types was based on the following criteria: (1) the latent period at threshold intensity and variations of the latent period as a function of stimulus strength; (2) dependence of the threshold of the response on sound duration (in the range of 1 to 100 msec); (3) dependence of the threshold tuning curve on sound duration; (4) dependence of the spike count in the response on the intensity of the signal. For numerous units these criteria were sufficient in establishing the type of the response.

The various response types were described in detail for neurons of the cochlear nuclei of the cat [10-12] and for neurons in the inferior colliculus of the rat [3, 8]. This chapter extends the studies to neurons of the inferior colliculus of the cat.

Many features of single unit responses to various sounds in the inferior colliculus of the cat are known in detail [5, 9, 13]. In the present work special attention was paid to the temporal characteristics of the neurons. This made it necessary to introduce some additional criteria for evaluation of the properties of the response.

Methods

Adult cats, weighing from 1.5 to 3.5 kg, free from external signs of otitis, were used in the experiments. The animals were anesthetized with an intraperitoneal injection of a mixture of chloralose and urethane (30 and 500 mg/kg, respectively). After the onset of narcotic sleep, the trachea was cannulated, and the cochlea, ipsilateral to the site of recording, was destroyed. The animal's head was then firmly fixed in a special headholder. After removal of the soft tissue, a trephine opening was made in the posterior part of the parietal bone, the tentorium forming its posterior border. The dura was dissected and the hemisphere was moved away from the midline. The resulting slit was tamponed in order to protect the inferior colliculus from injuries. The occipital pole of the hemisphere was then removed and the bleeding controlled with tampons soaked in soluble vitamin K.

The experiments were performed in a sound-deadened chamber. Tungsten microelectrodes with tip diameters of about 1 μ and coated with acetone varnish were used for recording. The electrodes were placed under visual control on the surface of the inferior colliculus. Further insertion was accomplished in steps of 2 to 4 μ by means of a hydraulic micromanipulator which was located outside the chamber. Tone bursts, 1 and 100 msec in duration, were used as stimuli. The acoustic signals were produced by an audiogenerator of the ZG-10 type with an electronic switch developed in our laboratory [6]. The intensity of the signals was regulated by an attenuator. Maximal sound intensity (zero attenuation) was equal to 80 dB above the level of 0.0002 dyn/cm^2, measured at 4 kHz. The following devices were used as sound emitters: (a) an electrostatic loudspeaker of the megaphone type with a frequency range from 2.8 to 20 kHz (the speaker was at a distance of 5 cm from the ear contralateral to the site of recording); (b) a dynamic loudspeaker (mounted with the backside of its cone in a sound-absorbing box). This speaker was located in the midline at a distance of 30 cm from each ear; the variations in its frequency characteristics were ±5 dB between 70 and 8000 Hz.

After a neuron responding to a sound signal was isolated, we first determined a threshold tuning curve. Tuning curves were determined for signals of 1- and 100-msec duration. The intensity of the sound, which caused a visually observed spike discharge with the probability of 0.5, in at least ten trials, was taken as threshold intensity. The frequency step in determining the tuning curve was 2 kHz; however, near the optimal (best) frequency it was equal to 25 to 30 Hz. After the determination of the threshold tuning curve, the spikes in a response were reduced to dots [17] on the tube face of the oscilloscope and the traces were photographed while the sound intensity varied for different series from a maximal to a threshold level; the duration of the signal in such a series was 1 and 100 msec. Two frequencies were examined in particular detail. One was the optimal frequency (f_0); the other will be referred to as nonoptimal (f_n). The latter is defined as that frequency for which the threshold of the response was 20 to 40 dB higher than for the optimal one. When the threshold tuning curve was relatively flat, the differences in thresholds were smaller. The tone bursts were presented once every 2 sec. Rectangular stimulus form for sound bursts was used. This was most important when the latent periods to the first spike were measured.

The experiments were performed on 22 cats and in all, 103 neurons were studied; in 78 neurons all the desired measurements were made.

In a number of experiments histological controls were carried out. After the experiment, the brain, with the electrode *in situ*, was fixed in 15% Formalin. The electrode tracks and the sites of recordings were determined from a series of sections by the method described by Fox and Eichman [1]. In the brains examined, the electrodes passed through the inferior colliculus obliquely in the anterior-posterior direction. In most cases, the recording sites were located among the cells of the central nucleus; only a few neurons were found to lie in the "lateral cortex"* of the inferior colliculus.

Results

CLASSIFICATION OF THE NEURONS ACCORDING TO THE RESPONSE TYPE

When evaluating the spike activity of the neurons, we concentrated our attention on those characteristics which were useful for neuron classification. These were (1) the value of the latent period at two intensities—at threshold intensity, at which the latent period has a maximal value (LP $_{thr}$) and at suprathreshold intensity, at which the latent period had a minimal value (LP$_{min}$); (2) the difference between threshold values (ΔI) when the signal was 1 and 100 msec in duration, respectively; (3) the number of spikes in the response to a signal 100 msec in duration at an intensity level at which the number of spikes was maximal (N_{max}). For the overwhelming majority of neurons this level was 80 dB. Only for a small number of neurons for which there was a decline in spike counts at higher intensities (the so-called nonmonotonic neurons [13]), was this level below 80 dB.

The evaluation of the material indicates that on the basis of the quantitative values for the above-mentioned characteristics, one can recognize two highly diverse groups of neurons as well as several intermediate groups. Basic Group a was established on the basis of the following characteristics:

* The authors are very grateful to G. N. Shmigidina for the morphological control of the material.

LP_{thr}=10 msec or less; ΔI, less than 8 dB; N_{max}, less than three impulses per stimulus of 100-msec duration. This group consisted of 32 neurons. Group b was established on the basis of the following values: LP_{thr}=over 20 msec; ΔI, more than 8 dB; N_{max}, over three impulses. This group consisted of 20 neurons.

Table 1 shows that the Group a neurons are characterized by (1) a short latent period over the entire range of sound intensities and small dispersion of these values not only at the maximal, but also at threshold intensity; (2) a small capacity for temporal summation, average 1.9 dB; (3) a small number of spikes in the responses (N_{max}=1.1). This, then, is a group of short-latency units without a pronounced capacity for temporal summation and discharging only a small number of spikes per stimulus (phasic neurons). We define these neurons as short-time constant neurons.

Group b neurons are characterized by (1) considerably longer latent periods at threshold intensity and considerable dispersion of these values. When sound intensity is high, the value of LP_{min} is small; the mean value of LP_{min} for the group was 11.0 msec [however, in one case (neuron 14), a very much longer latent period (44 msec) was observed]; (2) a very pronounced temporal summation capacity (the mean value of ΔI=24 dB); (3) a considerable number of spikes in response to a signal (N_{max}=9). This, then, is a long-latency, highly summating group of neurons with a tonic discharge. Such neurons are defined as long-time constant neurons.

Intermediate Groups ab_1 and ab_2 consist of neurons with intermediate characteristics. Group ab_1 (consisting of 16 neurons) differs from Group a only in its longer latencies. At threshold, the range of latent periods is 11 to 19 msec, while at maximal intensity it is 7 to 17 msec; these values compare with 7 to 10 and 4.5 to 8 msec, respectively, for the Group a neurons. In respect to all other parameters, Group ab_1 is close to Group a. Group ab_2 is characterized by latencies very similar to those of Group ab_1, but its neurons display a considerable capacity for temporal summation and there is a larger number of spikes in the discharge train. The character of the response itself is peculiar: the distribution of the spikes in time is limited to the first 20 to 40 msec from the onset of the sound. Such responses are defined as burst responses. The properties of the neurons in this group resemble those of Group b.

Six neurons in our sample could not be assigned to any of the four groups mentioned. One neuron had such a high level of spontaneous activity that it was difficult to ascertain its response characteristics. Two neurons exhibited habituation to repeated stimulation, which made it difficult to establish their modes of response. Two neurons had a long latent period (over 30 msec) both at threshold and at maximal intensity; their discharge consisted of one spike. One neuron had a short latency both at threshold and at maximal intensity and its response consisted of numerous spikes (N_{max}=9). One neuron finally

TABLE 1

Response Characteristics of Single Neurons to Sound Signals of Optimal (Best) Frequency[a]

Group	Latent period (msec)				Dif. in thresholds (ΔI in dB) for sound durations (t) of 1 and 100 msec		Max no. of spikes (N_{max}) in response to signal at $t=100$ msec		No. of neurons in each group[b]	Properties determining the group		
	Max (at threshold intensity, LP_{thr})		Min (at maximal intensity, LP_{max})							LP_{thr} at $t=100$ msec	Location of electrode	Distance from the surface (μ)
	$\bar{X} \pm \sigma/n^{1/2}$ and range of variation	sd	$\bar{X} \pm \sigma/n^{1/2}$ and range of variation	sd	$\bar{X} \pm \sigma/n^{1/2}$ and range of variation	sd	$\bar{X} \pm \sigma/n^{1/2}$ and range of variation	sd				
a	8.5 ± 0.1 7-10	0.9	6.5 ± 0.2 4.5-8	1.0	1.9 ± 0.5 -7 - +7.8	2.5	1.1 ± 0.1 0.8-2.9	0.5	32	<10	<8	<3
ab1	14.0 ± 0.6 11-19	2.5	10.0 ± 0.7 7-17	2.7	2.5 ± 0.7 -0.8 - +7.8	2.8	1.9 ± 0.2 1.0-3.0	0.8	16	$10 < LP_{thr} < 20$	<8	<3
ab2	13.6 ± 2.3 11-18	4.6	9.0 ± 1.7 7-15.6	3.5	14.0 ± 3.6 8-18	7.2	6.0 ± 2.5 3.0-11.0	5.0	4	$10 < LP_{thr} < 20$	>8	>3
b	45.0 ± 5.3 22-100	23.8	11.0 ± 1.9 5-44	8.5	24.0 ± 3.6 8-60	16.0	9.0 ± 1.2 3.0-20.0	5.4	20	>20	>8	>3

[a] $\bar{X}$ = mean; σ = standard deviation; n = number of items in the sample.
[b] Total number of neurons for all groups, 72.

displayed properties of a Group a neuron over a wide range of suprathreshold intensities (of the order of 30 dB) and the properties of a Group b neuron at still higher levels of stimulation (40 to 80 dB); such observations are more commonly made for neurons of the cochlear complex [10]. All these neurons may be assigned to an intermediate, heterogeneous group (ab_3 and ab_4).

Figure 1 presents distributions of threshold values for neurons of Groups a and b when the stimulus was the optimal frequency. The histograms indicate that thresholds for spike responses for Group a (short-time constant) neurons are distributed over a wide range of intensities from −20 to +70 dB, the mode falling between +20 and +30 dB. It is noteworthy that the histograms obtained for the short- and long-lasting sound signals are nearly the same. The histograms from Group b (long-time constant) neurons [Fig. 1(b)] show that at sound duration of 100 msec the threshold values are distributed over a range from −30 to +60 dB, with the mode between −10 and 0 dB. For sound signals of 1-msec duration, the distribution shifts towards higher intensities.

The distributions of the latent periods for the spike discharge at threshold and at high sound intensities are shown in Fig. 2. The distributions vary only

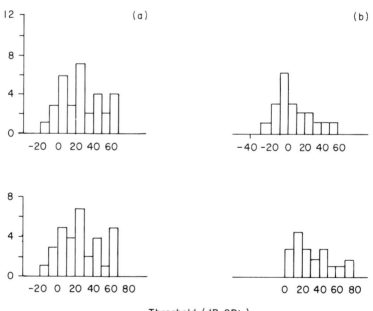

FIG. 1. Distribution of thresholds for short-time constant neurons (a) and long-time constant neurons (b). Ordinate: number of neurons; abscissa: intensity in decibels. Here and in all other figures, the intensity of the sound is given in decibels *re* 0.0002 dyn/cm^2. Upper graphs, thresholds for sound duration of 100 msec; lower graphs, thresholds for sound duration of 1 msec.

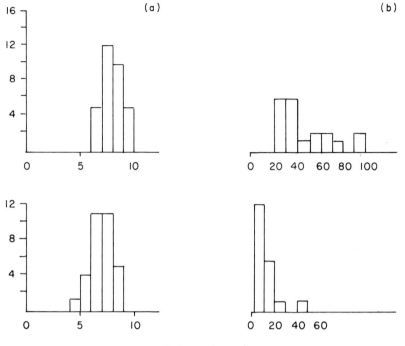

FIG. 2. Distribution of latent periods (LP) for short-time constant neurons (a) and long-time constant neurons (b). Upper graphs, latencies at threshold intensity (LP_{thr}); lower graphs, latencies at maximal intensity (LP_{min}). All LP values for sound duration of 100 msec.

within a narrow range for the neurons in Group a; they are markedly different at threshold and at maximal intensity for the neurons in Group b [Fig. 2(b)].

The tuning curves, despite their various shapes, also display some features which permit identification of a neuron as belonging to the Group a (and ab_1) or Group b (and ab_2). These features become particularly apparent when both brief and long-lasting sounds are used to determine the threshold tuning curve. It is characteristic for neurons of Group a (short-time constant neurons) that the tuning curves obtained for sounds of different duration are identical or nearly so (Fig. 3). This fact implies that the thresholds do not change significantly as a function of signal duration. It is characteristic for the neurons of Group b (long-time constant neurons) that an appreciable difference in threshold exists for brief and long-lasting sounds of the optimal frequency (Table 1; Fig. 1). Since the threshold changes, which are dependent on the sound duration, are, as stated, usually more pronounced at the optimal frequency than at other frequencies, the shapes of the tuning curves may be markedly different for the brief and for the long-lasting signals (Fig. 4).

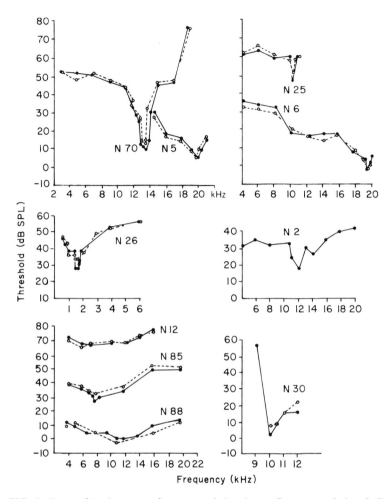

FIG. 3. Types of tuning curves for neurons belonging to Groups a and ab$_1$. Ordinate, intensity in decibels; abscissa, frequency of sound signals in kHz. Number of the corresponding neuron is given for each curve. Solid lines connecting filled circles represent sound duration of 100 msec; dashed lines connecting open circles represent sound duration of 1 msec. (For further explanation, see Table 2).

When the shape of the tuning curve is relatively regular and symmetric, it is possible to quantify the sharpness of the frequency selectivity by calculating the coefficient Q. Q is the ratio of the value of the optimal frequency (f_0) to the width of the frequency band (Δf) at a selected intensity level ($I_{\Delta f}$). The intensity level taken by us was 10 dB above the threshold at the optimal frequency ($Q = f_0/\Delta f$ with $I = 10$ dB). This method of evaluation makes it possible to classify the tuning curves according to the values of Q (the higher

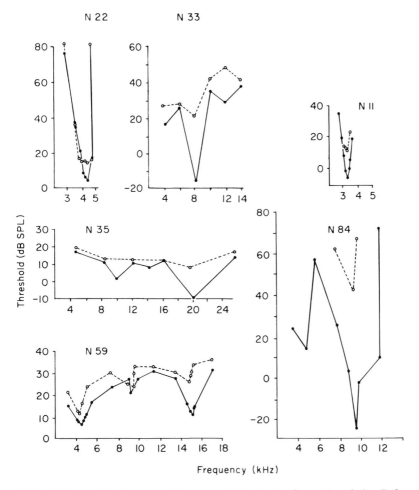

FIG. 4. Types of tuning curves for neurons belonging to Groups b and ab_2. Refer to Fig. 3 for explanations.

the value of Q, the sharper is the tuning curve). Figure 3 presents typical tuning curves with different Q values for neurons of Group a (short-time constant neurons) and neurons of Group ab_1. Some of these curves are characterized by substantial values of Q (9.1; 10.0; 15.0) both for brief and long-lasting signals (Fig. 3, neurons 5, 6, 70). However, a high-frequency selectivity, as defined by the value of Q, characterized only limited segments of the curves—at relatively low levels of the sound. Thus, e.g., when the sound intensity level is 11 to 15 dB above threshold, the tuning curve for neuron 5 becomes considerably more sloping. Particularly sharp changes in width of the tuning curves occur for neurons 6 and 25. The curve for neuron 70 makes a bend and becomes flattened when the intensity level is 33 dB above threshold. This intensity level, at which the frequency selectivity, expressed by a high value of Q (over 9.0), was still in evidence, was the highest among the 48 neurons that formed Groups a and ab_1.

Figure 4 depicts tuning curves for six neurons belonging to Groups b and ab_2 (long-time constant neurons). A high-frequency selectivity for sounds of long duration is characteristic for these neurons. If brief sounds are presented, there is a pronounced flattening of the tuning curve because of a rise in thresholds. However, on rare occasions (3 out of 20), even though the thresholds rose greatly, high Q values were observed also in response to brief sounds (neuron 84, Fig. 4). The shape of the tuning curve may be very diverse for neurons of either group, as can be seen in Figs. 3 and 4. Flat tuning curves are encountered more frequently for the short-latency neurons. Tuning curves with several maxima were observed (Fig. 4) more often for the long-latency neurons. Some of these curves display a pronounced asymmetry* (e.g., neuron 30, Fig. 3). The Q values for the tuning curves shown in Figs. 3 and 4 are assembled in Table 2.

An inspection of the tuning curves obtained for sounds of different duration indicates that for neurons in Group b, the greatest differences in threshold responses to brief and long-lasting signals occur for a frequency that is at or close to the optimal frequency (Fig. 4). Table 3 contains numerical data for five neurons of Group b and one of Group ab_2 (neuron 22) concerning the differences in thresholds at two durations for an optimal and a nonoptimal frequency. The mean threshold shift (ΔI) at an optimal frequency amounts to 18.6 dB, and at a nonoptimal frequency, to 1.36 dB. The table also presents data concerning the maximum number of spikes in the response to a sound 100 msec in duration. The mean number of impulses at the optimal frequency is 11.1 spikes, and at the nonoptimal frequency, 1.3 spikes. These data indicate that for a nonoptimal frequency, the responses of Group b neurons, as well as those of Group ab_2 (neuron 22) are similar to responses of neurons of the type a at the optimal frequency.

TONOTOPICAL ORGANIZATION AND ANATOMICAL DISTRIBUTION OF NEURONS WITH DIFFERENT RESPONSE TYPES

Histological examination reveals that our records were obtained from various parts of the central nucleus of the inferior colliculus. The locations of 38 neurons were established along seven electrode tracks. In five tracks (Fig. 5, tracks 3 to 7), there was a progression of optimal frequencies from low to

---

* Note the linear frequency scale in Figs. 3 and 4. If a logarithmic scale is used, most of the tuning curves display a steeper rise on the high-frequency side.

TABLE 2

Characteristics of the Tuning Curves of the Neurons[a]

Fig. no.	Neuron no.	Group	Q at $t=100$ msec	Q at $t=1$ msec	ΔI (dB) at f_0
3	26	ab_1	4.0	1.0	5.2
	12	a	0.55	0.5	-0.9
	85	a	0.9	0.8	5.0
	88	a	1.0	1.0	-2.0
	70	a	15.0	15.0	5.2
	5	a	9.1	9.1	0.0
	2	a	6.0	—	0.5
	30	a	12.5	—	4.3
	25	a	18.6	—	2.4
	6	a	10.0	10.0	1.7
4	22	ab_2	10.0	5.4	10.4
	33	b	16.0	1.6	39.0
	35^b	b	5.0	—	17.0
	59^b	b	7.5	6.0	15.0
	11	b	13.0	6.4	18.0
	84	b	32.0	16.0	68.0

[a] Refer to Figs. 3 and 4 and Table 1.
[b] For these neurons, only values for the larger optimum are listed.

high as the electrode advanced. These tracks clearly reveal the existence of a spatial frequency projection in the central nucleus, as has been described by other authors [13, 16]. An evaluation of the response types of the neurons encountered indicates that short-time constant neurons (Group a) and long-time constant neurons (Group b)—which greatly differ from each other in temporal characteristics—may be located close to each other along the same

TABLE 3

Characteristics of Temporal Summation and
Spike Activity of Neurons in Group b.[a]

No.	Neuron no.	f_o	ΔI (dB)		N_{max} at $t=100$ msec	f_o (kHz)	f_n (kHz)
			f_n	f_o	f_n		
1	22	10.4	0.0	2.9	2.0	4.2	3.2
2	31	19.0	0.0	14.0	1.0	12.0	9.0
3	35	17.0	2.6	12.0	1.0	20.0	4.0
4	41	40.0	3.5	13.0	1.0	2.5	2.55
5	48	18.4	0.0	5.0	1.0	10.0	14.0
6	83	7.0	2.0	20.0	2.0	3.0	4.0
Mean:		18.6	1.35	11.1	1.3		

[a] In response to a signal of an optimal (f_o) and a nonoptimal (f_n) frequency.
[b] Refer to Table 1 for legends.

electrode track. This is seen clearly when considering, for example, neurons along track 5 in Fig. 5. The electrode passed through the caudal part of the central nucleus and six neurons, whose optimal frequencies varied between 1.2 and 12 kHz, were studied along this track. Four of these neurons were Type b, one was a Group a neuron, and one was of an ab_1 type (which is similar to Type a). Two of these neurons (30 and 31, Table 4) with markedly different characteristics had optimal frequencies of 10 and 12 kHz, respectively, and were located in proximity to each other. An analysis of the characteristics of neurons in all seven punctures, located in various parts of the central nucleus, indicates that the only attribute that is topically organized is the optimal frequency of the neurons. We have never seen any indication of a topical arrangement according to latent period or capacity to summate (Table 4). In our sample, the short-time constant elements or Group a neurons were more often encountered in the anterior part of the central nucleus and in the region of entry of the lateral lemniscus fibers, while the long-time constant or Type b neurons were more often seen in the posterior sector of the nucleus (Fig. 5). However, the available sample is small and the difference is not statistically significant.

TABLE 4

Characteristics of Neurons and
Their Locations in the Inferior Colliculus.[a]

No. of electrode track	No. of neuron	Group	Optimal frequency (kHz)	LP[b] (msec)	ΔI (dB)	Threshold at $t=100$ msec	N_{max}	Location of electrode	Distance from the surface (μ)
5	26	ab_1	1.6	15-10	5.2	19.0	2.1	Caudal part of the central nucleus	1920
	27	b	1.2	45-10	18.0	16.0	6.0	Ventro-caudal part	2980
	28	b	2.8	30-10	8.0	15.0	6.0	of the central	3290
	29	b	8.0	70-11	60.0	-18.0	5.0	nucleus	3950
	30	a	10.0	9-7	4.3	3.0	1.0	Near the ventro-	4020
	31	b	12.0	38-7	19.0	8.6	14.0	caudal border of the central nucleus	4370
3	15	ab_4	5.3	58-32	8.7	56.0	1.0		3670
	16	ab_4	High spontaneous activity					Near the anterior	4130
	17	a	6.2	9-7	-7.0	47.0	1.0	pole of the	4640
	18	a	7.4	9-7	—	45.0	1.0	central nucleus	4740
	19	a	7.2	9-7	—	20.0	1.0		4850
1	2	a	12.0	9-7	0.0	19.0	1.0	Ventro-caudal	3890
	3	b	3.0	50-5	18.0	-11.0	6.0	part of the	3890
	4	a	2.8	9-7	0.0	27.0	1.0	central nucleus	3890
	5	a	20.0	9-7	0.0	4.0	1.0	near the entry of	4770
	6	a	19.7	9-7	1.7	-4.0	2.0	the lateral lemniscus	4950
	7	ab_4	20.0	35	36.0	44.0	5.0	fibers	5270

[a] Refer to Table 1 for legends.   [b] First number, LP_{thr}, second, LP_{max}.

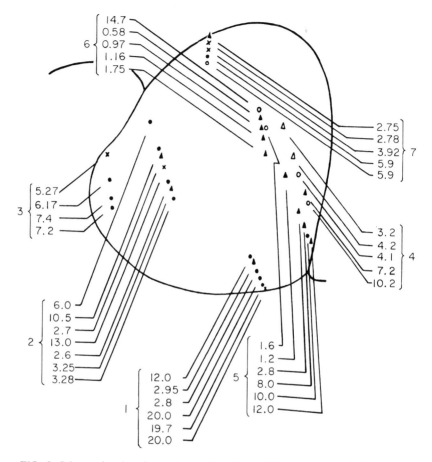

FIG. 5. Scheme showing the anatomical locations of the neurons studied in a sagittal outline of the inferior colliculus. Filled circles designate neurons of Group a; open circles, neurons of Group ab_1; filled triangles, neurons of Group b; open triangles, neurons of group ab_2; crosses, neurons of group ab_4. Each neuron is identified by the value of its optimal frequency in kHz. Seven electrode tracks are shown.

THE CHARACTER OF THE NEURAL DISCHARGE

Figures 6 and 7 present temporal spike patterns in the responses at different sound intensities for a short-time constant neuron or Group a neuron (Fig. 6) and for a long-time constant neuron or Group b neuron (Fig. 7). Neuron 17 (Fig. 6) hardly ever discharged more than one spike to stimuli of 100 and 1 msec in duration at all intensity levels; its latent period was short, and the dispersion was small at all intensity levels. A characteristic feature of this neuron was a "negative" temporal summation, i.e., a higher threshold for a

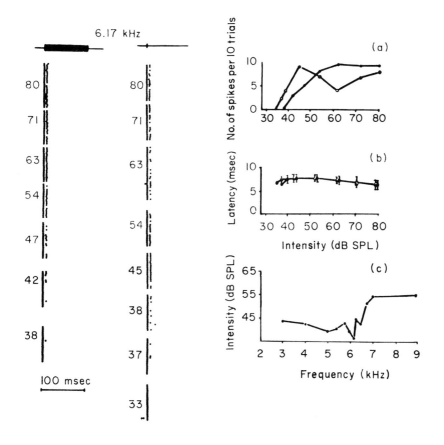

FIG. 6. Neuron 17 (Group a, short-time constant neuron). Left: discharge patterns to a sound of optimal frequency (6.17 kHz to signals of 100- and 1-msec duration. Duration of the signal is indicated at the top of each vertical column of records. Intensity of the signal was 1 msec (open circles) and 100 msec (filled circles), respectively. Ordinate: number of spikes per ten trials. Abscissa: sound intensity in dB. (b) Latent period as a occurrence of neural discharge. Right: (a) Spike-count functions when the duration of the signal was 1 msec (open circles) and 100 msec (filled circles), respectively. Ordinate: number of spikes per ten trials. Abscissa: sound intensity in dB. (b) Latent period as a function of sound intensity when the duration of the signal was 1 msec (open circles) and 100 msec (filled circles), respectively. Length of the vertical line at each point indicates the value of the standard deviation. (c) Threshold tuning curve for signals of 100-msec duration.

long-lasting sound. This phenomenon may result from the growth of inhibitory influences when the duration of the sound increases.

Neuron 31 (Fig. 7) belongs to Group b if its behavior is examined for its optimal frequency of 12 kHz. However, at a nonoptimal frequency (9 kHz),

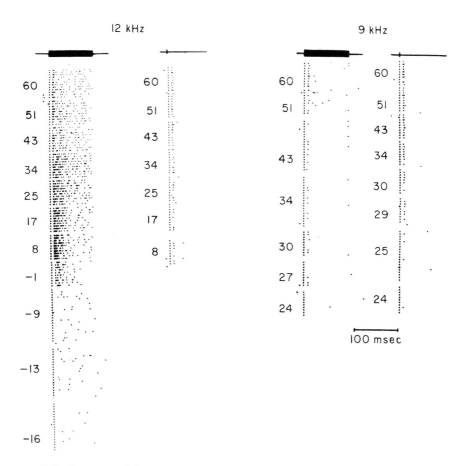

FIG. 7. Neuron 31 (Group b, long-time constant neuron with low spontaneous activity). Discharge patterns to sound signals of optimal (12 kHz) and nonoptimal (9 kHz) frequency. Duration of the signal is 100 and 1 msec, respectively. Intensity of the signal in dB is specified to the left of each block of records.

its discharge characteristics are markedly different (Figs. 7 and 8, Table 3). The spike-count intensity function for the optimal frequency tone of 100-msec duration reaches a maximum at a moderate intensity level [Fig. 8(a)]; the spike counts decline at still higher intensities. Thus, the neuron may be regarded as nonmonotonic. Neuron 31 was characterized by substantial differences in all its properties at the optimal and at a nonoptimal frequency. For the optimal frequency, the discharge train coincides with the duration of the signal; in response to a sound of nonoptimal frequency, the discharge is an "on" or "off" reaction.

It should be noted that the temporal impulse patterns of the neurons in the inferior colliculus are diverse; according to the data for the cat [13] and the rat [8], one can distinguish five or six types of discharge patterns for the

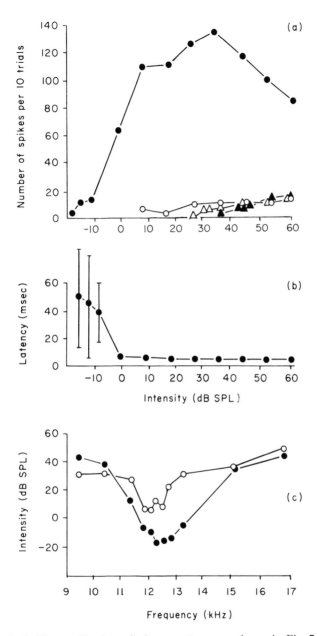

FIG. 8. Neuron 31 whose discharge patterns are shown in Fig. 7. (a) Spike-count functions for signals of different duration at the optimal frequency of 12 kHz (filled circles represent 100-msec duration; open circles, 1-msec duration), and at a nonoptimal frequency of 9 kHz (filled triangles, 100-msec duration; open triangles, 1-msec duration). (b) Latent period of the discharge as a function of sound intensity for signals of optimal frequency of 100-msec duration. Length of the vertical line indicates the value of the sd. No such values are shown for intensity levels of 0 to 60 dB since the sd for many of these points was less than 1 msec (0.42 to 0.88 msec). (c) Threshold tuning curves when the signals were 100 msec (filled circles) and 1 msec (open circles), respectively.

collicular neurons. Indeed, other neurons belonging to Group b differ essentially from neuron 31. For example, neuron 11 (Fig. 9) is characterized by marked spontaneous activity and by inhibition of this activity when the optimal-frequency stimulus, at moderate intensity, is presented. Moreover, at high sound levels there appear cyclic afterdischarges; an onset burst can be recognized. The number of impulses in the response increases monotonically with intensity for the overall spike count but is a nonmonotonic function for the onset burst. Nonetheless, the basic properties of the neuron which make it a Group b neuron (a marked change of the latency depending on the intensity, a pronounced temporal summation and a considerable number of impulses in the response) are fully maintained.

The response of neuron 35 (Fig. 10) is characterized by a burst which consists of a fair number of spikes and this response is similar for both a brief (1 msec) and a long-lasting (100 msec) sound. The spike-count function is monotonic. Its basic properties suggest that this neuron belongs to Group b.

Thus, it is clear that the functional classification based on temporal characteristics does not cover all the properties of the neuron. The question of how various types of responses relate to excitatory and inhibitory inputs, was considered by Maruseva (Chapter 11 of this volume).

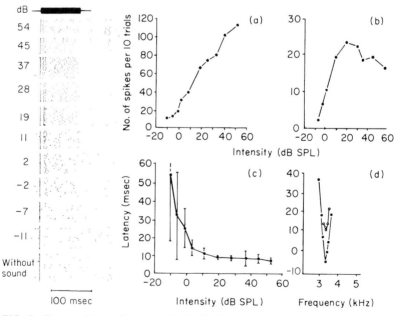

FIG. 9. Characteristics of neuron 11. Left, discharge patterns for signals of optimal frequency of 3.3 kHz at various stimulus intensities. (a) Spike-count function for the total time of stimulus duration (100 msec); (b) spike-count function for the onset burst only; (c) latencies at different intensity levels; (d) threshold tuning curves for sounds of 100 msec duration (filled circles) and 1-msec duration (open circles), respectively.

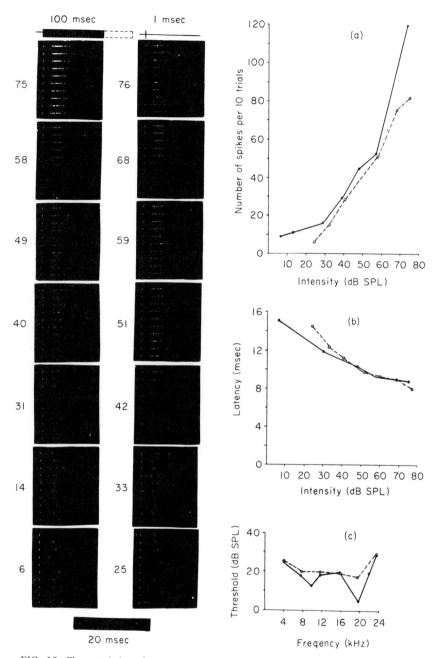

FIG. 10. Characteristics of neuron 35 when signals of different duration activated the neuron. Filled circles indicate values for 100-msec signals; open circles, values for 1-msec signals. (a) spike-count functions; (b) latencies at different intensity levels; (c) threshold tuning curves. Left, discharge patterns for signals of optimal frequency of 20 kHz for various stimulus intensities.

Discussion

The investigation of the temporal and temporal-frequency characteristics of the neurons makes it clear that the neurons that belong to Groups a and b form a large majority of all the neurons studied in the cat's inferior colliculus. Intermediate groups constitute about one-fourth of the neuron population. It was also observed that certain neurons may behave under some conditions as intermediate neurons of Types ab_1 or ab_2, and as belonging to the Groups a or b under other conditions of stimulation. It may be noted that some of the criteria used for classification of the neurons are not independent of each other. Thus, the value of the latent period at threshold intensity (LP_{thr}.) and the degree of temporal summation (ΔI) show for all neurons, irrespective of the groups to which the neurons belong, a high positive correlation ($r = 0.78$; $p < 0.001$). Therefore, there is little doubt that the maximal latency (LP_{thr})* and the degree of the temporal summation are interconnected phenomena, which, apparently, reflect the summation capacity of the neuron. This conclusion was drawn previously with respect to the neurons of the inferior colliculus of the white rat [7, 8], for neurons of the cochlear complex in the cat [10-12], as well as for some neurons in the primary auditory cortex of the cat [14, 15].

Whereas the latent period to the first spike at threshold intensity and the capacity for temporal summation are highly interdependent, the third criterion used in classification of the neurons, i.e., the average number of spikes in the response, is not correlated with the other two characteristics. It seems evident that the factors influencing the pattern of the response do not depend only on the phenomena that determine the summation capacity of the neuron.

In the auditory system, the existence of groups of neurons that differ in their temporal characteristics is essential for understanding how the system functions. The significance of such a differentiation was considered elsewhere in detail [3, 12]. Here, only the following may be briefly mentioned. The two groups of neurons, which differ in their temporal characteristics, apparently seem to perform different functions in the analysis of sound signals. One may assume that the short-latency neurons, which have practically no capacity for temporal summation and which often possess a well-defined frequency selectivity, irrespective of the duration of the sound, are primarily used to signal the beginning of the acoustic stimulation and to perform a short-time sound analysis. The capacity to achieve a sufficiently precise analysis in short time

---

* When considering the characteristics that reflect the summation properties of neurons in different parts of the auditory system in different animals, it is of great advantage to use as a criterion not only the absolute values of the latent period at threshold intensity, but also the difference or the ratio between the maximal (LP_{thr}) and minimal (LP_{min}) latent-period values.

periods and to preserve the short-time constants of cochlear processing reflect some of the remarkable properties of these neurons.

The long-latency neurons, which possess a very marked capacity for temporal summation and whose frequency selectivity sharpens with an increase of the sound duration, are adapted to accumulate information concerning the signal for a relatively long period of time. Such differentiation of the neurons enables the auditory system to operate within a wide temporal range, as well as within a wide range of intensity, with a sufficiently high frequency selectivity.

Conclusions

1. A quantitative evaluation of some characteristics of the neural discharges in the inferior colliculus in response to sounds makes it possible to suggest the existence of two basic groups of neurons.

2. The first group of neurons, Type a, is characterized by (a) short latent periods at threshold intensity (8.5 ± 0.12 msec) and a small decrease of these values (to 6.5 ± 0.16 msec) with an increase in signal intensity from threshold to a maximal level; (b) an insignificant fall of the threshold value (1.9 ± 0.45 dB) with an increase in the duration of the signal from 1 to 100 msec; (c) a tuning curve, which is independent of the signal duration (within the range of 1 to 100 msec); (d) slight dependence of the number of spikes in the response on the intensity and duration of the sound.

3. The second group of neurons Type b, is characterized by (a) long latent periods at threshold intensity (45 ± 5.3 msec) and a significant decrease of these values (to 11 ± 1.9 msec) with an increase in signal intensity from threshold to a maximal level; (b) a substantial decrease in thresholds (24 ± 3.56 dB) with an increase in the signal duration (from 1 to 100 msec); (c) a sharpening of the tuning curves with an increase of the signal duration from 1 to 100 msec; (d) pronounced dependence of the number of spikes in the response on the intensity and duration of the sound.

4. In addition to the two main groups of neurons, two intermediate groups are recognized with characteristics that are intermediate between those of the two basic groups. A small number of neurons exhibit a combination of characteristics of both basic groups.

5. Data have been obtained concerning the tonotopical organization of the cat's inferior colliculus.

6. On the basis of the experimental data, it is assumed that a multichannel system of neurons tuned to various frequency bands simultaneously accomplishes a frequency analysis along several channels, each of which possesses markedly different temporal characteristics (short-time constant and long-time constant neurons).

REFERENCES

1. Fox, C. A. and Eichman, J. A rapid method for locating intracerebral electrodes. Stain Technol., 34, 39-42, 1959.
2. Gersuni, G. V. On the time-place organization of the auditory system. *Proc. 18th Int. Congr. Psychol. Moscow*, 15. Symp., Publ. D-t, Moscow, 1966, pp. 112-118.
3. Gersuni, G. V. On the mechanisms of hearing (in connection with studies of time and time-frequency characteristics of the auditory system). *In* "Problems of Physiological Acoustics" (G. V. Gersuni, ed.), Vol. 6: Mechanisms of Hearing, pp. 3-32. Nauka, Leningrad, 1967 (in Russian).
4. Gersuni, G. V., Maruseva, A. M., Radionova, E. A., and Popov, A. V. Afferent inflow synaptic transformations on the neurons of the auditory system. *In* "Synaptic Processes" (P. G. Kostyuk, ed.), pp. 258-271, "Naukova Dumka," Kiev, 1968 (in Russian).
5. Hind, J. E., Goldberg, J. M., Greenwood, D. D., and Rose, J. E. Some discharge characteristics of single neurons in the inferior colliculus of the cat. II. Timing of the discharges and observations on binaural stimulation. *J. Neurophysiol.* 26, 321-341 (1963).
6. Lebedev, A. P. Electronic gate with a low level of disturbances and the possibility of smooth phase control. *J. Higher Nervous Activity (USSR)* 16, 742-746 (1966) (in Russian).
7. Maruseva, A. M. On the temporal characteristics of the auditory neurons in the inferior colliculus of rats. *Proc. 18th Int. Congr. Psychol. Moscow,* 15. Symp., Publ. D-t, Moscow, 1966, pp. 162-164.
8. Maruseva, A. M. On the time characteristics of neurons of different types in the inferior colliculus of the rat. *In* "Problems of Physiological Acoustics" (G. V. Gersuni, ed.), Vol. 6: Mechanisms of Hearing, pp. 50-62. Nauka, Leningrad, 1967 (in Russian).
9. Nelson, P. G., and Erulkar, S. D. Synaptic mechanisms of excitation and inhibition in the central auditory pathway. *J. Neurophysiol.* 26, 908-923 (1963).
10. Radionova, E. A. Correlation between some characteristics in the response of the auditory system neurons to sound stimuli. *Biophysics (USSR)* 11, 478-487 (1966) (in Russian).
11. Radionova, E. A. The temporal characteristics of the reaction of the cochlear nucleus neurons. *Proc. 18th Int. Congr. Psychol. Moscow,* 15. Symp., Publ. D-t, Moscow, 1966, pp. 156-158.
12. Radionova, E. A. On the significance of time characteristics of the response of the chochlear nucleus neurons. *In* "Problems of Physiological Acoustics" (G. V. Gersuni, ed.), Vol. 6: Mechanisms of Hearing, pp. 32-50. Nauka, Leningrad, 1967 (in Russian).
13. Rose, J. E., Greenwood, D. D., Goldberg, J. M., and Hind, J. E. Some discharge characteristics of single neurons in the inferior colliculus of the cat. I. Tonotopical organization, relation of spike counts to tone intensity, and firing patterns of single elements. *J. Neurophysiol.* 26, 294-320 (1963).
14. Vardapetian, G. A. Dynamic classification of single unit responses in the auditory cortex of the cat. *J. Higher Nervous Activity (USSR)* 17, 95-106 (1967) (in Russian).
15. Vardapetian, G. A. The characteristics of single unit responses in the auditory cortex of cat. *In* "Problems of Physiological Acoustics" (G. V. Gersuni, ed.), Vol. 6: Mechanisms of Hearing, pp. 74-90. Nauka, Leningrad, 1967 (in Russian).

16. Vartanian, I. A., and Ratnikova, G. I. Frequency localization and temporal summation in the auditory centers of the midbrain. *In* "Problems of Physiological Acoustics" (G. V. Gersuni, ed.), Vol. 6: Mechanisms of Hearing, pp. 62-74. Nauka, Leningrad, 1967 (in Russian).
17. Wall, P. D. Repetitive discharge of neurons. *J. Neurophysiol.* **22**, 305-320 (1959).

11
Temporal Characteristics of the Auditory Neurons in the Inferior Colliculus

A. M. Maruseva

Numerous published data indicate that auditory neurons differ greatly in their firing patterns in response to acoustic signals [1-5, 7, 11, 16-18, 22, 26]. The significance of such patterns for the functioning of the auditory system as a whole may be elucidated by studying the properties of different neurons. Despite abundant data pertaining to the activity of single elements in various parts of the auditory system, it is very difficult to systematize them because of substantial differences in the experimental conditions of different investigations. It is thus advisable to develop a single experimental program in order to obtain comparable data for the various levels of the auditory system.

The complex structure of natural sounds, in which modulations of amplitude and frequency occur, suggests that temporal characteristics of the analyzing system are of great significance in the evaluation of such sounds. We may therefore assume that investigations of temporal properties of separate groups of neurons in the auditory system are of particular importance for understanding how the system works.

In this chapter, the author has examined the relation of the latent period (LP) to changes in the intensity of the sound signals; the relations of threshold and character of the impulse activity to changes in the duration of the signal; the recovery time of single elements.

Methods

Most of the experiments were performed on neurons of the inferior colliculus of the rat; a few were also carried out on the inferior colliculus of the cat.

The animals were anesthetized with a mixture of chloralose (30 mg/kg) and urethane (500 mg/kg), intraperitoneally; some experiments were carried out under sodium amytal (70 mg/kg). All the animals were tracheotomized. In half of the experiments, the cochlea was destroyed on one side. The body temperature was maintained within the limits of 36.5° to 37.5°C. The animals were placed in a sound-deadened chamber. All recordings were made on units in the right inferior colliculus. Tungsten electrodes with a tip diameter of about 1 μ were used. The resistance of the electrodes, at a frequency of 1000 Hz, fluctuated between 15 and 60 MΩ. At the beginning of the experiment, the electrode was placed on the surface of the colliculus, in its posterior part. The electrode was advanced by means of a hydraulic micromanipulator.

A generator of white noise served as a source of noise signals; a ZG-10 sound generator, as a source of tonal signals. The characteristics of the high-frequency emitter used in the experiments were uniform from 4 to 20 kHz. The emitter was placed to the left of the animal at a distance of 5 cm from the base of its pinna. The intensity of the sound signals was regulated by an attenuator. The maximal intensity of the stimulation was 80 dB above the level of 0.0002 dyn/cm^2. Signals, which ranged in duration between 100 and 1 msec, were applied every 2 to 3 sec. An amplifier of the UBP1-02 type with a cathode follower was used for amplication of the signals displayed. In most experiments, the unit discharges were reduced to dots [30] for photographic recording.

The electrode track was determined from a series of sections according to the method of Fox and Eichman [6]. The brain of the animal was fixed in 15% Formalin with the electrode *in situ*.

Results

GENERAL CHARACTERISTICS OF THE NEURONS OF THE INFERIOR COLLICULUS

Altogether, 400 neurons in the inferior colliculus of the white rat and 35 neurons in the cat were studied. The responses of the units to noise signals (which had a duration of 50 to 100 msec) differed for different units as regards both the duration of the spike train and the temporal distribution of the impulses.

The responses may be divided into the following types: (I) impulse activity throughout the time of stimulus presentation with cessation of the activity when the stimulus is turned off; (II) impulse activity which persists for some time after the sound signal is turned off; (III) spike train with a pronounced pause after the initial spike burst (silent period); (IV) impulse activity only to the onset and turning off of the sound signal; (V) impulse activity which stops prior to the termination of the stimulus; (VI) responses to the onset of the stimulus consisting of one or two spikes at any signal intensity (Fig. 1). Elements with regular spontaneous discharges which responded to the acoustic stimulation by inhibition of their activity were also observed. Similar types of reactions have been described by Rose *et al.* [26] for neurons of the inferior colliculus of the cat.

The data indicate that various neurons of the inferior colliculus of the rat may have widely different thresholds and a wide range of thresholds is observed for neurons of any response type. It may be pointed out that elements that are physically close to each other, i.e., neurons which are

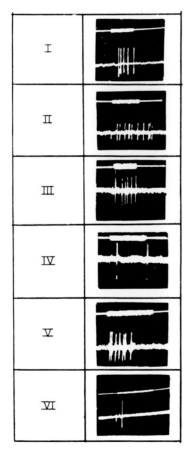

FIG. 1. Various types of neural responses in the inferior colliculus to noise signals of 100-msec duration. Upper trace in each record represents stimulus form. Intensity of the stimulus: 45 dB above threshold for the respective neuron. Data in this and all subsequent figures refer to responses of the rat.

detected as a result of a very small displacement of the microelectrode, often have similar thresholds and similar optimal frequencies. Nonetheless, the discharge pattern of such neurons may be substantially different.

A detailed study of the latent period, when the signal intensity is varied systematically, reveals great differences in the responses between various neurons. In some of them, a decrease of stimulus strength toward the threshold level results in a three- to fivefold increase of the latent period in comparison with its minimal value (the greatest increase is usually observed near threshold). For other neurons, the changes in latent period are more uniform, and the latency increase is usually not more than 50% over the minimal value.

The measurements of threshold intensity for stimuli of different duration (1 to 100 msec) reveal that a change in stimulus duration also has different effects for different neurons. For some neurons, a diminution of signal duration from 20 to 1 msec causes a very marked shift in threshold intensity (up to 50 dB), while for other neurons the change in threshold is small (not more than 5 dB), or is absent altogether.

It can be concluded, therefore, that the neurons studied may be divided into two basic groups on the basis of latency changes—which may occur with variations of the intensity of the sound signals—and on the basis of threshold changes, which may result with variations of stimulus duration. The first group consists of neurons for which highly significant latency and threshold changes occur; the second group consists of neurons for which such changes are small under similar experimental conditions.

Close scrutiny of the discharge patterns indicates that neurons which produce responses belonging to types I, II, III, and V (Fig. 1) form the first, larger group. The second group consists predominantly of neurons responding only to the onset of the acoustic stimulation (type VI) and of a rather small number of units which produce an on-off response (type IV). A detailed description of this material was presented previously [20, 21].

Statistical evaluation of the data reveals a positive correlation between the magnitude of the latent period changes, when the intensity of the stimulus varied, and the magnitude of the threshold changes with variation of stimulus duration.

Figure 2 illustrates these relations. The data pertain to two neurons which are typical representatives of the two different groups. For the neuron with sustained discharges, the latent period increased sharply near threshold (the maximal latent period value exceeded the minimal value more than five times). With a decrease of the duration of the noise signal from 100 to 1 msec, the threshold increased for the same neuron by 39 dB. For the neuron of the second group—with an onset discharge pattern—the changes in the latent period and thresholds were small (3 msec and 5 dB, respectively).

The different character of the shifts in the latent period and of the threshold in responses of the various collicular neurons is demonstrable for both noise and tonal signals. For tonal signals, however, these shifts are most

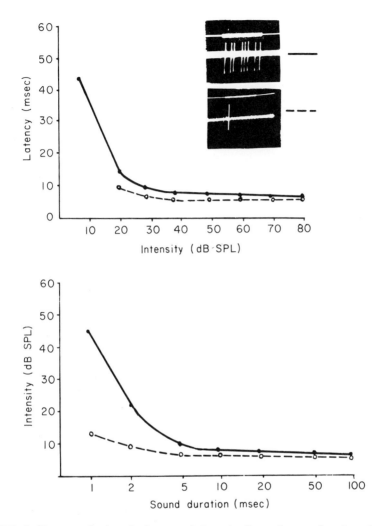

FIG. 2. Upper graph plots the latent period to the first spike as a function of signal intensity. Abscissa, intensity of the sound in dB SPL (sound pressure level *re* 0.0002 dyn/cm^2); ordinate, latent period in msec. Lower graph plots the threshold intensity as a function of signal duration. Abscissa, duration of the noise burst in msec; ordinate, threshold in dB SPL. Solid curves are plots for a neuron of the first group; dashed curves are plots for a neuron of the second group. Samples of discharge patterns of both neurons shown in the inset.

distinct at the optimal (best) frequency of the neuron. With intensity changes of sound signals of a markedly different (nonoptimal) frequency, the latent periods and thresholds of the responses were not substantially affected.

An examination of the data for the individual neurons belonging to the

first, numerically larger group shows that the magnitude of the shifts in the
latent period and threshold may be very different for the various neurons.
This finding provided a basis for a better estimate of the dynamics of impulse
activity of neurons in this group. We thus conclude that first, for a considerable number of these neurons, the number of spikes produced, with variation
in the intensity of the signal, is a nonmonotonic intensity function. Moreover,
the duration of the latent period may often also be a nonmonotonic function
of stimulus strength (Fig. 3). In the auditory system of mammals, the
existence of neurons whose discharge numbers are a nonmonotonic function

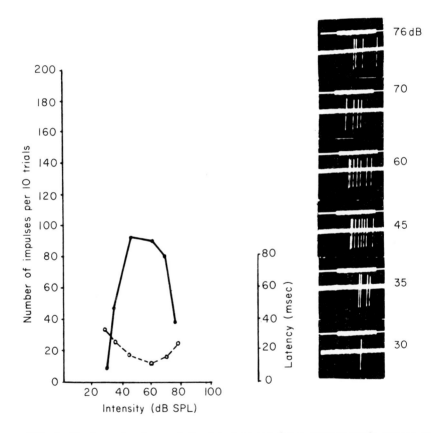

FIG. 3. Number of spikes and the latent period for a nonmonotonic neuron as
functions of stimulus strength. Stimulus: noise bursts of 50 msec duration. Abscissa,
intensity of the signals in dB SPL. Left ordinate represents the number of spikes in 10
trials; right ordinate represents the value of the latent period in msec. Solid curve plots
spike counts; dashed curve plots values of the latent period. Column at right records
responses of the neuron at different intensities of the signal. Actual intensity used, in dB
SPL, is indicated to the right of each plot.

of stimulus strength has been described by a number of authors [12-15, 25-27]. According to Greenwood and Maruyama [14], occasional neurons of this type are encountered in the dorsal cochlear nuclei. The results of several studies [2, 12, 15, 26, 27] warrant the conclusion that the number of nonmonotonic elements increases markedly in the higher synaptic regions of the auditory system. This conclusion together with the results of the present study, namely, that shifts in the latent period and threshold are greatest for nonmonotonic neurons, suggested a further study of their functional characteristics.

RESPONSES OF NEURONS WHOSE SPIKE-COUNT INTENSITY FUNCTIONS BE-COME NONMONOTONIC FOR SIGNALS OF CERTAIN DURATION

The impulse activity of 50 nonmonotonic neurons was thoroughly investigated. The data indicate that these neurons display important pecularities as regards the number of spikes in the individual response, the temporal distribution of impulses, as well as in the changes in the spike patterns when the intensity and duration of the signals varies.

It should be stressed, first, that an exact correspondence between the duration of the stimulus and the duration of the spike train was observed for only a very small number of nonmonotonic neurons [Fig. 4(a)]. The bulk of such neurons responded with sustained discharges only within a narrow range of intensities (not more than 20 dB above threshold) [Fig. 4(b) and (c)]. For some neurons, the duration of the impulse activity was manifestly shorter than that of the signal at all intensity levels [Fig. 4(d)]. When the stimulus intensity exceeded the level that was optimal for spike counts the responses of some neurons consisted of initial bursts of impulses, while responses of others became reduced usually to one or two discharges [Fig. 4(c)].

Irrespective of the pattern of their impulse activity all nonmonotonic neurons exhibited marked changes in their response when other parameters of the sound signals, and particularly their duration, was varied. Figure 5 illustrates this point for neuron 19 which was stimulated by noise pulses of 50 and 5 msec, respectively. The upper graph in Fig. 5 shows that for signals which were 50 msec in duration, the optimal intensity level for the spike counts of the neuron was 17 dB SPL. For higher intensities there were fewer spikes; the onset response became irregular, or disappeared altogether. Patterns on the right indicate that a shortening of the duration of the stimulus to 5 msec had two results: the discharges became more stable in time, and there were more spikes per trial. The upper graph illustrates that with shortening of the stimulus there is not only a shift in the optimal intensity toward higher values, but also a broadening of the intensity range over which the neuron responds vigorously. It is noteworthy that for brief signals the shifts in the

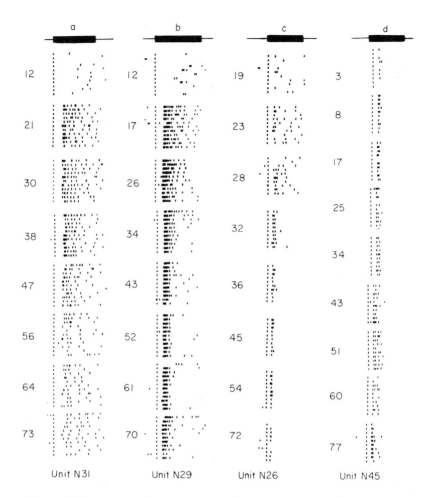

FIG. 4. Different types of changes in the discharge patterns for four nonmonotonic neurons when the intensity of the noise burst varies. (a) Duration of the discharge train corresponds to the duration of the stimulus; (b) and (c) different degrees of shortening of the discharge train when stimulus intensity increases beyond that which causes the optimal number of discharges; (d) duration of the discharge train is shorter than the duration of the stimulus over the whole effective intensity range. Numbers to the left of each pattern represent intensity in dB SPL. Duration of the noise burst was 50 msec.

latent periods approximate those seen for the monotonic neurons (lower graphs, Fig. 5).

Figure 6 presents records and spike-count intensity functions for another nonmonotonic neuron. The duration of the noise burst was 50, 5, and 2 msec, respectively. Records pertaining to the signals of 50 msec duration show that the maximal number of spikes in a response of this neuron was two, even at

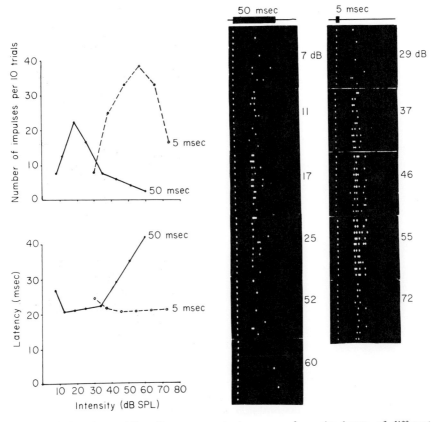

FIG. 5. Impulse activity of a nonmonotonic neuron for noise bursts of different duration. Stimulus intensity in dB SPL plotted against number of spikes per ten trials (upper graphs) and against latent period (in msec), lower graphs. Dashes indicate signal duration of 5 msec; solid lines, signal duration of 50 msec. Right: discharge patterns in response to noise bursts of different duration at various intensities. Intensity in dB SPL is indicated for each block of records. String of dots on the left of each data block indicates the onset of the stimulus. Note that the optimal intensity for the maximal number of spikes is 17 dB for signals of 50-msec duration, and 55 dB for signals of 5-msec duration.

the optimal intensity (60 dB). When the duration of the signal was shortened to 5 msec, the number of impulses in the response increased and the character of the response pattern changed for stimuli at higher intensity. For signals of 2-msec duration the spike-count intensity function approximated that for monotonic neurons. The records in Fig. 6 imply that the rise in the number of impulses in the response, when signals of short duration are presented, is due to lengthening of the time during which discharges occur, as well as to a greater density of spikes in the initial burst.

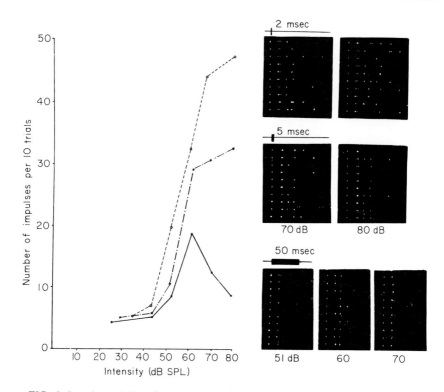

FIG. 6. Impulse activity of a nonmonotonic neuron to noise bursts of 50 msec (solid line), 5 msec (dots and dashes), and 2 msec (dashes), respectively. Optimal intensity for 50-msec signals was 60 dB. For further explanation, see Fig. 5.

Evaluation of all the available material suggests that a specific feature of all neurons, which produce nonmonotonic spike-count intensity functions in response to long-lasting signals (50 msec and over), is a pronounced afterdischarge in response to brief sounds. In some neurons of this type the spike trains, in response to brief signals, assuméd a cyclic character, i.e., there was a series of successive groups of impulses (Fig. 7). The duration of such a cyclic impulse activity was different for different neurons. The maximal duration of brief signals, for which the cyclic activity could still be detected, did not exceed 5 msec. The phenomenon was most pronounced at moderate intensities of the signals (from 40 to 60 dB). When the intensity of the stimulation exceeded 60 dB, the cyclic character of the spike trains became less distinct because of an increase in the duration of the separate bursts.

Among all the neurons studied in the inferior colliculus, we encountered three which responded only to very brief signals; a lengthening of the stimulus beyond 5 msec led to a disappearance of the responses. This suggests that for such neurons there is a sharp decline in threshold when the signal duration

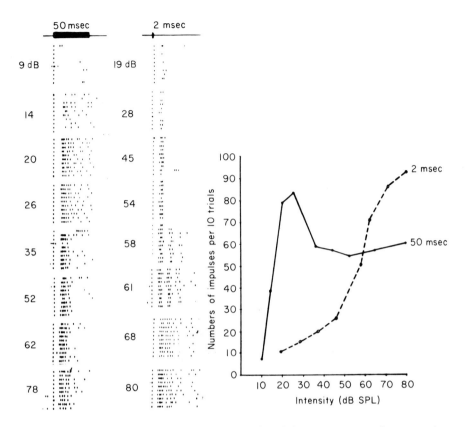

FIG. 7. Cyclic character of spike trains produced by a nonmonotonic neuron in response to brief signals. Graphs plot the intensity of the signal against the number of spikes per 10 trials. Solid line indicates signal duration of 50 msec; dashes, signal duration of 2 msec. For further explanation, see Fig. 5.

decreases. A study of one neuron of this type is shown in Fig. 8. It is of great interest that as the duration of the noise burst becomes reduced, the neuron responds over a wider intensity range. Unfortunately a more detailed description of neurons of this type cannot be given at the present time. It is also unknown how common such neurons may be, since the search stimulus for the responsive neurons was, as a rule, of considerable duration in our experiments.

RECOVERY TIME OF THE RESPONSE

Measurements of the recovery time were made for 45 neurons whose discharge patterns varied. All measurements pertain to the collicular neurons

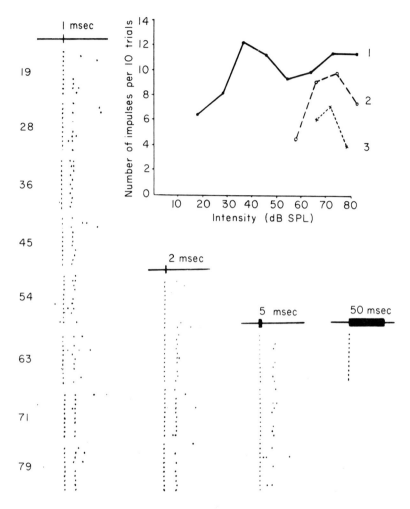

FIG. 8. Impulse activity of a nonmonotonic neuron which responded only to short signals. Numbers 1, 2, and 3 identify, respectively, the curves for signals of 1-, 2-, and 5-msec duration. For further explanation, see Fig. 5.

of the rat. The recovery time was estimated from presentation of a pair of clicks or a pair of short noise bursts, the second member of the pair being presented with varied delay. Both signals were always of equal intensity. The intensity level varied for different neurons; the choice of a suitable intensity level was determined not only by the threshold value, but also by changes in impulse activity which accompanied a change in stimulus strength.

Data obtained from these experiments indicate that the recovery time of various neurons may differ substantially. This observation agrees with the results of other authors [2, 14, 28]. According to Suga, the recovery time of the neurons in the inferior colliculus in bats ranges from several msec to 100 msec. When comparing the available data pertaining to the recovery time of various neurons in the auditory system, it is well to remember that the process of recovery can be evaluated according to any of the three stages: (a) an occasional response to the second signal of the pair; (b) a regular occurrence of a response to the second signal; and (c) a full identity of both responses (an equal number of impulses in the responses and an equal latent period). Thus, different criteria may be used for defining the recovery process.

Our own data suggest that the differences between individual neurons in the time required for a complete recovery are determined mainly by the time at which the responses to the second signal become regular [stage (b)]. The time interval, which characterizes the beginning of the recovery [stage (a)], does not always allow to predict its further course. On the basis of the data obtained, three groups of neurons may be distinguished (1) neurons with a recovery time not exceeding 10 msec; (2) neurons requiring a recovery time of 15 to 40 msec; and (3) neurons for which regular responses to the second signal arise at delays of the order of 50 msec (Fig. 9).

It may be mentioned that neurons with short recovery time are similar in a number of other properties. Thus, for elements with the shortest recovery time (up to 10 msec) the latent period changes as a function of signal intensity, and the threshold changes as a function of stimulus duration are very small. For most neurons of this group, the number of spikes per stimulus did not exceed two impulses. However, a small number of neurons with a short recovery time responded to signals of 50-msec duration with sustained discharges. A characteristic feature of these neurons was a correspondence between the duration of the stimulus and the duration of the discharge train; the spike-count intensity functions were always strictly monotonic.

Neurons with a recovery time ranging from 15 to 40 msec responded to signals (of 50 to 100 msec in duration) with an initial burst of impulses; the discharge train ended prior to the end of the signal at all intensities of the stimulus. The threshold changes in the neurons of this type did not exceed 10 dB. The latent period changes were similar to those in group 1.

Neurons with a nonmonotonic character of the spike-count intensity functions had the longest recovery time. It must be emphatically stressed that for such neurons the recovery time was markedly dependent on the intensity of the sound signals used. At intensities below the optimal level, the recovery time of the nonmonotonic neurons was quite short, whereas at intensities exceeding this level, the recovery time increased greatly (Fig. 10).

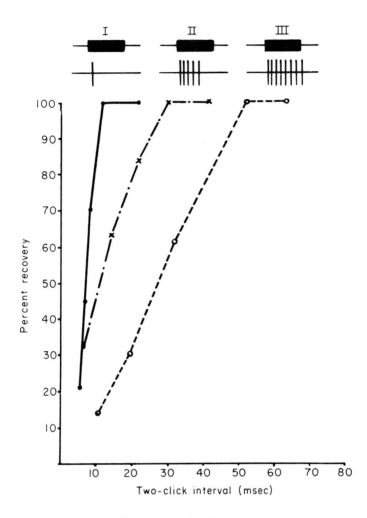

FIG. 9. Recovery process in neurons of different types. Abscissa represents time intervals between delivery of the two signals in msec; ordinate, number of responses to the second signal divided by the number of responses to the first signal ×100. Signal intensity was 20 dB above the threshold. The signals were clicks of 0.2-msec duration. Signal duration and response type is indicated for each graph.

Discussion

Parametric studies of neurons in the inferior colliculus of the rat (and also some experiments on the inferior colliculus of the cat) suggest that several

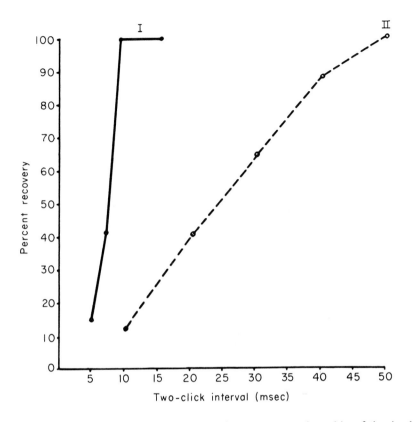

FIG. 10. Recovery process in a nonmonotonic neuron at two intensities of the signal. I, below the optimal level; II, above the optimal level. For further explanation, see Fig. 9.

functionally different groups of neurons exist in this synaptic station of mammals [19-21]. A similar conclusion was drawn by Radionova [23, 24] as regards the neurons in the cochlear nuclei of the cat, and by Vardapetian [29] who studied the neurons in the primary auditory cortex of the same animal.

A comparison of experimental data, obtained in a number of studies carried out according to the same research design, has been made by Gersuni [8] as well as by a group of workers in the Laboratory of Physiology of Hearing at the Pavlov Institute of Physiology of the USSR Academy of Sciences [9, 10].

Measurements of the recovery time in neurons with different types of responses and data obtained in the study of neurons whose spike-count intensity functions are nonmonotonic suggest a division of neurons in the auditory system into two basic groups: (1) neurons with relatively constant properties, and (2) neurons whose functional capacities can undergo substantial changes. An evaluation of the properties of the neurons of the second group indicates that the capacity of the neuron to change its functional properties may be quite diverse for different neurons. This is apparent since the latent period values may be quite different for different neurons for the same changes of stimulus intensity; the changes in the discharge patterns may be of different character; there may be different threshold shifts as a function of signal duration; neurons may differ greatly in their recovery time. The greatest variability in all parameters of the responses was observed for non-monotonic neurons.

Of special interest are the measurements of the recovery time since this interval may differ for the same neuron when the intensity of the signal used for this measurement varies. It seems to hold that the recovery time of nonmonotonic neurons is short when signals of low intensity (below that for the optimal spike count) are used; when signal intensity increases, the recovery time is longer. When we relate this finding to spike-count intensity functions, it seems obvious that, for the nonmonotonic neurons, the recovery time increases when the intensity level of the signal becomes sufficiently high to provoke inhibitory events.

This observation and the results of the studies of impulse activity, when signals of different duration are presented, lead to the conclusion that inhibitory influences may play an important role not only in forming discharge patterns, but also in changing the functional properties of the neuron. This is illustrated in Fig. 11, which summarizes the dynamics of the responses for neurons of different types. As already stressed, a complete correspondence between the duration of a spike train and the duration of the stimulus was found only for a small number of neurons in the inferior colliculus (Group a). Typical for these elements are a monotonic character of the spike-count intensity function; small changes in the latent period; and a short recovery time. Neurons of Type a may be regarded as elements for which no inhibitory influences are apparent.

A characteristic feature of the Group b neurons in Fig. 11 is a marked similarity of their responses to signals of different duration. For stimuli of 50 to 100 msec in duration, the spike train ends before the signal is turned off, while in response to brief signals (1 to 2 msec), these neurons produce pronounced afterdischarges. In either case, the response consists of a compact burst of impulses which lasts about equally long over a wide range of stimulus intensities. The spike-count intensity function remains monotonic in the entire range of intensities; the latent period changes are small; the recovery time does not exceed 30 msec. The presence of inhibitory influences in such neurons is reflected in the pattern of the impulse activity (the impulse train is limited in time and the response is of the "burst" type), as well as in an increase of the recovery time in comparison with that for neurons belonging to group A. The neurons of group B can apparently transmit information

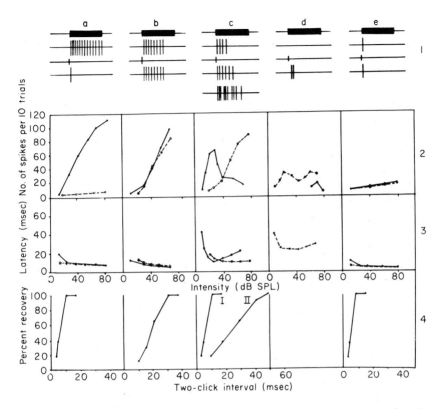

FIG. 11. Variations in number of spikes, latent period, and recovery time as a function of stimulus strength and its duration in neurons of different types. Pattern 1 demonstrates discharge patterns for stimuli of different duration (a to e); pattern 2, spike-count intensity functions for stimuli of 50-msec duration (solid line) and 2-msec duration (dashes) (a, b, c, and e); spike-count intensity functions for stimuli of 5-msec duration (solid line) and 1-msec duration (dashes) (d); pattern 3, latent period values (a to e). Signal durations as in pattern 2. Pattern 4 demonstrates recovery time. Intensity of the clicks was 20 dB above threshold value (a, b, e). Intensity of the clicks below the optimal level (CI); click intensity above the optimal level for maximum number of spikes (CII) (nonmonotonic neuron).

concerning changes in the intensity of both the short and the long-lasting signals.

Group c in Fig. 11 represents nonmonotonic neurons that respond with long spike trains within a narrow intensity range. At intensities exceeding the optimal level, most of these neurons respond with a shorter spike train, although in some cases a decline in discharge rate is observed while the duration of the train remains constant. The degree of reduction in spike activity and the intensity range over which this reduction occurs are different for various elements of Group c. The neurons of this group are the most likely ones to undergo functional reorganization when the parameters of the sound signal change. The responses of the neurons of Type c to short signals often consist of a greater number of impulses than do the responses to long-lasting signals, and the spike train is of a similar or longer duration. The spike counts for short signals approach or become a monotonic intensity function. For some neurons the afterdischarges occur rhythmically. Because of these properties, Type c neurons may be regarded as specialized elements adapted to analyze sound signals of short duration.

Type d neurons in Fig. 11 respond only to short signals, less than 5 msec in duration. Signals of a longer duration remain ineffective. Characteristic for the small sample available were the irregularity of the response, the variability of the latent period and, for some, a nonmonotonic character of the spike-count intensity function. The full recovery of d neurons could not be measured. The appearance of a response to the second signal was recorded for one such neuron at a delay of 30 msec. All these observations suggest that considerable inhibitory influences interact to produce the discharge pattern of these neurons.

On the basis of the data at hand, one may classify the neurons belonging to Types b, c, and d as a group of elements which may change their functional properties. The degree and character of the changes are the result not only of the strength of the inhibitory influence, but also of its relation in time to the onset of the excitatory events.

Type e neurons, shown in Fig. 11, may be characterized as elements with stable properties. The changes in the latent periods of their responses as a function of signal intensity are small. The thresholds remain constant when the stimulus duration varies. The patterns of the impulse activity in response to signals of different frequencies do not exhibit any essential differences. The time of full recovery does not exceed 10 msec. These observations suggest that inhibitory influences are probably absent. The capacity of neurons of this type to transmit information concerning changes in the character of the sound signals seems limited. It should be noted that the data obtained for the recovery time of neurons of Type e somewhat contradict the results obtained by Suga [27] who concluded that neurons with a phasic response type possess a longer recovery time than do neurons responding with long spike trains. In the present study, it was found that not all elements responding to the onset of an acoustic stimulus have similar properties. For a considerable number of neurons responding with an initial burst of impulses, the spike counts bear a nonmonotonic relation to stimulus strength which probably indicates the presence of inhibitory influences. It was also found that there is a relationship between the recovery time and the presumed strength of the inhibitory activity.

In conclusion, it should be stressed that in the auditory system, the existence of neurons, which electively respond to sound signals of different intensity, duration, and frequency, is presumably significant in the formation of differentiated responses of animals to sound signals of various structures.

REFERENCES

1. Aitkin, L. M., Dunlop, C. W., and Webster, W. R. Click evoked response patterns of single units in the medial geniculate body of the cat. *J. Neurophysiol.* **29**, 109-123 (1966).
2. Aitkin, L. M., and Dunlop, C. W. Interplay of excitation and inhibition in the cat medial geniculate body. *J. Neurophysiol.* **31**, 44-61 (1968).
3. Chang, H. T., and Wu, C. P. Unit responses to sound stimulation and an inhibitory mechanism in nucleus *corpus trapezoideum. Sci. Sinica.* **13**, 937-957 (1964).
4. Erulkar, S. D. The responses of single units of the inferior colliculus of the cat to acoustic stimulation. *Proc. Roy. Soc. (London) Ser.* **B150**, 336-355 (1959).
5. Evans, E. F., and Whitfield, I. C. Classification of unit responses in the auditory cortex of the unanesthetized and unrestrained cat. *J. Physiol. (London)* **171**, 476-493 (1964).
6. Fox, C. A., and Eichman, J. A rapid method for locating intracerebral electrode tracts. *Stain. Technol.* **34**, 39-42 (1959).
7. Galambos, R., Rose, J. E., Bromiley, R. B., and Hughes, J. R. Microelectrode studies on the medial geniculate body of the cat. II. Response to clicks. *J. Neurophysiol.* **15**, 359-380 (1952).
8. Gersuni, G. V. On the time-place organization of the auditory system. *Proc. 18th Int. Congr. Psychol.* Symp. 15, Publ. D-t, Moscow, 1966. pp. 112-118.
9. Gersuni, G. V. On the mechanisms of hearing (in connection with studies of time and time-frequency characteristics of auditory system). *In* "Problems of Physiological Acoustics" (G. V. Gersuni, ed.), Vol. 6: Mechanisms of Hearing, pp. 3-32. Nauka, Leningrad, 1967 (in Russian).
10. Gersuni, G. V., Altman, Y. A., Maruseva, A. M., Radionova, E. A., Ratnikova, G. I., and Vartanian, I. A. Chapter 10.
11. Gerstein, G. L., and Kiang, N. Y.-S. Responses of single units in the auditory cortex. *Exp. Neurol.* **101**, 1-18 (1964).
12. Grinnell, A. D. The neurophysiology of audition in bats: intensity and frequency parameters. *J. Physiol. (London)* **167**, 38-66 (1963).
13. Grinnell, A. D. The neurophysiology of audition in bats: temporal parameters. *J. Physiol. (London)* **167**, 67-96 (1963).
14. Greenwood, D. D., and Maruyama, N. Excitatory and inhibitory response areas of auditory neurons in the cochlear nucleus. *J. Neurophysiol.* **28**, 863-892 (1965).
15. Hind, J. E., Goldberg, J. M., Greenwood, D. D., and Rose, J. E. Some discharge characteristics of single neurons in the inferior colliculus of the cat. II. Timing of the discharges and observations on binaural stimulation. *J. Neurophysiol.* **26**, 321-341 (1963).
16. Katsuki, Y., Watanabe, T., and Maruyama, N. Activity of auditory neurons in upper levels of the brain of the cat. *J. Neurophysiol.* **22**, 343-359 (1959).
17. Katsuki, Y., Sumi, T., Uchiyama, H., and Watanabe, T. Electric responses of auditory neurons in the cat to sound stimulation. *J. Neurophysiol.* **21**, 569-588 (1958).

18. Kiang, N. Y.-S., Watanabe, T., Thomas, E. C., and Clark, L. F. Stimulus coding in the cats auditory nerve. *Ann. Otol. Rhinol. Laryngol.* **7**, 1009-1026 (1962).
19. Maruseva, A. M. On the temporal characteristics of the auditory neurons in the inferior colliculus of rats. *Proc. 18th Int. Congr. Psychol.* Symp. 15, Publ. D-t. Moscow 1966. pp. 162-164 (in Russian).
20. Maruseva, A. M. On the time characteristics of neurons of different types in the inferior colliculus of the rat. *In* "Problems of Physiological Acoustics." (G. V. Gersuni, ed.), Vol. 6: Mechanisms of Hearing, pp. 50-62. Nauka, Leningrad, 1967 (in Russian).
21. Maruseva, A. M. On the dynamics of inhibitory phenomena in the auditory system for signals of different duration. *Proc. 6th Acoust. Conf. Moscow, 1968*, Sect. JI5, pp. 4-8 (in Russian).
22. Nelson, P. G., and Erulkar, S. D. Synaptic mechanisms of excitation and inhibition in the central auditory pathway. *J. Neurophysiol.* **26**, 908-923 (1963).
23. Radionova, E. A. The temporal characteristics of the reaction of the cochlear nucleus neurons. *Proc. 18th Int. Congr. Psychol. Moscow,* Symp. 15, Publ. D-t, Moscow, 1966. pp. 156-158.
24. Radionova, E. A. Correlation between some characteristics in the response of the auditory system neurons to sound stimuli. *Biophysics (USSR)* **11**, 478-487 (1966) (in Russian).
25. Rose, J. E., Galambos, R., and Hughes, J. R. Microelectrode studies of the cochlear nuclei of the cat. *Bull. Johns. Hopkins Hosp.* **104**, 211-251 (1959).
26. Rose, J. E., Greenwood, D. D., Goldberg, J. M., and Hind, J. E. Some discharge characteristics of single neurons in the inferior colliculus of the cat. I. Tonotopical organization, relation of spike counts to tone intensity, and firing patterns of single elements. *J. Neurophysiol.* **26**, 294-320 (1963).
27. Suga, N. Single units activity in cochlear nucleus and inferior colliculus of echolocating bats. *J. Physiol. (London)* **172**, 449-474 (1964).
28. Suga, N. Recovery cycles and responses to frequency modulated tone pulses in auditory neurons of echo-located bats. *J. Physiol. (London)* **175**, 50-80 (1964).
29. Vardapetian, G. A. The temporal characteristics of cortical auditory neurons of cat. *Proc. 18th Int. Congr. Psychol. Moscow,* Symp 15., Publ. D-t, Moscow, 1966. pp. 174-175.
30. Wall, P. D. Repetitive discharge of neurons. *J. Neurophysiol.* **22**, 305-320 (1959).

12

Impulse Activity of Neurons of the Rat's Inferior Colliculus in Response to Amplitude-Modulated Sound Signals

I. A. Vartanian

Studies of auditory neurons in response to frequency- or amplitude modulated sound signals began only rather recently. A number of investigations were carried out on neurons of the auditory cortex [2, 17, 21] and inferior colliculus in various animals [8, 9, 12, 16]. The data reported mainly concern responses to frequency-modulated signals; only limited observations have been made regarding the activity of neurons in the inferior colliculus when amplitude-modulated (am) sound signals are presented [12].

This chapter describes some results obtained in a study of single neurons in the inferior colliculus of the rat when am sound signals are applied. Such signals approximate certain biologically emitted sounds [5]. Moreover, studies of neural responses to various modulation rates are of importance for determination of the capacity of neurons of different types [4, 10, 13, 14] to transmit information concerning slow and rapid intensity changes in time. Such studies may also detect single units which may be specialized for handling certain parameters of the signal.

Methods

The experiments were performed on rats under chloralose-urethane anesthesia (30 and 500 mg/kg, intraperitoneally). The cochlea, contralateral to the side of the stimulation, was destroyed. The surgical procedure to expose the inferior colliculus was described previously [19]. Tungsten electrodes with a tip diameter of about 1 μ and a resistance of 10 to 20 MΩ, or glass microelectrodes filled with Wood's alloy with a platinum tip of 1 to 3 μ in diameter and resistance of 800 kΩ to 1.5 MΩ were used for recording. In most experiments the location of the electrode tip was estimated from the depth of the electrode insertion; in some cases histological controls were exercised by the method of Fox and Eichman [3].

The impulse activity of the neurons was recorded with a MEZ-28-A magnetic tape recorder. A reliable separation of the impulse activity from the background activity was achieved with the aid of a threshold device. Subsequently, an automatic analysis of the impulse activity [18] was performed. The usual display was a poststimulus time histogram (PST) which graphs the occurrence of spikes in time from the moment of the stimulus presentation. Such histograms are usually based on responses to 25 to 50 successive stimuli. In some experiments, the spike discharges were photographed from the tube face of the oscilloscope as "dot patterns" [20] or as a conventional display while the data were simultaneously recorded on tape.

Broadband white noise, tones of different frequency (3 to 20 kHz) and clicks (of 2.5-msec duration and delivered 30 times per second) were used as amplitude-modulated signals. The signals were produced by a white-noise generator, a ZG-10 generator of pure tones, and an "Alvar" impulse stimulator. A special switch modulator, at the input of which the carrier and the modulating frequency were available, was used for sinusoidal symmetrical amplitude modulation. The amplitude of the carrier changed proportionally to the modulating signal. The output of the modulator was connected to the input of the transistor switch which cut out sections of the amplitude-modulated signal in zero phases of the modulation rate. The electrical form of one cycle of the modulated stimulus is shown in Fig. 1. The modulation rates ranged from 1 to 100 Hz. The signal duration fluctuated within the limits of one period of the modulation rate. The modulation depth in all experiments was 90 to 100%.

The sound signals were presented by an electrostatic loudspeaker whose output was flat within ±1.5 dB from 4 to 20 kHz. The loudspeaker was located at a distance of 5 to 10 cm from the animal's ear contralateral to the operated side. As the modulated signal was switched on with a very fast risetime, a click was heard. The intensity of the sound was measured in decibels of attenuation relative to a maximal level (zero dB attenuation) which corresponded to 71 dB SPL *re* 0.0002 dyn/cm^2, when measured with a microphone situated at a distance of 10 cm. The sound signals were presented every 3 sec. The experiments were conducted in a sound-deadened, screened chamber.

The responses of 140 neurons of the inferior colliculus were recorded; for 80 of them, amplitude-modulated signals were used.

The following characteristics of the impulse responses were studied. (1) The thresholds to a noise and to tones of different frequencies for signals of 2 and

0° 90° 180° 270° 360°

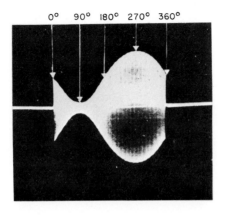

FIG. 1. Electrical form of the amplitude-modulated signal. The numbers indicate the phases of the modulation cycle.

100 to 200 msec in duration. On the basis of these data we determined the optimal (best) frequency, the threshold tuning curves for two sound durations, and the capacity for temporal summation.* The threshold for a spike response was taken as that intensity of the stimulus, at which the response occurred with a probability of 0.5. (2) The discharge pattern (duration of the spike train, distribution of the discharges in time, number of impulses). A noise or tone of optimal frequency, at an intensity of 40 to 50 dB above unit threshold, were used for studying responses to amplitude-modulated signals. The duration of the stimuli was 80 to 100 and 600 to 1000 msec. PST-histograms, in some cases unit records, as well as data abtained by the "dot pattern" method were evaluated. (3) in 25% of the experiments, the latent period of the responses at threshold and at the maximal stimulus intensity was measured.

Results

GENERAL CHARACTERISTICS OF SPIKE ACTIVITY IN THE INFERIOR COLLICULUS

When evaluating the discharge patterns of the neurons to signals with a duration of 80 msec [Fig. 2(A)] and 600 to 1000 msec [Fig. 2(B)], it is possible to recognize two extreme types of spike responses. (1) A type for which

* The capacity for temporal summation was expressed by the value of the threshold shift (in dB) when the signal duration changed from 2 to 100 msec.

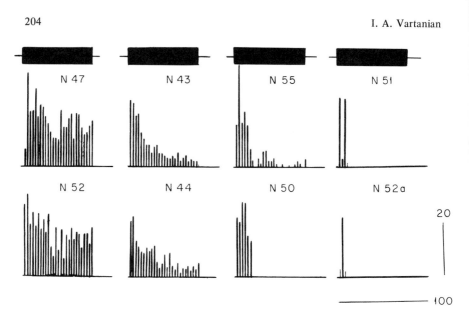

FIG. 2. Poststimulus histograms for 16 neurons of the inferior colliculus in response to noise signals of 80-msec duration (a) and 600- to 1000-msec duration (b), see facing page. Intensity of the sound signals in all cases was 40 to 60 dB above the threshold for the spike. Poststimulus histograms, shown in this and subsequent figures (except Fig. 11) are based on a sample which consists of responses to 25 consecutive stimuli. Each neuron is identified by a number. Abscissa, time in milliseconds; ordinate, number of spikes. Values for the abscissa and ordinate given in the right-hand corner apply to all histograms.

sustained discharges occur during the entire period of stimulation. The temporal distribution of spikes in such responses may be relatively homogeneous [Fig. 2(a), neurons 47 and 52; Fig. 2(b), neurons 87 and 101]; or a densely spaced initial burst of impulses may occur [Fig. 2(a), neurons 43 and 44; Fig. 2(b), neurons 104 and 117]. (2) A type for which an on-discharge (and sometimes on-off discharge) consisting of 1 to 2 impulses occurs [Fig. 2(a), neurons 51 and 52a; Fig. 2(b), neurons 129 and 96]. Neurons with a discharge burst consisting of four to eight impulses at the signal onset [Fig. 2(a), neurons 50 and 55; Fig. 2(b), neurons 123 and 118] occupy an intermediate position between neurons that respond only with one or two impulses to the onset of a sound of any duration, and neurons that produce sustained discharges with a densely spaced initial burst.

A decrease in signal intensity from the maximal to a near-threshold level, in steps of 5 to 10 dB, resulted in a regular decrease in spike numbers. Thus, all the neurons here described displayed monotonic spike-count intensity functions [7, 15]. The responses of nonmonotonic neurons will be considered in another paper.

It should be noted that neurons of the inferior colliculus vary markedly in the degree and rate of adaptation [Fig. 2(b)]. There are neurons that show

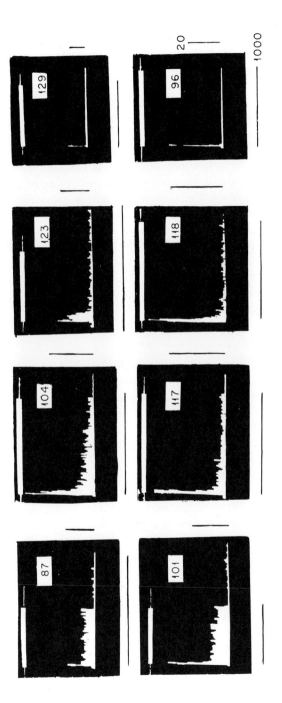

FIG. 2(b).

only an insignificant adaptation (87 and 101) and those which adapt greatly during the first 20 to 100 msec from the onset of the discharges (104 and 117). Among the examined neurons those which adapt strongly form the majority, while neurons showing insignificant adaptation are relatively seldom encountered (5 out of 32).

Figure 3 presents data concerning the capacity for temporal summation for neurons with different discharge patterns. For neurons with sustained discharges [Fig. 3(a)], the values range widely but temporal summation values of less than 10 dB were found only for two neurons (their response patterns approximated burst responses). Most of the neurons with an on-discharge pattern are characterized by a temporal summation value not exceeding 5 dB [Fig. 3(b)]. Only a small number in this sample had values close to those of more than 5 dB, which occur for neurons with burst responses [Fig. 3(c)]. For all the neurons investigated there was a high positive correlation, as previously described [6, 10, 13, 14], between the capacity for temporal summation and the relation of the latent period to sound intensity.

RESPONSES OF NEURONS OF DIFFERENT GROUPS TO AMPLITUDE-MODULATED SOUND SIGNALS

Significance of the Modulating Frequency

Neurons with Sustained and Burst Discharges. All neurons with sustained and burst discharges respond to signals which are modulated with a low frequency (1 to 5 Hz), with an impulse activity reproducing the rhythm of the modulation [Figs. 4 and 9(b)]. When the modulation rate increases, the response of the neuron is synchronized with each period of the modulation cycle up to a certain modulation rate, which may be different for different neurons. Figure 4 indicates that a modulation rate up to 30 Hz is reproduced by the discharges of neurons 117 and 103 and up to 50 Hz by neuron 120. The burst responses of neuron 123 (Fig. 5) follow a modulation rate up to 20 Hz. A further increase of the modulation rate results in irregular discharges and in a decline of the general activity level. It seems possible, finally, to modulate at such a rate that only an initial response arises with a complete or partial suppression of the subsequent discharges (Figs. 4 and 5).*

It can be shown that even when responses to steady sound signals are similar (e.g., Fig. 4, neurons 117 and 120, upper histograms) and the capacity to summate is almost the same (8 and 9 dB, respectively, for neurons 117 and 120), the distribution of the discharges at the same modulation rates may differ greatly. The maximal modulation rhythm which these two units followed was also different (30 and 50 Hz, respectively).

---

* For neuron 120 (Fig. 4), this rate has not been reached presumably due to the limited range of the modulation rate (100 Hz) in our experiments.

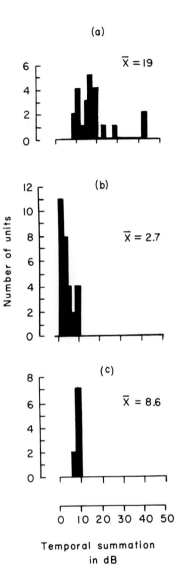

FIG. 3. Distributions of neurons with different discharge patterns according to the capacity for temporal summation. (a) Neurons with a sustained discharge (35%); (b) neurons with an onset discharge (52%); (c) neurons with burst discharges (13%). Abscissa, capacity for temporal summation in decibels; ordinate, number of neurons. The capacity for temporal summation was measured by the value of the threshold shift when the duration of the signal was changed from 2 to 100 msec in duration. $\overline{X}$ represents mean value.

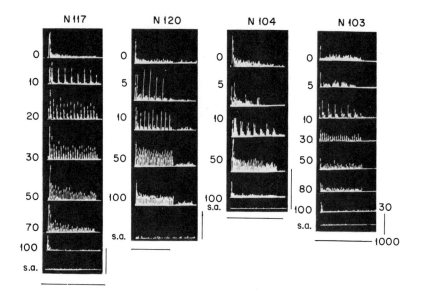

FIG. 4. Poststimulus histograms for four neurons with a sustained discharge. Responses to amplitude-modulated noise with different frequency. Numbers on the left represent modulation rate in Hz. Intensity of the signals, 55 dB SPL *re* 0.0002 dyn/cm². Values for ordinate and abscissa shown at lower right apply to all histograms in the figure. In this and all subsequent figures, s.a. designates a sample of spontaneous activity.

Close scrutiny of the available material reveals that the maximal modulation rate which a neuron can follow and the capacity to summate are not correlated.

Neurons with an On-Discharge. Unlike neurons with sustained and burst discharges, most neurons with onset discharges, whose temporal summation capacity was 0 to 5 dB, did not respond to the modulation rates used in our experiments. These neurons discharged in response to a click produced by the modulated signal, when it was switched on [Fig. 6(a) and 6(b)], or to an amplitude-modulated series of clicks [Fig. 6(c)].

However, 13% of the neurons whose temporal summation capacity was 0 to 5 dB reacted selectively when sufficiently high modulation rates were applied (Fig. 7). This selectivity was expressed by the neuron following the modulation rate (Fig. 7, neuron 138), or by an increase in the general level of activity (Fig. 7, neurons 137 and 133).

Among the neurons with an onset discharge pattern and temporal summation capacity of more than 5 dB, some units were encountered which re-

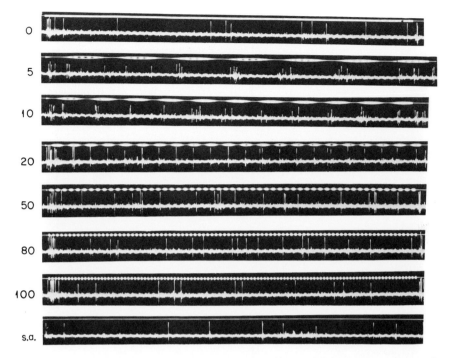

FIG. 5. Impulse activity of neuron 123 in response to an amplitude-modulated tone of optimal frequency (6 kHz). Numbers to the left represent the modulation rate. Intensity, 50 dB SPL.

sponded to low rates of modulation. Thus, neuron 84 (Fig. 8) was unresponsive to a modulation rate of 2 Hz; however, in response to a signal modulated with a frequency of 5 Hz, discharges appeared locked to a definite phase of the modulation cycle. Neuron 120a responded with a reproduction of the modulation rhythm of 10 Hz and higher [Fig. 11(A)]. No onset neuron responded to a modulation rate of less than 5 Hz. With an increase of the modulation rate, the neurons of this group, like the neurons with sustained and burst discharges responded within a given frequency range, with discharges following the rhythm of modulation; a further increase in the modulation rate led to a disturbance in the rhythm of neural discharges and, finally, to the appearance of an initial response only with subsequent occasional spikes (Fig. 5, 8, 11).

Significance of the Carrier Frequency

The studies of responses to modulated sounds were conducted with due regard for the frequency sensitivity of the neurons which was ascertained by

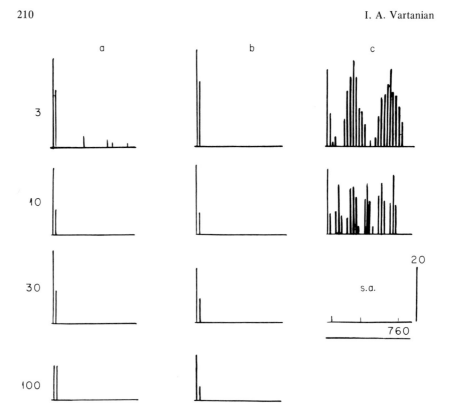

FIG. 6. Poststimulus histograms for neuron 34. Responses to modulated signals. (a) Carrier frequency of 4 kHz (optimal frequency); (b) noise, (c) clicks (30/sec). Intensity of the signals: 45 dB above the threshold for the response. For further information, see Fig. 4.

determination of the frequency-threshold curves. Optimal and nonoptimal* frequencies were used.

Neurons with Sustained Discharges. The data suggest that for neurons in this group the responses to modulated signals of optimal and nonoptimal frequencies differ substantially (Fig. 9). While in response to a modulated signal of optimal frequency [Fig. 9(a), left column] the discharges of the neuron follow a modulation rhythm of up to 30 Hz, a modulated signal of nonoptimal frequency [Fig. 9(a), right column] evokes an on-response and causes discharges that are not synchronized with the modulation rate and whose number does not exceed the level of spontaneous activity. The re-

* A nonoptimal frequency is a frequency for which the threshold of the response exceeded the threshold at the optimal frequency by not less than 20 dB. In cases where the threshold difference in the examined frequency range was less than 20 dB, we regarded as a nonoptimal that frequency which differed from the optimal one by the greatest number of cycles.

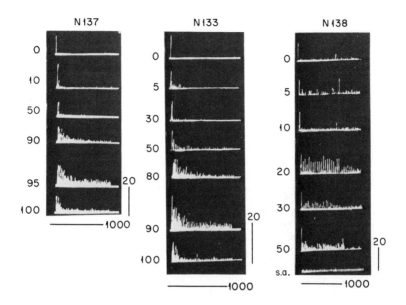

FIG. 7. Poststimulus histograms produced by three onset neurons in response to amplitude-modulated signals. Carrier for neurons 137 and 133: noise. Stimulus intensity 55 dB SPL; temporal summation capacity, 1 and 2 dB, respectively. Carrier for neuron 138: 20 kHz (optimal frequency). Stimulus intensity, 50 dB SPL; temporal summation capacity, 5 dB. For further information, see Fig. 4.

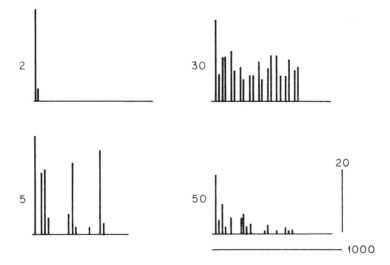

FIG. 8. Poststimulus histograms for neuron 84 responding to an amplitude-modulated tone of 7 kHz (optimal frequency). Stimulus intensity, 50 dB SPL; temporal summation capacity, 9 dB. For further explanation, see Fig. 4.

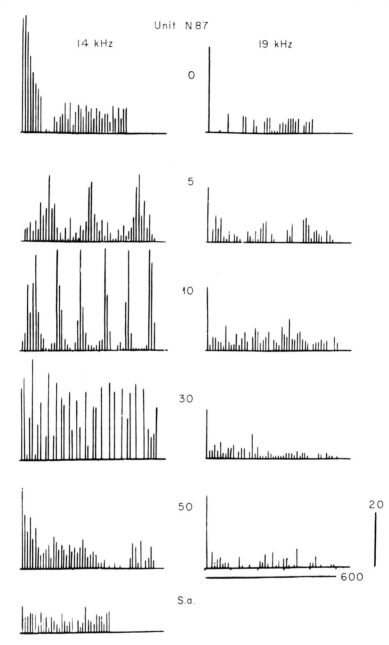

FIG. 9. Poststimulus histograms for two neurons with a sustained discharge pattern responding to modulated tones of optimal and nonoptimal frequency. (a) Data for neuron 87. 14 kHz is the optimal frequency; 19 kHz is the nonoptimal frequency. Stimulus intensity, 50 dB SPL; temporal summation capacity, 16 dB for 14 kHz signals and 4 dB for 19 kHz stimuli. Numbers between the histograms represent modulation rate.

sponses to nonmodulated sound signals for these frequencies [first horizontal histogram row in Fig. 9(a)] are also markedly different. An overwhelming majority of neurons, in the sample studied, behaved as neurons with a sustained discharge pattern when the optimal frequency was modulated, and as neurons with an on-discharge pattern when the nonoptimal frequency was modulated.

That differences between the responses to modulated signals of optimal and nonoptimal frequencies are not determined by the differences in signal intensity is attested by the results shown in Fig. 9(b). Clearly, the responses to the modulated optimal frequency signals (left column) and nonoptimal signals (right column) are different when the sound pressure level for both signals is the same (upper histograms) or when both signals are at the same level above threshold (lower histograms).

Figure 10 presents another example of responses (for neuron 139), when different signals are modulated. The responses to modulated signals of optimal (b) and nonoptimal (c) frequencies are similar to those described above. However, signals of optimal frequency (b) evoke responses within a considerably wider range of modulating frequencies (more than 100 Hz) than is the case for responses to a modulated noise (a).

Unit N 70

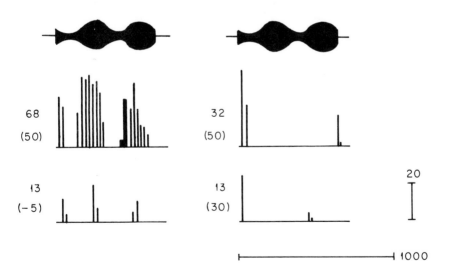

FIG. 9(b). Data for neuron 70. Left column indicates poststimulus histograms for responses to a modulated tone of optimal frequency of 19 kHz; right column shows poststimulus histograms for responses to a nonoptimal frequency of 5 kHz. Modulation rate, 3Hz. Upper numbers on the left indicate stimulus intensity in dB above the threshold for the response to nonmodulated signals; numbers in brackets indicate intensity in dB re 0.0002 dyn/cm^2. Temporal summation capacity, 18 dB for 19 kHz and 4 dB for 5 kHz signals.

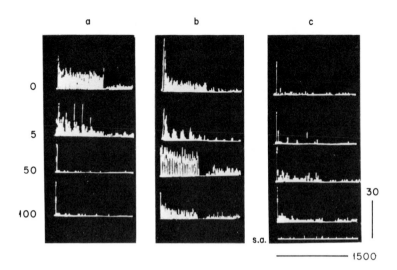

FIG. 10. Poststimulus histograms for neuron 139 when noise (a), optimal frequency of 17.5 kHz (b), and nonoptimal frequency of 7 kHz (c) were presented. Stimulus intensity in all cases was 40 dB above the threshold for the response. Temporal summation capacity for noise, 12 dB; for 17.5 kHz, 13 dB; for 7 kHz, 0 dB.

Neurons with an Onset Discharge. Neurons with onset discharge patterns and low capacity for temporal summation (0 to 5 dB) (Fig. 6) did not respond to modulated signals of optimal and nonoptimal frequencies within the examined range of modulation rates (12 neurons).

For some neurons with onset discharge patterns and a capacity for temporal summation of more than 5 dB there were substantial differences between the responses when signals of optimal and nonoptimal frequencies were applied. As shown in Fig. 11, there is no difference (upper histograms) in the responses to nonmodulated tones of different frequencies (10 and 20 kHz). The response pattern was also the same for all intensities of the stimuli. The temporal summation capacity varies only slightly for different frequencies [Fig. 11(c)]. Nonetheless, the responses to the am sounds of different frequencies differ in that the reproduction of the rhythm begins at different frequencies of modulation, and the limit to which the modulation rhythm is followed is considerably higher when the optimal frequency is modulated.

Amplitude-Modulated Clicks

Short, impulsive signals which are slowly amplitude-modulated are a widespread phenomenon in biological sound emission [5]. In the present work am impulsive signals (clicks) were utilized on the one hand as equivalent to

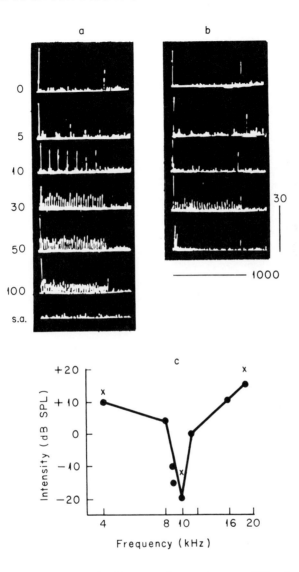

FIG. 11. (a) and (b) Poststimulus histograms for onset neuron 120a when modulated tones of optimal frequency of 10 kHz (a) and a nonoptimal frequency of 20 kHz were presented (b). Stimulus intensity, 40 dB above the threshold for the response. Each histogram based on responses to 50 stimulus presentations. (c) Threshold tuning curve for stimulus of 200-msec duration. Crosses indicate thresholds for response for signals 2-msec duration.

natural signals, and on the other hand as test signals to determine the capacity of the neuron to respond to a rhythmical stimulus with a very fast risetime.

Neurons with Sustained and Burst Discharges. When clicks (rate, 30/sec; frequency of modulation 2 to 10 Hz) were used as stimuli, most neurons responded with a reproduction of the rhythm of modulation. Records in Fig. 12 indicate that neuron 120 responded with a reproduction of the rhythm of modulation to a modulated train of clicks (b) and to modulated noise (a). Some differences are observed in the discharge rate and in the distribution of discharges relative to the phase of the modulation cycle. The response to a nonmodulated train of 30 clicks/sec is similar to the response when modulated noise with a frequency of 30 Hz is presented. Only two "burst" neurons failed to respond to a train of 30 clicks/sec, regardless of whether or not the stimuli were modulated. When the frequency of the clicks was decreased to 20/sec, these neurons responded to each click and reproduced the modulation rhythm of 2 to 5 Hz. It should be noted that the maximal modulation rhythm of the signal which was reproduced by these neurons was 20 Hz. The response of one of these neurons is shown in Fig. 5.

Neurons with an Onset Discharge. Most neurons of this group (80%) responded with a reproduction of the modulation rhythm of 2 to 10 Hz, the carrier being a train of 30/sec clicks [Fig. 6(c)]. It should be emphasized that a rhythm of 30 Hz was not reproduced by the same neurons for sinusoidal modulation of a tone or noise [Fig. 6(a), 6(b)]. Some neurons reproduced the modulation rhythm only when the frequency of the clicks in the series did not exceed 20/sec (20% of the neurons).

Thus, information concerning slowly modulated impulsive signals, which are very common natural sounds, can be transmitted by an overwhelming majority of neurons of the inferior colliculus.

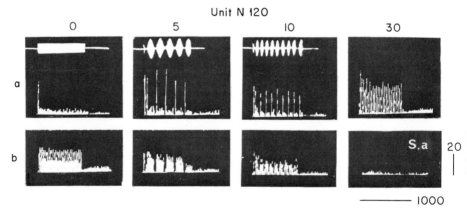

FIG. 12. Poststimulus histograms for neuron 120 in response to a modulated noise (a) and to a train of 30 clicks/sec (b). Modulated rate is indicated above each histogram. No responses to a train of 30 clicks/sec, modulated with a frequency of 30 Hz, were recorded since such a modulated rate would correspond to the frequency of the clicks in the train.

Discussion

Two widely different groups of neurons can be distinguished among the units of the inferior colliculus on the basis of their discharge characteristics. The first group consists of neurons with a sustained response pattern and pronounced capacity for temporal summation (average, 19 dB). The second group consists of elements with an onset discharge pattern and insignificant capacity for temporal summation (0 to 5 dB). Intermediate groups with a sustained or burst discharge patterns and temporal summation capacity of 5 to 10 dB, as well as neurons with an onset discharge pattern and a similar magnitude of temporal summation capacity overlap the range of temporal characteristics of the two extreme groups (Fig. 3). The neurons of the intermediate groups combine some properties which are peculiar to each extreme group, i.e., the independence of the discharge from the duration of the signal (burst discharge or onset discharge), but the temporal summation capacity for these neurons is considerably highly than is the case for typical on-neurons. These findings are in accord with previous studies [10, 15].

A question of interest is: Which neural groups are involved and in what way can the properites of the am sound signals be transmitted?

Our results imply that tonic neurons with sustained discharge patterns and pronounced capacity for temporal summation respond to slow modulation rates with a reproduction of the rhythm of the modulation cycle. The capacity to reproduce low modulation rates may result from the capacity of these neurons to accumulate information about the signal in time (pronounced temporal summation) and from their low sensitivity to the risetime changes of the signal.*

Neurons with burst discharge patterns and some neurons with sustained discharge patterns but with densely spaced initial spikes also respond with a reproduction of slow modulation rhythms. However, their spike activity reached, as a rule, a maximal level at the phase of the modulation cycle, close to 180° (Fig. 4, neurons 120 and 104; Fig. 5).

Neurons with sustained and burst discharges respond with a reproduction of the modulation rhythm up to a certain frequency; above that frequency a disturbance of the rhythm reproduction is in evidence; for still higher frequencies a complete suppression of the discharges may occur (Figs. 4, 5). It may be assumed that the limit of reproduction of the modulation rhythm is determined by the recovery period of the neuron. This assumption is supported by the data in Fig. 12. The neuron responded to each click delivered

---

* Our data show that for neurons with sustained discharges and pronounced capacity for temporal summation (more than 10 dB) the thresholds do not change significantly even if the time constant of the sound signal becomes as large as 70 msec.

at a rise of 30/sec [Fig. (b)] as well as to a noise modulated with a frequency of 30 Hz [Fig. (a)]. Similarly, for neurons which could follow only 20/sec clicks, the maximal frequency of reproduction of the modulation rhythm was 20 Hz (Fig. 5).

In contrast to neurons with sustained discharges, a considerable number of neurons with an on-discharge pattern did not respond to the modulation frequencies used in our experiments. Some neurons of this group, however, responded selectively within a certain range of modulation frequencies (Figs. 7, 8, and 11). One may suppose that a selective response arises when such a combination of the modulation rate and of the risetime of each oscillation is present so that the recovery time allows the unit to respond to each oscillation, and the risetime of amplitude is sufficiently high to evoke a discharge. The data in Fig. 6 suggest such an interpretation. For a train of clicks at 30/sec [Fig. 6(c)], sustained activity is present; a tone of optimal frequency and a noise modulated with a frequency of 30 Hz do not evoke such activity [Figs. 6(a) and 6(b)]. The occurrence of a response exclusively in the region of sufficiently high modulation frequencies for data shown in Fig. 7 presumably required a combination of a rapid recovery of the response and a high sensitivity to changes in the risetime of the sound oscillation. Our data show that the threshold for some neurons with an onset discharge pattern sharply increases for sound signals even with a small time constant (2 to 5 msec).

Apparently, the combination of the recovery time and of the sensitivity to the risetime of the signal determines the selective response to modulated sounds (Figs. 7, 8, and 11). Such a response may be regarded as a manifestation of a functional specialization of a neuron which reacts to some combination of stimulus parameters.

One can envisage that an assembly of neurons possessing different properties accomplishes the analysis of very slow as well as rapid intensity fluctuations, the slow fluctuations being handled by the tonic neurons, the rapid ones by the phasic elements. The intermediate neural groups assure the function of the auditory system within a wide range of changing rhythms.

Our data make it evident that the introduction of modulation augments in some cases the capacity of the neuron to transmit information concerning the characteristics of a sound signal [Fig. 10 (a) and (b); Fig. 11]. While the patterns of the responses to nonmodulated sounds need not differ, the responses to modulated signals may differ significantly.

In the final analysis, the greater capacity of neurons of various types to detect modulation rhythms, if the carrier is the optimal frequency, is presumably the result of a complex interaction of the excitatory and inhibitory events [1, 7, 11]. A particularly clear manifestation of the excitatory and inhibitory interactions, when modulated signals are presented, can be observed in the responses of nonmonotonic neurons. However, the description of these findings will be given elsewhere.

Conclusions

Neurons of the inferior colliculus are divided into groups according to the pattern of their response to long-lasting sound signals (noise, optimal frequency) and other temporal characteristics of the response. Neurons with sustained discharges and pronounced capacity for temporal summation (more than 10 dB), on the one hand, and neurons with an on-discharge and insignificant capacity for temporal summation (0 to 5 dB), on the other, form the two extreme groups. Neurons with sustained and burst discharges and a capacity for temporal summation of 5 to 10 dB, as well as neurons with a similar temporal summation capacity but with a phasic discharge, occupy an intermediate position. Neurons of the inferior colliculus differ greatly in their characteristics. They range widely from neurons with a pronounced capacity for a temporal summation of up to 45 dB and insignificant adaptive properties to neurons with an on-discharge pattern consisting of one impulse, which have no capacity for temporal summation.

Neurons with sustained and burst discharges respond to slow modulation rates with synchronized impulse activity which reproduces the rhythm of the modulation cycles. They reproduce the modulation rate up to a definite limit; when this limit is exceeded, a disturbance of the reproduction of the rhythm and, subsequently, a suppression of the responses occur.

Most neurons with an on-discharge and insignificant capacity for temporal summation (0 to 5 dB) did not respond to the modulation rates used in the present experiments. However, some of these neurons did respond selectively within a certain range of high modulation frequencies either by following the modulation rhythm or by a general increase of impulse activity. Neurons of this group with a capacity for temporal summation of over 5 dB respond to a modulated signal with rhythmic discharges. The synchronization starts with a definite modulation frequency, which in no case was lower than 5 Hz. The rhythmic activity, which corresponds to the modulation rate, persists up to a definite limit, after which only an initial response is produced.

The neurons of the inferior colliculus respond to a wider range of modulation frequencies, if the optimal frequency of the neuron is the modulated stimulus.

REFERENCES

1. Erulkar, S. D. The responses of single units of the inferior colliculus of the cat to acoustic stimulation. *Proc. Roy. Soc. (London) Ser.* **B 150**, 336-355 (1959).
2. Evans, E. F., and Whitfield, I. C. Classification of unit responses in the auditory cortex of the unasthetized and unrestrained cat. *J. Physiol. (London)* **171**, 476-493 (1964).

3. Fox, C. A., and Eichman, Y. A rapid method for locating intracerebral electrodes. *Stain Technol.* **34**, 39-42 (1959).
4. Gersuni, G. V. On the mechanisms of hearing (in connection with studies of time and time-frequency characteristics of the auditory system). *In* "Problems of Physiological Acoustics." (G. V. Gersuni, ed.) Vol. 6: Mechanisms of Hearing, pp. 3-32. Nauka, Leningrad, 1967 (in Russian).
5. Gersuni, G. V. Hearing in its connection with biological sound production. *Vestn. Akad. Nauk USSR* **7**, 69-77 (1968) (in Russian).
6. Gersuni, G. V., Altman, I. A., Maruseva, A. M., Radionova, E. A., Ratnikova, G. I. and Vartanian, I. A. Chapter 10.
7. Greenwood, D. D., and Maruyama, N. Excitatory and inhibitory response areas of auditory neurons in the cochlear nucleus. *J. Neurophysiol.* **28**, 863-892 (1965).
8. Grinnell, A. D. The neurophysiology of audition in bats: intensity and frequency parameters. *J. Physiol. (London)* **167**, 38-66 (1963).
9. Grinnell, A. D., and McCue, I. I. G. Neurophysiological investigations of the bat *Myotis lucifugus*, stimulated by frequency-modulated acoustical pulse. *Nature (London)* **198**, 453-458 (1963).
10. Maruseva, A. M. On the time characteristics of neurons of different types in the inferior colliculus of the rat. *In* "Problems of Physiological Acoustics." (G. V. Gersuni, ed.), Vol. 6: Mechanisms of Hearing, pp. 50-62. Nauka, Leningrad, 1967 (in Russian).
11. Nelson, P. G., and Erulkar, S. D. Synaptic mechanisms of excitation and inhibition in the central auditory pathway. *J. Neurophysiol.* **26**, 908-923 (1963).
12. Nelson, P. G., Erulkar, S. D., and Bryan, I. S. Responses of units of the inferior colliculus to time-varying acoustic stimuli. *J. Neurophysiol.* **29**, 834-860 (1966).
13. Radionova, E. A. Correlation between some characteristics in the response of the auditory system neurons to sound stimuli. *Biophysics. (USSR)* **11**, 478-487 (1966) (in Russian).
14. Radionova, E. A. On the significance of time characteristics of the response of the cochlear nucleus neurons. *In* "Problems of Physiological Acoustics" (G. V. Gersuni, ed.), Vol. 6: Mechanisms of Hearing, pp. 32-50. Nauka, Leningrad, 1967 (in Russian).
15. Rose, J. E., Greenwood, D. D., Goldberg, J. M., and Hind, J. E. Some discharge characteristics of single neurons in the inferior colliculus of the cat. I. Tonotopical organization, relation of spike counts to tone intensity and firing patterns of single elements. *J. Neurophysiol.* **26**, 294-320 (1963).
16. Suga, N. Recovery cycles and responses to frequency modulated tone pulses in auditory neurons of echo-locating bats. *J. Physiol. (London)* **175**, 50-80 (1964).
17. Suga, N. Functional properties of auditory neurons in the cortex of echo-locating bats. *J. Physiol. (London)* **181**, 670-700 (1965).
18. Vaitulevich, S. F., and Likhnitsky, A. M. Use of impulse analyzer AI-100 for temporal analysis of impulse activity. *J. Higher Nervous Activity (USSR)* **16**, 747-752 (1966) (in Russian).
19. Vartanian, I. A., Lebedeva, Z. P., and Maruseva, A. M. Electrical responses in the inferior colliculus of the rat to brief sound signals (clicks). *Bull. Exp. Biol. Med. (USSR)* **61**, 3-6 (1966) (in Russian).
20. Wall, P. D. Repetitive discharge of neurons. *J. Neurophysiol.* **22**, 305-320 (1959).
21. Whitfield, I. C., and Evans, E. F. Responses of auditory cortical neurons to stimuli of changing frequency. *J. Neurophysiol.* **28**, 665-672 (1965).

13
Neurophysiological Mechanisms of Sound-Source Localization

J. A. Altman

In the localization of a sound source in space, at least two basic tasks must be solved by animals—localization of the sound at its onset (an orienting reaction to the sound) and following the sound when its source is displaced from the midline. One of the common methods for exploring the neurophysiological mechanisms subserving spatial hearing is to take advantage of the phenomenon of lateralization. Lateralization of brief sound signals (e.g., clicks) allows study of the neural responses during localization of the sound at its onset, while lateralization of long-lasting sound signals makes it possible to investigate the specific features of the neural activity when the auditory system accumulates information concerning a sound source displaced from the midline.

The neural activity of the superior olive [6-8, 13], the first level in the auditory system where convergence of afferents from both ears is known to occur [13, 17], was thoroughly explored as regards lateralization of brief sound signals (clicks). Other investigations also disclosed pronounced changes in the activity of neurons of the inferior colliculus and the superior olive in connection with lateralization of long-lasting tone signals [10, 14, 16].

The purpose of the present work was a systematic study of the neural responses of the inferior colliculus of the cat as they may bear on lateralization of both single clicks and long-lasting sounds. Trains of clicks were used as long-lasting sound signals since, according to the literature [4, 15], rhythmical series of brief sound bursts are preferred localization signals in biological sound emission. It might therefore be assumed that a series of brief sound stimuli is particularly suited to detect the characteristics of neural activity of the inferior colliculus when long-lasting sound is lateralized.

Methods

The experiments were carried out on cats, weighing 1.5 to 3.5 kg, anesthetized with a mixture of chloralose and urethane (30 mg/kg of chloralose +
500 mg/kg of urethane, given intraperitoneally). After the onset of narcotic
sleep, tracheotomy was performed, and the animal's head was firmly fixed in
a special headholder. After removal of the soft tissues, the bone over the
occipital pole was removed and the dura was dissected. The hemisphere was
carefully displaced forward and the resulting slit, through which the inferior
colliculus was clearly seen, was tamponed, the tampons having been soaked in
a physiological salt solution. Then the occipital pole of the hemisphere was
removed and the bleeding stopped with soluble vitamin K.

The experiments were performed in a sound-deadened chamber. The recordings of the impulse activity of the neurons were done with tungsten microelectrodes (the diameter of the electrolytically ground tip, coated with acetone
varnish, was about 1 μ); the equivalent resistance of the electrodes, measured
at a frequency of 1000 Hz, was 10 to 40 MΩ. With the aid of a manipulator,
the electrode was placed into contact with the surface of the inferior colliculus. After this was done, the surface of the nucleus was covered with warm
vaseline oil. Insertion of the electrode into the tissue was accomplished in
steps of 1 to 2 μ by means of a hydraulic manipulator that was located outside
the chamber. The number of insertions into the nucleus did not exceed three in
any one experiment; as a rule, one or two insertions were made. During the
experiments, the body temperature of the animal was maintained at a constant
level 37° to 38°C (as measured in the pit of the animal's extremity). In addition,
when the depth of the anesthesia decreased (as judged by the rate of respiration,
as well as by the pupillary reaction and muscular tremor), 100 mg/kg of
urethane were injected.

Co-phasic single clicks, with a duration of the main oscillation of 0.2 msec,
or trains of such clicks delivered at a rate of 10 to 30 clicks/sec for 500 to
700 msec were used as stimuli. The clicks were produced by a generator of
rectangular electrical pulses with two independent outputs and with a wide
range of control of the time intervals between the outputs. Two transducers
of the TD-6 type served as sound emitters; they possessed relatively similar
frequency characteristics within the range of 600 to 5000 Hz. In order to
prevent the transmission of the sound from one ear to the other, the phones
were wrapped in several layers of Porolon and placed into hollow metallic
spheres. Metallic funnels were attached to the emitting surfaces of the phones
(before the latter were placed into the spheres), and metallic tubes were
connected to these funnels. The tubes were led through openings in the
spheres and firmly placed in the animal's auditory meatus. The deadening of
the transmission of the sound from one ear to the other, measured in four

animals by the magnitude of the neural response at the round window (N_1), was equal to 40 to 42 dB. In view of this, the intensity of the binaural stimulation was not allowed to exceed 30 to 35 dB above the threshold for the response.

A UBP-1-02 amplifier was used. The impulse activity was recorded on a film from the screen of an oscilloscope, as a rule, by the dot method [19]. The stimuli in each series were repeated from 10 to 20 times. During recording, the stimulus repetition rate was not more than once per 2 sec. In some experiments, the discharges were recorded on tape. The subsequent processing of the material was done with the aid of an automatic device which made it possible to obtain poststimulus-time histograms [18].

After detecting a neuron that responded to sound, the threshold for the response was determined, and then the dependence of the response character- istics on the intensity of the monaural and binaural stimuli was studied. The lateralization was caused either by varying the time intervals (ΔT) between the binaurally presented signals (intervals ranged from 11 to 2000 μsec) or by varying the intensity of one of them (ΔI). By varying the ΔT, we investigated the neural reactions when one signal led the other and also when the order of stimuls presentation was changed. When the ΔI was varied, one ear was stimulated by a click (or a train of clicks) of constant intensity, while the intensity of stimulation of the opposite ear was varied, as a rule, within the limits of 18 dB ($\pm$ 9 dB relative to the initial level) in steps of 1.5 to 2.5 dB. After that was accomplished, a click of constant intensity was presented to the ear that was previously stimulated by various sound intensities, while the intensity of the stimulus to the opposite ear was varied. Control responses (to binaural stimulations at ΔT and $\Delta I = 0$) were recorded several times during the experiment. Histological controls carried out in most experiments, which consisted of a series of sections on a freezing microtome, established that the tracks of the electrode were located in the central nucleus of the inferior colliculus.

Results

Altogether about 200 neurons were studied. The unit response to brief clicks is characterized in the overwhelming majority of cases by a brief discharge burst consisting of one to five impulses, and the response to a train of clicks by rhythmical discharges, synchronous with the rhythm of the stimuli. The characteristics of the impulse activity in response to monaural and binaural stimulations (to single clicks, as well as to click trains) have been previously described in greater detail [2, 3].

VARIATION OF THE TIME INTERVAL BETWEEN BINAURALLY PRESENTED
CLICKS (114 NEURONS)

When ΔT varies, the responses of the neurons of the inferior colliculus may
be divided into several types.

The first type of response (16 neurons) is characterized by an augmentation
or decrease of the impulse activity for several (two to four) definite values of
ΔT. If the order of stimulus presentation is reversed, a given ΔT, which
previously caused an augmentation of the responses, now causes their decline
and, vice versa, a ΔT, which caused a decline of the impulse activity with a
given separation of the stimuli, provokes its augmentation when the order of
stimulus presentation is reversed. Data for one such neuron are shown in Fig.
1. When the ipsilateral stimulation [Fig. 1 (e)] leads, a decline of the impulse
activity is observed at ΔT=170 and 700 to 1000 μsec and a rise at ΔT=70 and
200 to 300 μsec. When the contralateral stimulation leads [Fig. 1 (f)], reverse
changes are observed. At ΔT=40 to 70 and 200 to 300 μsec the response
markedly declines, whereas at ΔT=170 and 700 to 1000 μsec the response
does not appreciably differ from the initial level and even becomes somewhat
augmented. Simultaneous to augmentation of the reaction, changes occur in
the latent period. When the impulse activity increases, the latent period
shortens, whereas a decline in spike numbers leads to a considerable increase
of the latency values.

The second type of reaction (30 neurons) is similar to the first. A rise in
impulse activity for a definite range of ΔT's and a depression in this activity
for the same time intervals, when the order of presentation of the clicks is
reversed, is characteristic for this type. The second type differs from the first
by the absence of alternating phases of augmentation and decrease in the
impulse activity when the time intervals between the signals are varied.
Records for one such neuron are presented in Fig. 2. When the ipsilateral
stimulation [Fig. 2 (d)] leads by 11 μsec, an almost complete suppression of
the discharges occurs. The suppression persists up to an interval of 1300 μsec.
However, when the contralateral stimulation [Fig. 2 (e)] leads within the
same range of ΔT's, an impulse activity is present and even shows some
increase. A characteristic feature of this type of reaction is the absence of a
negative correlation between the latent period values and the magnitude of the
reaction. Figure 2 shows that the latency of the reaction does not change with
a decline in impulse activity when the contralateral stimulus leads. However,
when the ipsilateral stimulus leads, the appearance of spikes (ΔT=1520 μsec)
is accompanied by a marked increase of the latent period in comparison with
the initial value (it exceeds the latter twice). Considering that the response of
the neuron in question consisted of two impulses to simultaneous binaural
stimulation [Fig. 2 (a)], a comparison of the magnitude of the reaction with
its latent period suggests that the decline in spike numbers, when the contra-

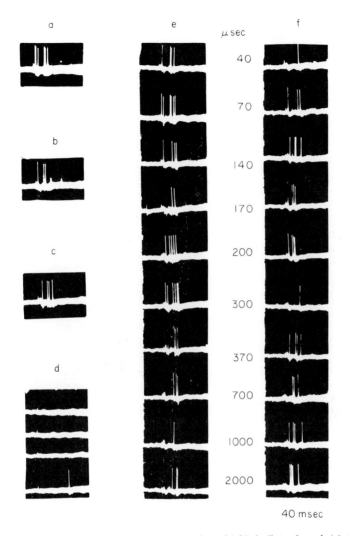

FIG. 1. Neuron 29. Responses to (a) contralateral, (b) ipsilateral, and (c) binaural stimuli. Sound intensity is 30 dB above threshold for binaural stimulation. (d) Spontaneous activity of the neuron. (e) contralateral stimulus applied first; (f) ipsilateral stimulus applied first. Numbers between oscillograms represent values of ΔT in μsec. Small vertical deflections in the oscillograms indicate the onset of stimulation here and in all other similar figures.

lateral ear leads (ΔT=1300 to 2000 μsec), is caused by a suppression of the second spike in the response, while with the ipsilateral ear leading (ΔT=1500 to 2000 μsec), it is the first impulse that is inhibited.

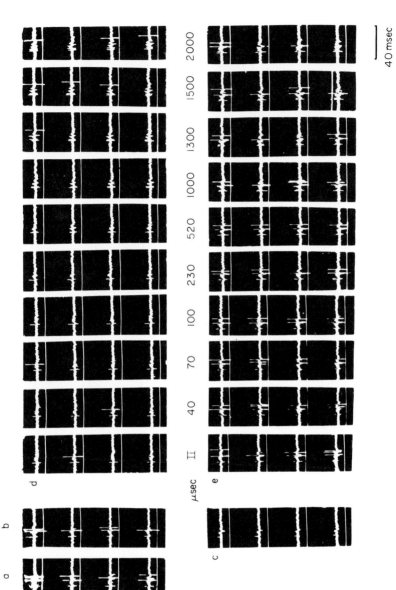

FIG. 2. Neuron 60. Responses to (a) binaural, (b) contralateral, and (c) ipsilateral stimuli. (d) Ipsilateral stimulus applied first; (e) contralateral stimulus applied first. Numbers between oscillograms represent values of ΔT in μsec. Sound intensity is 22 dB above threshold for binaural stimulation.

The next two types of reaction are characterized by an augmentation (3rd type, 24 neurons), or a depression (4th type, 22 neurons) in the impulse activity when the stimulus to one ear leads, without corresponding changes in this activity, if the order of stimulus presentation is reversed. Such reaction types occur when either the ipsilateral or the contralateral stimulus leads. The necessary ΔT values are specific for a given neuron, but are different for various neurons and may actually exceed the range of the ΔT's used. These types of reaction are schematically presented in Figs. 3 (c) and (d).

The last (5th) type of reaction (six neurons) is characterized by a gradual augmentation of the reaction relative to the initial value, when ΔT increases, and by a similarly gradual decline of the reaction, when the order of stimulus presentation is reversed; such changes were observed in the entire range of the ΔT used [Fig. 3 (e)].

For 16 neurons (out of 114) the variations of ΔT did not cause any changes in the response. A scheme of the reactions of all types detected by means of varying ΔT is presented in Fig. 3 [(a) to (f)]; summary data relating to this series of experiments are assembled in Table 1.

VARIATION IN THE INTENSITY OF ONE OF THE BINAURALLY PRESENTED SIGNALS

Such variations were studied for 103 neurons. The study revealed several types of reactions quite similar to those that had been established by varying ΔT.

The most numerous group of neurons (31), which responded to the variation of ΔI by changes in their response, is characterized by the following. Within a certain range an increase of stimulus strength to one ear causes a rise (or decline) in the number of spikes in the response in comparison with the control level. An increase in stimulus strength in the opposite ear provokes opposite effects—a decline (or rise) in spike activity over the same intensity range. In 19 neurons (out of 31 belonging to this type), the spike activity changes not only when the monaural stimulus is strengthened, but also when it is attenuated. In such cases, an increase in the intensity of the stimulus to one ear augments the reaction, while a weaker stimulus decreases it. When the intensity of the stimulus to the opposite ear increases, the response becomes depressed, and when it decreases, the response is augmented. This type of reaction is shown in Fig. 4.

The second (16 neurons) and the third (15 neurons) type of reaction is characterized either by an augmentation or by a decrease in spike numbers in the response over a certain intensity range of ΔI for one of the binaurally presented stimuli. They differ from the first type by the absence of the opposite changes when ΔI is varied for the other ear [Figs. 5 (b) and (c)].

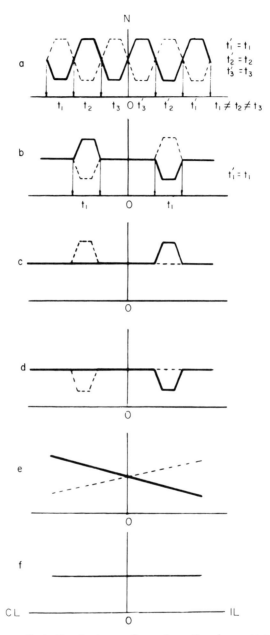

FIG. 3. Scheme illustrating the types of neural reactions in response to variations of ΔT values. Abscissa, ΔT; ordinate, magnitude of the reaction (N). O represents $\Delta T=0$; CL, contralateral stimulus applied first; IL, ipsilateral stimulus applied first. Solid and dashed lines indicate variants of the reaction. Schemes (a) to (f) demonstrate types of neural reactions.

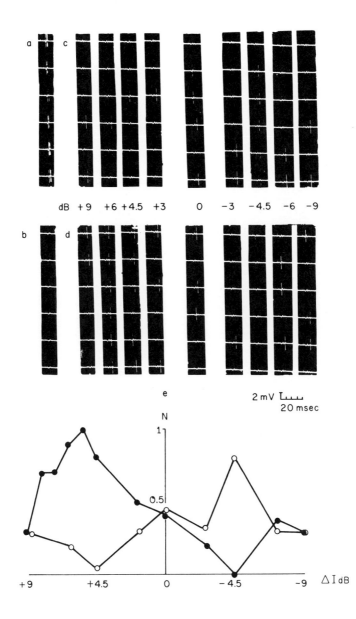

FIG. 4. Neuron 177. Responses to (a) ipsilateral and (b) contralateral stimuli. (c) Responses when the intensity of the contralateral stimulus varied relative to the ipsilateral stimulus. (d) Responses when the intensity of the ipsilateral stimulus varied. Numbers between oscillograms represent increase (+) or decrease (−) of the respective monaural stimulus in comparison to the control level when ΔI between the two ears = 0 dB. (e) Graph plotting ΔI (abscissa) against the average number of spikes in the response (ordinate). ΔI varies from +9 to −9 dB in relation to the control level of 22 dB above threshold for the binaural stimuli and ΔI=0. Filled circles indicate ΔI values for ipsilateral ear; open circles, ΔI values for contralateral ear.

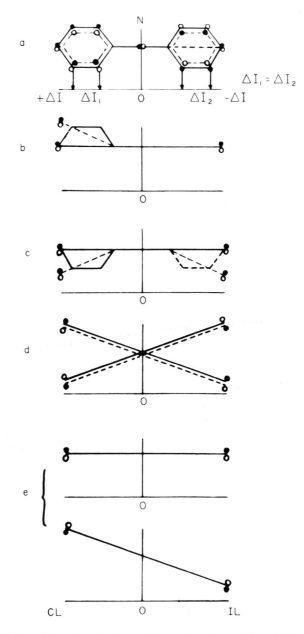

FIG. 5. Scheme illustrating the types of neural reactions with variation of ΔI values. Abscissa, intensity changes ($\pm\Delta I$); ordinate, magnitude of the reaction (N). O represents $\Delta I = 0$. Solid and dashed lines indicate variants of the reaction. (a) to (e) Types of neural reactions. Filled circles show variations of the intensity of the ipsilateral stimulus; open circles, variations of the intensity of the contralateral stimulus.

Four neurons, for which a diminution in the impulse activity—in comparison with the control level—was observed, both when the intensity of the monaural stimulus was increased and when it was decreased, were also related to the third type of reaction. A characteristic feature of these neurons is that they respond in different ways to ipsilateral, contralateral and binaural stimuli. Data for one of these neurons are shown in Fig. 6.

The fourth type of reaction (eight neurons) is characterized by gradual augmentation of the impulse activity when the intensity of the stimulation at one ear increases and by decrease in this activity when this intensity declines. Opposite changes are observed when ΔI is varied for the other ear. This type of reaction differs from the reaction of neurons which belong to the first type by gradual changes in activity over the entire range of ΔI variations, while for neurons of the first type, changes are observed only for specific values of ΔI [Figs. 5 (c) and (d)].

For 33 neurons no change in spike numbers was observed when ΔI was varied. For 12 of them, an increase in the intensity of both ipsilateral and contralateral stimuli caused a similar increase of the response, while a decrease in the intensity of monaural stimuli caused a similar decrease [Fig. 5 (e)].

The types of neuronal reactions occurring with variations of ΔI are schematically presented in Figs. 5 (a) to (e); summary data relating to this series of experiments are given in Table 1.

For 68 neurons, changes in impulse activity were studied when both ΔI and ΔT varied. No correlation was found between the types of reactions described for ΔI and ΔT variations. Only for nine neurons was it found that if a stimulus to one ear leads and evokes an augmentation (or decrease) of the impulse activity, then an increase of the stimulus intensity in the same ear resulted also in augmentation (or decrease) of spike activity. For all other neurons, which responded with changes in their activity to the variation of both ΔT and ΔI, varied combinations of the reaction types occurred. However, observations on neurons, for which variations of ΔT and ΔI were studied, made it possible to distinguish two neural groups. For one of them only the variations of ΔT provoke pronounced changes in the impulse activity according to one of the described types, whereas variations of ΔI do not produce any appreciable changes in the response (22 neurons). The other group (36 neurons) responds with pronounced changes in spike activity when both parameters (ΔT and ΔI) are varied. The remaining ten neurons were not affected by variations of either ΔT or ΔI. Examples illustrating the two groups are shown in Figs. 7 and 8. One more specific feature of the neural behavior may be pointed out. It was true for a number of neurons that, when one of the stimuli leads and its intensity is increased, the effects of variations of ΔT and ΔI become considerably more pronounced [Figs. 8 (e) and (f)].

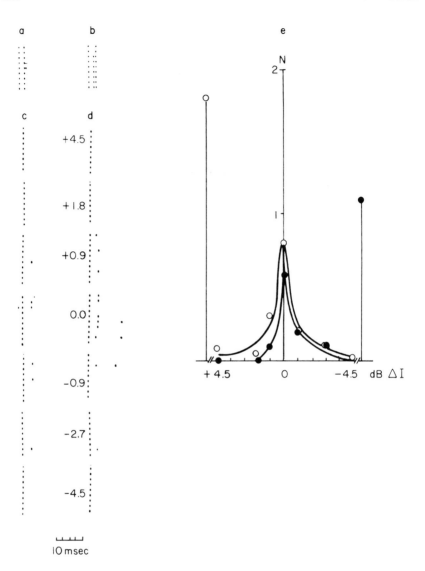

FIG. 6. Neuron 189. Responses to (a) contralateral and (b) ipsilateral stimuli. (c) Intensity of the ipsilateral stimulus varies; (d) intensity of the contralateral stimulus varies. Left string of dots in the oscillograms indicate here and in Figs. 7 and 8 the onset of the stimulus. Other dots indicate the time of occurrence of the discharges. Numbers between oscillograms represent increase (+) or decrease (−) in the intensity of the monaural stimuli in dB in comparison with the control level (control level, 35 dB above the threshold for binaural stimuli). (e) Graph plotting changes in the intensity (ΔI) of the ipsilateral (filled circles), and contralateral (open circles) stimuli in dB (abscissa) against the average number of spikes (N) (ordinate). Vertical bar with open circle at top represents magnitude of the response to ipsilateral stimulus; vertical bar with a filled circle at top, magnitude of the response to contralateral stimulus.

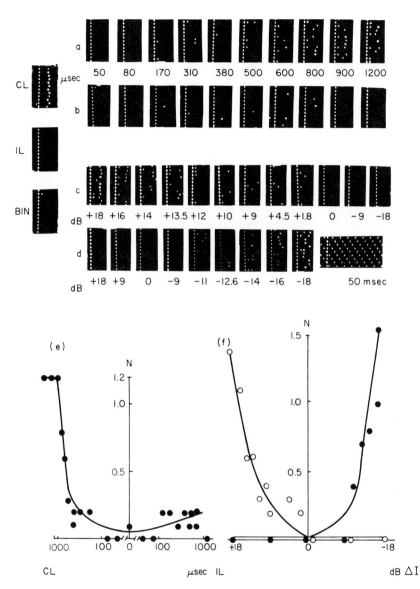

FIG. 7. Neuron 261. CL indicates responses to contralateral stimuli; IL, responses to ipsilateral stimuli; BIN, response to binaural stimulation. (a) Contralateral stimulus leads; (b) ipsilateral stimulus leads. Numbers between oscillograms represent ΔT in μsec. (c) intensity of the contralateral stimulations varies. (d) intensity of the ipsilateral stimulus varies. Numbers under the oscillograms indicate increase (+) or decrease (−) of the intensity of the monaural stimulus in dB relative to the control level ΔI=0. (e) average number of spikes as a function of ΔT. Abscissa, ΔT in μsec. To the left of O, (CL) contralateral stimulus leads; to the right of O, (IL) ipsilateral stimulus leads. Ordinate, number of spikes (N). (f) Average number of spikes as a function of ΔI. Abscissa, change of intensity of monaural stimulus (ΔI) in dB relative to the control level; ordinate, number of spikes (N). Dots: variation in intensity of the ipsilateral stimulus; circles: variation in intensity of the contralateral stimulus. Control level of intensity is 28 dB above the threshold for the response to binaural stimuli (for ΔI=0).

TABLE 1

Summary Data Concerning the Types of Neural Responses when Single Clicks Are Presented Binaurally[a]

| Types of reaction | ΔT | | | | | | Δ^c | | | | | |
| | No. of neurons | % | Contralateral stimulus leads | | Ipsilateral stimulus leads | | No. of neurons | % | Contralateral stimulus increased | | Ipsilateral stimulus increased | |
			Aug. of the response	Dim. of the response	Aug. of the response	Dim. of the response			Aug. of the response	Dim. of the response	Aug. of the response	Dim. of the response
First	16	14.0	_b_	_b_	_b_	_b_	31	30.0	24	7	7	24
Second	30	26.3	19	11	11	19	16	15.6	9	—	7	—
Third	24	21.0	14	—	10	—	15	14.6	—	5	—	10
Fourth	22	19.4	—	9	—	13	8	7.8	2	6	6	2
Fifth	6	5.3	3	3	3	3	—	—	—	—	—	—
No changes	16	14.0	—	—	—	—	33	32.0	—	—	—	—
	114	100.0					103	100.0				

[a] The time interval between them (ΔT) or their intensity ΔI varies.

[b] Not included in this table since both augmentation (Aug.) and diminution (Dim.) in impulse activity occurs repeatedly for these neurons with either ear leading.

[c] An increase in the intensity of the monaural stimulus as well as a decrease in the intensity of the stimulus to the opposite ear are regarded as an increase of the monaural stimulus.

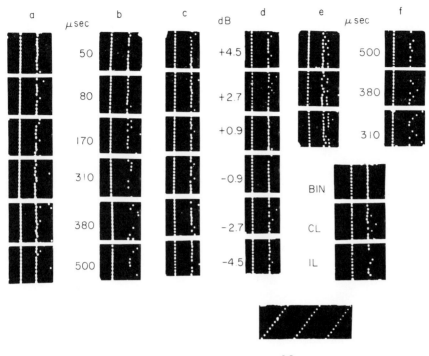

20 msec

FIG. 8. Neuron 276. (a) Contralateral stimulus leads; (b) ipsilateral stimulus leads. Numbers between oscillograms represent ΔT in μsec; (c) intensity of the ipsilateral stimulus varies; (d) intensity of the contralateral stimulus varies. Numbers between oscillograms show increase (+) or decrease (−) of one of the monaural stimuli. (e) Contralateral stimulus was increased by 4.5 dB relative to the control level (ΔI=0) and leads in time (μsec), as indicated between the oscillograms. (f) Ipsilateral stimulation was increased by 4.5 dB and leads in time (μsec), indicated between the oscillograms. BIN stands for response to binaural stimuli; CL, response to contralateral stimuli; IL, responses to ipsilateral stimuli. Control level of intensity is 22 dB above the threshold for binaural stimuli (ΔI=0).

LATERALIZATION OF A CLICK TRAIN

As already mentioned in the Methods section, trains of clicks delivered at a rate of 10 to 30/sec (for a duration of 500 to 700 msec) were used as long-lasting sound signals. We examined 47 neurons of varying ΔT between the binaurally presented trains; but only 39 of these neurons could be studied by varying the ΔI. Four of these neurons (out of 39) did not respond with any changes of their impulse activity to variations of ΔT or ΔI; 21 neurons responded with changes in spike numbers to a variation of ΔT as well as of ΔI; 14 neurons responded only to variations of ΔT. Out of eight neurons which were studied by varying only ΔT, four responded to such variations while four did not. It should be noted that the responses to trains of clicks did not reveal any types of reactions which were different from those described with lateralization of a single click.

However, when one compares the effect of variation of ΔT and of ΔI on the response to the first clicks in the stimulus train with the effect on the response to the remaining clicks, a number of observations can be made which are characteristic for a rhythmic stimulation. With this in mind, all the neurons studied may be divided into two groups: (a) neurons reacting with unidirectional changes in spike activity (augmentation or depression) both in the initial segment of the response and in its subsequent segment, and (b) neurons for which only the later part of the response undergoes changes, while the initial part of the response remains unaltered. Out of 43 neurons which responded with changes in their impulse activity to variations of ΔT, only 27 neurons showed changes in spike activity both in the initial and in the later segment of the response. For the remaining 16 neurons, the spike activity underwent changes only in the later segment of the response. Similar observations were made for neurons which respond to a variation of ΔI—15 neurons (out of 21) responded with changes of the impulse activity both in the initial and the later segment of the response, and six neurons changed their activity only in the later response segment. This observation is illustrated in Fig. 9. It can be seen that a considerable lead of the contralateral stimulus [Fig. 9 (a)] was required to make the neuron gradually reproduce the rhythm of stimulation, whereas a response to the first click in the train was observed at all the delays used. With variations of ΔI, a large increase in the intensity of the contralateral stimulus (45 dB) was necessary to obtain late discharges [Fig. 9 (c)]. Summary data concerning the lateralization of a train of clicks are presented in Table 2.

Since the neurons of the inferior colliculus are able in time to accumulate information about sound signals displaced from the midline, it may be assumed that in the auditory system neurons exist which react specifically to the direction of movement of the sound source. In order to verify this assumption, a sound signal modeling a given direction of the sound movement was used. The signals consisted of trains of clicks presented binaurally (duration of the train was 1.68 sec; click repetition rate, 8 to 30/sec). At the beginning of the presentation, a given maximal delay between stimuli (ΔT_{max}) was used; this delay was decreased linearly and in the middle of the presentation (i.e., at the 0.84th sec), it reached a minimal value. Then the delays were gradually increased so that at the end of the presentation (i.e., at the 1.68*th* sec), the delay again reached its initial value. When such signals were presented to human subjects, they were perceived as a gradual displace-

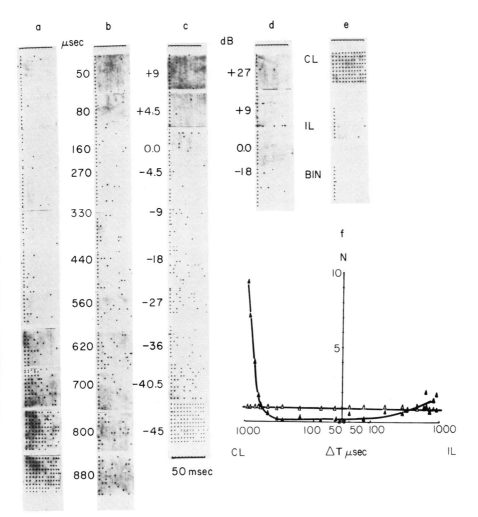

FIG. 9. Neuron 330. Stimulation by a train of clicks (rate of stimulation, 20 Hz; duration of the stimulus, 600 msec; intensity, 30 dB above the threshold for binaural stimuli). (a) Contralateral stimulus leads; (b) ipsilateral stimulus leads. Numbers between oscillograms represent ΔT in μsec; (c) change in intensity of the ipsilateral stimuli; (d) change in intensity of the contralateral stimuli. Numbers to the left of the oscillograms represent increase (+) or decrease (−) in dB in one of the monaural stimuli relative to the control level when ΔI=0. (e) Responses to contralateral (CL), ipsilateral (IL) and binaural (BIN) stimuli when ΔI=0 and ΔT=0. The lines above the oscillograms indicate stimulation marks. Each dot in the oscillograms indicates time of occurrence of an impulse. (f) Average number of spikes as a function of ΔT. Abscissa, time in μsec (ΔT) by which the contralateral (CL) or the ipsilateral (IL) stimulus leads; ordinate, average number of impulses (N). Open triangles indicate first spike in the response; filled triangles, number of spikes in the response minus the initial spike.

TABLE 2

Summary Data Concerning the Types of Neural Responses
to Binaurally Presented Trains of Clicks

Type of response	Change in the initial and late segment of the response (number of neurons)	Change in the late segment of the response only (number of neurons)
Variation of Time Intervals (Δt)		
Reciprocal changes of the response	5	3
Augmentation of the response		
(a) Contralateral stimulus leading	5	3
(b) Ipsilateral stimulus leading	2	2
Diminution of the response		
(a) Contralateral stimulus leading	5	3
(b) Ipsilateral stimulus leading	10	5
	27	16
Variation of Intensity (ΔI)		
Reciprocal changes of the response	2	4
Augmentation of the response		
(a) Intensity increase of contralateral stimulus	3	2
(b) Intensity increase of ipsilateral stimulus	1	—
Diminution of the response		
(a) Intensity increase of contralateral stimulus	3	—
(b) Intensity increase of ipsilateral stimulus	6	—
	15	6

ment of a fused acoustic image from the ear to the midline and back to the ear. A use of different ΔT_{max} made it possible to modify the rate of displacement of the acoustic image since the magnitude of the growth (or diminution) of ΔT for each subsequent click increased (or decreased). These facts, as well as the data of Masterton et al. [12], who have shown that cats are able to discriminate the degree to which one of the clicks leads the other, suggest that the above-described signal models one of the important parameters that we use to localize the sound source during its displacement. The application of these signals disclose the existence in the inferior colliculus of neurons which may be regarded as detectors of the direction of the sound source movement. Poststimulus-time histograms of the activity of one such neuron are presented in Fig. 10. At the intensity of stimulation used, the neuron responded to monaural and binaural stimuli [Figs. 10 (a), (b), and (c)]. A decrease of the ΔT, when the contralateral stimulation was leading, resulted in a suppression of the impulse activity within a certain range of changes of ΔT and in augmentation of this activity when ΔT was gradually increased. The increase in impulse activity depended also on the rate of change of ΔT. A change in ΔT, when the ipsilateral stimulus was leading (two histograms on the right in Fig. 10), caused only some augmentation in the impulse activity which was evenly distributed in the entire range of ΔT and did not depend on the decrease or increase of the interval between the binaurally presented clicks. Thus, these data imply the existence of neurons that respond with specific changes of spike activity to definite changes of ΔT, as well as to the rate of such changes. In view of this, it may be supposed that in the auditory system there exist neurons which specifically react to the direction of movement of the sound source.

Discussion

The results of the present work confirm the data obtained by Hind et al. [10] and by Rose et al. [16] who studied the activity of neurons in the inferior colliculus of the cat by varying ΔI (long-lasting tone signals were used). These investigations established in most of the neurons a depression of the impulse activity when the intensity of one of the binaurally presented signals was varied; consequently, these neurons may be related to the third type of reaction mentioned in the present work. Only for one of the neurons described by Rose et al. [16] were the changes of impulse activity investigated by varying ΔI for ipsilateral and contralateral stimuli (in the latter case, an increase in spike activity was established). However, the diverse initial levels of intensity (the differences reaching 30 dB) used by these authors when varying the intensity of stimulation of the right and left ear, do not allow us

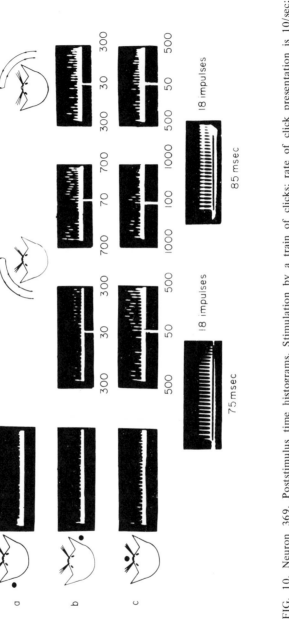

FIG. 10. Neuron 369. Poststimulus time histograms. Stimulation by a train of clicks; rate of click presentation is 10/sec; intensity, 10 dB above the threshold for binaural stimuli (at ΔT=0); duration of the stimulus, 1.68 sec. Histograms are based on responses to 20 repetitions of the stimulus. Bin width is 10 msec. Response to (a) contralateral, (b) ipsilateral, and (c) binaural stimuli (at ΔT=0). Four oscillograms on the left show contralateral stimulus leads; two oscillograms on the right: ipsilateral stimulus leads. Numbers under the oscillograms represent ΔT_{max} – ΔT_{min} – ΔT_{max} (see text). White bar indicates the time at which ΔT is at a minimal value (ΔT_{min}). Calibration signal on the left pertains to the five oscillograms on the left (distance between bars = 75 msec); calibration signal on the right pertains to the remaining four oscillograms (distance between bars = 85 msec). The duration of the stimulus is marked by a black line in the calibration oscillograms.

to regard the given neuron as belonging to the first type of reaction with any confidence. As for the variation of ΔT, Hind *et al.* [10] and Rose *et al.* [16] detected changes in spike activity which are close to the first type of reaction described here. The fact that in our work (see also Ref. [1]) there is no periodicity in the changes of the impulse activity is apparently due to the character of the acoustic stimulation; when varying ΔT, we used clicks, whereas Rose and his co-workers made use of a phase shift between binaurally presented low-frequency tone signals.

A comparison of the results of the present investigation with data obtained from studies of neurons of the superior olive [6, 7, 13] permits us to establish some similarities as well as essential differences in the changes of impulse activity under conditions of lateralization of the sound. The changes are similar in that most of the investigated neurons of the superior olive and a considerable number of the neurons of the inferior colliculus manifest reciprocal changes in spike activity for variations of both ΔT and ΔI. The differences are very substantial because as far as we know, under conditions of lateralization, the spike activity of most neurons of the superior olive manifests a gradual change in spike activity over the whole range of ΔT and ΔI [7], whereas it is a characteristic feature of neurons of the inferior colliculus that their impulse activity changes only over a limited range of ΔT and ΔI which is strictly specific for a given neuron. Only 14 neurons (six for variations of ΔT and eight for variations of ΔI) belong to the type of reaction that is characteristic of neurons of the superior olive [Fig. 3 (e); Fig. 5 (d)].

The differences we have described between the reactions of the neurons of the inferior colliculus and the superior olive indicate the essential transformations in spike activity which may occur in these two divisions of the auditory system under conditions of lateralization of the sound. It would appear that the predominant result of these transformations is a transition from gradual changes of the impulse activity over the whole range of variations of ΔT and ΔI (superior olive) to nonlinear changes of this activity limited by definite time intervals between the binaurally presented signals or by definite intensities of one of the monaural stimuli (inferior colliculus). In view of this, the latter transformation may be characterized as leading to a sharpening of the response in time or intensity. It may be stressed once more that the ranges of ΔT and ΔI, which provoke changes in the impulse activity, are strictly specific for a given neuron; they differ for various neurons and may exceed the ranges of ΔT or ΔI used in this investigation. For a given neuron, the specificity of the range of ΔT, which produces a change in spike activity was described by Rose and his co-workers [16] who designated this interval as a "characteristic delay of the unit."

A quantitative evaluation of the response sharpening indicates that the effect on spike activity in a nonlinear type of reaction is about ten times greater than the effect observed for neurons of the superior olive under similar experimental conditions, as well as for neurons of the inferior colliculus which respond with linear changes in their impulse activity. The described transformations must therefore raise the capacity of the auditory system for detecting at which ear the stimulus arrives earlier, at which ear it is more intense, the rate of change of time differences, and the rate at which the stimulus to one ear becomes more intense.*

The experimental data pertaining to trains of clicks reveal that the types of responses to such stimuli are the same as those which appear to single clicks. This implies that only a finite number of transformations of the impulse activity occurs at the level of the inferior colliculus when signals significant for localization are applied.

The application of trains of clicks disclosed some peculiarities in the behavior of neurons when ΔT and ΔI were varied. Thus, in more than one-third of the neurons studied, the change of the impulse activity affected only the later segment of the response, while its initial segment remained unaltered with ΔT or ΔI varied. In other words, rhythmical trains of clicks substantially extend the capacity of the neurons of the inferior colliculus to respond with changes in spike activity which contribute to the localization of a long-lasting sound source. This explains why rhythmic bursts of acoustic sounds are preferred localization signals in nature. It should also be noted that the discussed responses to rhythmic click trains are concordant with a number of psychophysical observations, which have established that the differential thresholds for lateralization decline for rhythmical trains of clicks in comparison with the thresholds for single clicks [9, 11].

The existence of neurons detecting the direction in which the sound moves shows that the neural net of the auditory system includes receptive areas that may respond with specific reactions to a property of the acoustic signals such as the direction of the sound movement.

Conclusions

Variations in the impulse activity of neurons of the inferior colliculus were studied in anesthetized cats under conditions of lateralization, which were

---

* The values of the latent period of the response may serve, along with the magnitude of the response, as an additional factor for localization of sound. As shown above, the latency values are dependent on the number of impulses in the response. The probable role of latency changes for localization of the sound has been discussed in the literature [5, 10, 13].

generated by varying the time intervals between binaurally presented signals or the intensity of one of them. Several types of reactions were observed under these conditions. A comparison of the results of the present investigation with data in the literature, which pertain to responses of neurons in the superior olive, suggests that a substantial transformation of spike activity occurs between these two divisions of the auditory system. The main effect of this transformation is a transition from gradual (linear) changes of spike activity for the entire range of time intervals and intensities to nonlinear changes which are strictly limited to definite time intervals or definite intensities.

Under conditions of lateralization of rhythmical trains of clicks, it was shown that in time, neurons are able to accumulate information concerning the sound source as it is displaced from the midline. Two-thirds of the studied neurons responded with similar changes of spike activity both to the initial and to the later segments of the stimulus train. For one-third of the neurons only the response to the later segment of the stimulus train was subject to change, while the response to the first clicks of the series remained unaltered in comparison with the control level.

The study revealed the existence of neurons detecting the direction in which the sound source moves. This suggests the existence of complex receptive areas in the neural net of the auditory system which determine this property of the acoustic signals.

REFERENCES

1. Altman, J. A. Responses of the inferior colliculus neurons of the cat when time intervals between binaurally presented stimuli vary. *Biophysics (USSR)* 11, 488-497 (1966) (in Russian).
2. Altman, J. A. Characteristics of impulse activity of neurons in the inferior colliculus of the cat when monaural and binaural stimuli are presented. *In* "Problems of Physiological Acoustics" (G. V. Gersuni, ed.), Vol. 6: Mechanisms of Hearing, pp. 158-173. Nauka, Leningrad, 1967 (in Russian).
3. Altman, J. A. Responses of the inferior colliculus neurons of the cat to lateralization of rhythmic acoustic stimuli. *J. Higher Nervous Activity (USSR)* 19, 59-70 (1969) (in Russian).
4. Busnel, R. G. (ed.) "Acoustic Behaviour of Animals." Elsevier, Amsterdam, 1963.
5. Erulkar, S. D. The responses of single units in the inferior colliculus of the cat to acoustic stimulation. *Proc. Roy. Soc. (London) Ser.* B150, 336-355 (1959).
6. Galambos, R., Schwartzkopff, J., and Rupert, A. Microelectrode study of the superior olivary nuclei. *Amer. J. Physiol.* 197, 527-536 (1959).
7. Hall, J. L., II. Binaural Interaction in the Accessory Superior Olivary Nucleus of the Cat-an Electrophysiological Study of Single Neurons Techn. Rep. 416 M.I.T. Press, Cambridge, Massachusetts, 1964.
8. Hall, J. L., II. Binaural interaction in the accessory superior-olivary nucleus of the cat. *J. Acoust. Soc. Amer.* 37, 814-823 (1965).

9. Harris, G. G., Flanagan, J. L., and Watson, B. J. Binaural interaction of a click with a click pair. *J. Acoust. Soc. Amer.* **35**, 672-678 (1963).

10. Hind, J. E., Goldberg, J. M., Greenwood, D. D., and Rose, J. E. Some discharge characteristics of single neurons in the inferior colliculus of the cat. II. Timing of the discharges and observations on binaural stimulation. *J. Neurophysiol.* **26**, 321-341 (1963).

11. Klumpp, R. G., and Eady, H. R. Some measurements of interaural time difference thresholds. *J. Acoust. Soc. Amer.* **28**, 859-864 (1956).

12. Masterton, J., Jane, J. A., and Diamond, I. T. Role of the brainstem structures in sound localization. I. Trapezoid body, superior olive, and lateral lemniscus, *J. Neurophysiol.* **30**, 341-359 (1967).

13. Moushegian, G., Rupert, A., and Whitcomb, M. A. Medial superior-olivary unit responses to monaural and binaural clicks. *J. Acoust. Soc. Amer.* **36**, 196-202 (1964).

14. Moushegian, G., Rupert, A., and Whitcomb, M. A. Brain-stem neuronal response patterns to monaural and binaural tones. *J. Neurophysiol.* **27**, 1174-1191 (1964).

15. Möhres, F. P., and Neuveiler, G. Die Ultraschallorientierung der Grossblatt-Fledermäuse (Chiroptera-Megadermatidae). *Z. Vergl. Physiol.* **53**, 195-227 (1966).

16. Rose, J. E., Gross, N. B., Geisler, C. D., and Hind, J. E. Some neural mechanisms in the inferior colliculus of the cat which may be relevant to localization of a sound source. *J. Neurophysiol.* **29**, 288-314 (1966).

17. Stotler, W. A. An experimental study of the cells and connections of the superior olivary complex of the cat. *J. Comp. Neurol.* **98**, 401-431 (1953).

18. Vaitulevich, S. F., and Likhnitsky, A. M. Use of the impulse analyzer AI-100 for temporal analysis of impulse activity. *J. Higher Nervous Activity (USSR)* **16**, 747-752 (1966) (in Russian).

19. Wall, P. D. Repetitive discharge of neurons. *J. Neurophysiol.* **22**, 305-320 (1959).

14

Some Characteristics of Single Unit Responses of the Auditory Cortex in the Cat

G. A. Vardapetian

Microelectrode studies of unit responses in the auditory cortex and in the more peripheral synaptic regions of the auditory chain are important for the understanding of the functional organization of the neural mechanisms of the auditory system. Data from cortical studies may be expected to disclose the final transformations concerning the afferent information about an external signal and may yield some knowledge about the complex integrative processes that occur at the cortical level of this sensory system.

However, the available data [5-8, 12, 14, 16-18, 22, 30] are limited and are often contradictory as regards both the frequency selectivity of cortical units and the general characteristics of their response. It is unlikely that the contradictory findings are the result of different experimental conditions, particularly the presence or absence of general anesthesia, since contradictory observations were reported for data obtained in anesthetized and unanesthetized preparations. The controversial results may be partly due to technical problems. However, they must be attributed mainly to difficulties in the evaluation of the inconstant activity of the cortical units. A sizable fraction of isolated units in the primary auditory cortex of the cat produce inconstant responses as noted by some workers [5, 6, 8, 16] both in anesthetized and unanesthetized preparations. Inconstancy of the response and variability of its characteristics sharply distinguish cortical neurons from those in the relay nuclei of the auditory system. Nevertheless, the criteria for response evaluation and classification of neurons, generally employed in studies of auditory cortical units, do not differ from those employed in studies of the auditory relay nuclei. Therefore, the criteria for a stable response, while adequate for description of regularly driven units ("securely driven units" of some authors [5]), do not apply to a sizable fraction of cortical units whose responses are very variable.

In this chapter, apart from studies of the response characteristics of securely driven units, we attempt a definition of the response properties of insecurely driven units by repeated application of the sound signal. Although no adequate quantitative estimate of the dynamics of the variable response can be given at the present time, it seems possible to establish, at least for some units, a functional trend which may have some bearing on such complex processes as "memory" and "learning."

Moreover, it should be noted that in the previous studies of cortical units, no effort was made to examine the effect of sound duration on the characteristics of the response. However, the significance of the temporal characteristics of the acoustic signal for the various functions of the auditory analyzer is known not only from psychophysical investigations, but also from systematic investigations carried out in the laboratory of Gersuni [2, 10, 11, 20, 23, 28, 29, 31, and others].

Consequently, the objectives of the present study were (a) to investigate the response properties of the auditory cortical units and to classify them according to the stability of their response, and (b) to obtain information about the characteristics of auditory unit responses to acoustic signals of different duration.

Methods

The experiments were carried out on cats under chloralose anesthesia. Responses of single units in the primary auditory cortex were studied to tonal and noise bursts of different duration at various intensity levels. Single clicks and pairs of clicks of equal intensity but with a varying time interval between them were employed as stimuli as well. The sound stimuli were presented repeatedly with a frequency of 1/3 sec. Maximum available intensity of the stimulus was 60 dB sound pressure level (SPL) *re* 0.0002 dyn/cm^2 for noise, and 80 dB for tones.

The surgical techniques and the setup for recording and stimulation were previously described in detail [27]. In order to minimize the respiratory and pulsation movements of the brain tissue, cisternal drainage was carried out through the cisterna magna, and the cortex was covered with an agar-agar solution (3-4% agar in physiological saline). An electrode drive system (a modification of Hubel's chamber [15]) was mounted on the skull. Single unit activity was recorded extracellularly with tungsten microelectrodes with tip diameter of less than 1 μ and an impedance of 30 to 50 MΩ at a frequency of 1000 Hz. Single unit discharges were displayed on the oscilloscope screen and photographed. Simultaneously, the discharges were also registered on tape for subsequent automatic processing with the aid of an impulse analyzer to plot poststimulus time (PST) histograms.

Results

GENERAL REMARKS

As the electrode was advanced through the cortex and a unit isolated, an acoustic "search" stimulus was presented. Usually, the search procedure took about 30 to 45 min. It soon became apparent that responsiveness of a unit as well as its response pattern were affected by the length of the stimulus application. Therefore, after the isolation of a unit, and after the optimal adjustment of the electrode position, the sound stimulus was turned off (usually for 10 to 15 min) in order to restore the initial response capacity of the unit under study. The frequency of presentation of the stimulus did not exceed 0.3/sec. At faster rates of stimulus delivery a spike-count reduction (occasionally followed by a total extinction of the response) was observed for a great majority of the units. The unit discharge consisted of two-phasic spikes of 0.5 to 0.8 msec in duration. The potentials were of equal amplitude, frequently initially negative, rarely initially positive.

DYNAMIC CHANGES IN RESPONSES OF CORTICAL UNITS

Cortical auditory units, when repeatedly stimulated by an acoustic signal, may remain unresponsive to sound (12%) or fall into two groups if constancy of the response and stability of its properties are taken as criteria. Units of the first group (37% of a total of 72 units studied) regularly responded to a signal and had reasonably stable response characteristics. On the other hand, responses of units in the second group (51%) were very unstable and the response underwent substantial changes if the same stimulus was applied over a period of time. However, when the responses were studied for a sufficiently long time, a regular pattern could be observed in the reactions of some "unstable" units (29% of the total)—with repetition of the stimulus, the responses of these units became either extinguished or they became intensified and stabilized.

Units that ceased to respond with stimulus repetition, became responsive again, either after a period of silence or when the characteristics of the stimulating signal were changed. In some cases when the characteristics of the stimulus were changed the response was not only restored to its initial magnitude, but it was increased. Figure 1 illustrates an extinction of a response that consisted of two spikes with repeated application of an identical stimulus and the recovery of the responsiveness with subsequent modifications of the discharge pattern which gradually stabilized and became tonic rather

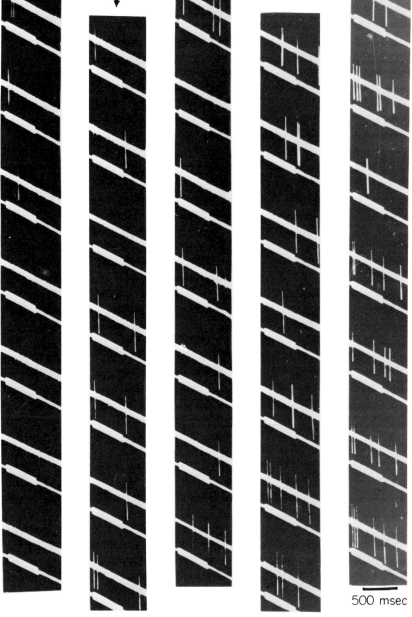

FIG. 1. Successive records demonstrating extinction of the unit response when an identical stimulus is repeated (left vertical column) and recovery of the response with a subsequent modification of the discharge pattern when the frequency of the stimulus was changed continually within the range of 3 to 20 kHz (onset of these stimuli marked by an arrow). Upper trace indicates response of the unit; lower trace, stimulus form.

than phasic. This was accomplished by shifts in the stimulus spectrum (continuous rotation of the indicator of the audiofrequency generator within a frequency range of 3 to 20 kHz).

Units whose discharges were facilitated with repetition of the stimulus retained their response patterns long after the stimulus was turned off, or when another stimulus with different parameters was presented. The newly evoked response pattern was superimposed on the response traces which were preserved from the previous response pattern. However, in contrast to extinction of the response, which occurred after a few applications of the stimulus and was therefore clearly demonstrable in a few successive records, facilitation of the response and preservation of its pattern developed relatively slowly, i.e., a prolonged application of the stimulus was necessary. Hence, the dynamics of the response pattern in the latter case were demonstrable only if an adequate number of successive responses were summated.

In Figs. 2-4 PST histograms are shown pertaining to discharges of three units in response to noise bursts of different duration at constant intensity. The level of spontaneous activity before stimulation is indicated for each unit

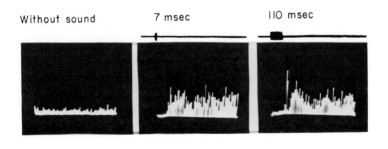

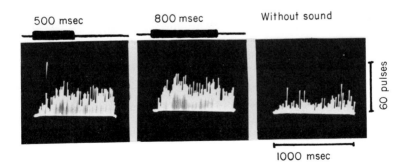

FIG. 2. Poststimulus-time (PST) histograms (from upper left to lower right) plotting discharges of a unit to noise bursts of differnt duration specified for each record. Stimulus intensity: 60 dB SPL *re* 0.0002 dyn/cm^2. The histograms demonstrate preservation of traces of past response when activity is recorded in absence of stimulation. Histograms based on responses to 60 stimuli which were applied once every 3 sec over a period of 3 min. Time between histograms, 20 to 30 sec.

by a histogram at the upper left. A histogram at the lower right shows the level of spontaneous activity after each respective series of stimuli.

In Fig. 2 the unit responds regardless of stimulus duration (7, 110, 500, and 800 msec) with a prolonged train of discharges which are distributed throughout the time of analysis (1000 msec) of the histograms; these are based on responses to 60 successive sound bursts. It is clear from Fig. 2 that the background activity before stimulation is low. With stimulation of noise bursts of different durations there is not only a considerable rise in the number of impulses but an emergence of a characteristic time pattern as well. This discharge pattern is preserved in the record obtained after cessation of the stimuli (lower right histogram). It is most likely that the discharges recorded in the absence of acoustic stimulation indicate a preservation of traces of the past response rather than of a mere increase in the level of spontaneous activity after prolonged stimulation of the neuron. This is suggested by the similarity between the configuration of this histogram and the histograms obtained during stimulation of the neuron.

In Fig. 3 the preservation of traces of the past response is seen for another neuron which had a more complex discharge pattern than that shown in Fig. 2. The level of spontaneous activity of this unit before the beginning of stimulation was much higher than that for the unit in Fig. 2. The pattern of spontaneous activity recorded after the entire stimulation series* is quite different from that obtained before the beginning of the stimulation since some features of the past response patterns to sound stimuli are preserved. PST histograms in Fig. 4 demonstrate the same phenomenon of retention of a previous response pattern for still another unit. The histogram obtained after the stimulation series (Fig. 4, lower right) bears all the features of the unit response to sound stimuli, i.e., there is an initial burst of impulses and subsequent discharges are separated by an inhibitory pause. This fact suggests that after cessation of stimulation there existed a rhythmic afterdischarge which tended to preserve the pattern of the previous stimulation.

In Figs. 3 and 4 the responses of the units to sound bursts of different durations consist of an initial short-latency discharge, a pause, and subsequent discharges which group around one or two peaks; a second peak arises in response to stimuli of long duration (300 and 800 msec). The time pattern of these responses shows some interesting features when latency to the first peak is measured from the termination of the sound burst. For the data in Fig. 3, the values of these off-latencies for sound bursts of 7, 14, 28, and 110 msec are 493, 486, 472, and 470 msec, respectively; for durations of 300 and 800

* The series consisted of stimuli of six different sound durations. Sixty successive sound bursts for each duration were presented at a rate of one stimulus per three seconds over a period of 3 min in order to obtain data for one histogram. The entire series consisted of 360 sound bursts (total time of stimulation was 18 min; pauses between records lasted 30 sec).

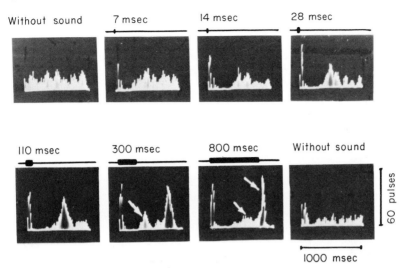

FIG. 3. PST histograms for responses of a unit demonstrating preservation of traces of the pattern of past responses. The basic response pattern consists of discharges at the onset and at the termination of noise bursts of different duration. (Duration of noise indicated for each histogram.) Stimulus intensity, 60 dB SPL. The second group of impulses arising as an off-response is displaced to the right with an increase in duration of the stimulus. The arrows indicate the additional peaks. Histogram plots as in Fig. 2.

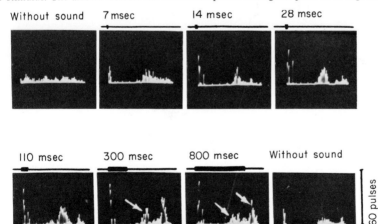

FIG. 4. PST histograms for responses of a unit demonstrating preservation of traces of the pattern of past responses. Stimulus, noise bursts of different duration, which is indicated for each histogram; Intensity, 60 dB SPL. A second group of impulses arising as off-response is displaced to the right with an increase in duration of the stimulus and is preserved in the form of traces after the stimulus has ceased. The arrows indicate the additional peaks. Histogram plots as in Fig. 2.

msec a second peak is present. For the 300-msec burst the off-latency is 480 msec for the second larger peak (which is nearly the same value as the latency to the first peak for the shorter noise bursts), and 120 msec for the first peak. For the 800-msec sound burst there are also two peaks. The second (larger) one occurs with an off-latency of 35 msec; the first peak occurs 200 msec before the termination of the sound burst. For the unit in Fig. 4 the off-latencies to the first peak for the 7, 14, 28, and 110-msec sound bursts, and the off-latency to the second peak for the 300-msec sound burst are 583, 596, 582, 530, and 560 msec, respectively. Evidently, for the patterns of these two units the off-latency values are of the same order of magnitude for sound bursts of different durations. This is a rather peculiar timing for sound-burst cessation. Another feature of the pattern of these two units is the appearance of additional peaks preceeding the larger off-peaks. Such peaks appear for long-duration stimuli of 300 and 800 msec. In our series, the long-duration stimuli were preceded by numerous bursts of shorter duration. The existence of rhythmic afterdischarges which occur with a definite time pattern after cessation of the entire series of stimuli (i.e., after 360 presentations) makes it highly probable that a rhythmic afterdischarge with a pattern appropriate for the last stimuli presented may have also arisen in the earlier records of the series. An assumption seems justified that the additional earlier peaks observed for stimuli of 300- and 800-msec durations reflect rhythmic afterdischarges caused by the preceding stimuli (the 110-msec-long stimuli for the 300-msec record, and the 300-msec-long stimuli for the 800-msec record). In the latter record, the time of analysis is actually too short to determine whether the proper off-response to this stimulus occurred, since the time of analysis was only 1000 msec, while the expected time of appearance of the off-peak is 1300 msec. It may be assumed that the last well-defined peak, as shown in this histogram (Fig. 4) represents traces from the pattern of the previous response of the unit to a stimulus of 300-msec duration.

Hence, we may assume that information concerning the stimulus, which is reflected by the discharge pattern of the unit, is preserved by some cortical neurons in the form of traces for some time after the stimulus has ceased. The character of the response of these neurons (the temporal configuration of impulses) is thus determined not only by the parameters of the stimulus applied at a given time, but also by the past "experience" of the neurons and the state of this "experience." Accordingly, the relationship between the response characteristics such as latent period, number of impulses, and the temporal configuration of the impulses, on one side, and the parameters of the acting stimulus, on the other, is to some extent variable.

The response patterns of the remaining neurons (22%), in the group of "unstable units," were also very variable. However, in contrast to the responses described above, no regular patterns of behavior could be found for responses in this group of neurons. PST histograms and successive records of the discharges for one such unit are shown in Fig. 5. Perhaps a more

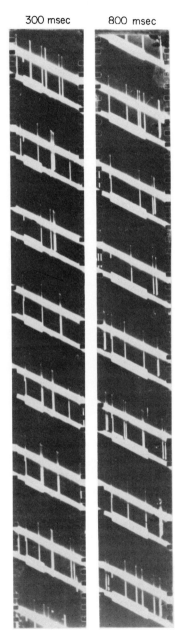

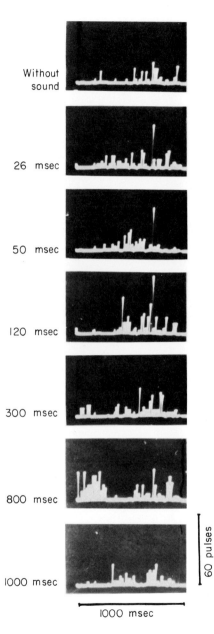

FIG. 5. Successive records and PST histograms for a "variable" unit. No regular trend in the response variability is demonstrable. Stimulus: noise bursts of different duration, indicated for each record. Intensity: 60 dB SPL. Oscillograms upper trace: unit response; lower trace: stimulus form. Histogram plots as in Fig. 2.

sophisticated method for estimation of response variability than the crude criteria, used in the present investigation, is necessary for an adequate evaluation of the responses of these units.

RESPONSE CHARACTERISTICS OF CORTICAL "STABLE UNITS"

The "stable" units responded rather regularly to sequential presentations of sound bursts and displayed reasonably stable response characteristics. Their response consisted either of sustained discharges or phasic discharges arising at either the onset or termination of a sound burst, or at both. A response area was obtainable for them. The latent periods ranged from less than 7 to 20 msec; occasional units responded with latencies of more than 100 msec. Within limits, the number of spikes evoked tended to be proportional to the intensity as well as to the duration of the stimulus [28].

When the intensity of the stimulus was increased from threshold value to 20 to 25 dB above threshold, an increase in spike count (N) and a decrease in latent period (LP) were observed. A maximal rate of increase in the value of N and a maximal rate of decrease in LP took place within 10 dB above threshold. An intensity increase over 25 to 30 dB above threshold had no appreciable effect on these response parameters.

With an increase in the duration of a noise burst, threshold intensity (defined as that intensity at which an impulse occurred in a response with the probability of 0.5) decreased by almost 9 dB, with a critical time of summation of the order of 10 to 12 msec. During the temporal summation process, increase in the value of LP was insignificant. The summation curves for four units are shown in Fig. 6.

In order to determine the range of intensities within which the duration of the stimulus influenced the magnitude of the response, noise bursts of increasing duration (from 1 msec to durations exceeding the latent period of the response) were used. With an increase in the duration of the stimulus, the spike count increased. The effect of stimulus duration on the number of initial spikes was restricted to the range of intensities less than 15 dB above threshold and was at a maximum at threshold intensity. For the spikes occurring later, the effect of stimulus duration was demonstrable up to intensities of 25 to 30 dB. These phenomena are illustrated in Fig. 7, which pertains to a unit whose response consisted of an initial burst and late discharges separated by a pause of 120 to 160 msec.

For some units with sustained discharges, the histograms for the late responses were more complex. An increase in the duration of the stimulus up to a certain value caused an increase in the magnitude of the response. A further increase in the duration of the stimulus was followed by depression of the response.

The importance of stimulus duration for both the initial and later segments of the response is demonstrated in the PST histograms of Fig. 8. Here, the

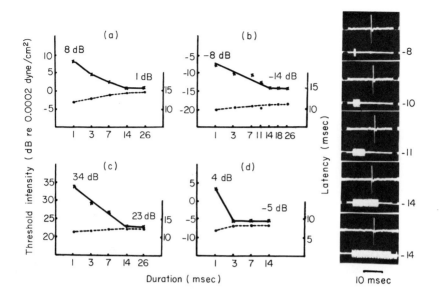

FIG. 6. Relation of threshold intensity (solid line) and latent period (dashes) to the duration of the noise burst. (a-d) Plots for four different units. Each plotted value is the mean for 20 responses. Threshold defined as that intensity at which one impulse occurred in the response with the probability of 0.5. Ordinate on left represents intensity in dB SPL; ordinate on right, latency (msec). Abscissa, duration of the stimulus in msec. Patterns on the right indicate threshold responses of unit B for different durations and intensities of the stimulus. Intensity of the stimulus in dB is indicated for each record. Upper trace shows unit response; lower trace, stimulus form.

initial discharge burst arising after a latent period of 20 msec increased in magnitude as the duration of the stimulus was increased from 7 to 14 msec. A further increase in the duration had no effect on that segment of the response. The late discharges arising at a fixed interval of 150 msec after the initial discharge increased in number with an increase in the duration of the stimulus up to 26 msec; their number decreased with a further increase of stimulus duration beyond 100 msec. The histograms further show that when prominent, the first group of late discharges is followed by a second pause lasting 100 msec (histograms for stimuli of 14 and 26 msec in duration). Concurrently with depression of the late discharges, the second pause became shorter (histograms for stimuli of 100, 200, and 300 msec in duration). It may be postulated that these pauses and periods of depression following the unit discharges are probably due to "recurrent" inhibitory effects.

The PST histograms in Fig. 9 demonstrate the importance of the duration of tonal burst (10 kHz) for the off-discharges of a neuron. Discharges arising with a latent period of 50 msec after switching off the stimulus are displaced

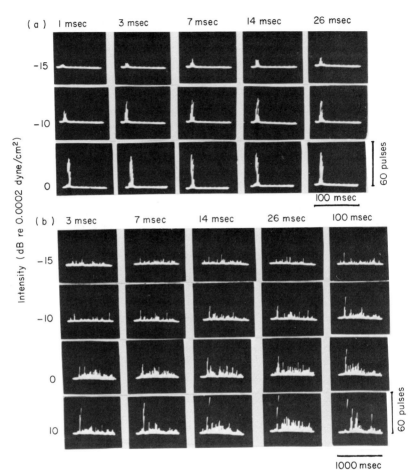

FIG. 7. PST histograms for a unit responding with sustained discharges to noise bursts of different duration at different intensity levels. Response consists of an initial burst and late impulses separated by a pause of 120 to 160 msec. (a) Histograms for initial burst, time of analysis, 100 msec; (b) histograms for late discharges, time of analysis, 1000 msec. Histograms based on responses to 60 stimulus presentations.

to the right in accordance with the duration of the stimulus. For a stimulus of 500 msec (the time of analysis of the histogram is also 500 msec) the expected response lies outside of the histogram display time. It is clear from Fig. 9 that no response occurred to a burst of 26-msec duration. A response was present when the duration of the stimulus was 50 msec, and it increased in magnitude with an increase in the duration up to 150 msec. It remained

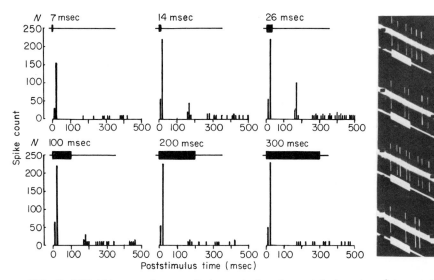

FIG. 8. PST histograms for a unit demonstrating the varied character of temporal summation in the late segment of the response. Stimulus: noise bursts of different duration. Duration of the stimulus is indicated for each histogram. Stimulus intensity: -1 dB SPL. On the right: four successive records of unit responses; upper trace: unit discharge; lower trace: noise stimulus of 500-msec duration. Histograms are based on responses to 60 presentations of the stimulus.

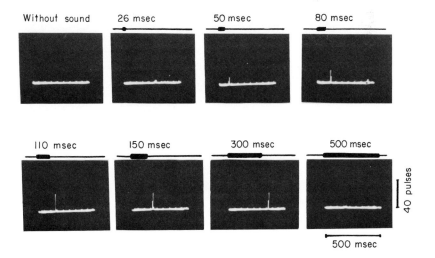

FIG. 9. PST histograms of a unit with an off-response pattern responding to tonal stimuli of different duration. Frequency: 10 kHz; intensity: 80 dB SPL. Histograms are based on responses to 40 presentations of the stimulus. Other explanations in text.

unchanged thereafter, despite a further increase in stimulus duration. However, an increase in magnitude of the response for this neuron cannot be regarded as the result of temporal summation since the time of 150 msec during which the effect of stimulus duration could be observed was much longer than the latent period of this particular response (50 msec). The absence of a response to a stimulus of 26-msec duration, its appearance at a duration of 50 msec, and the gradual increase in the response until the stimulus duration was 150 msec may have been due to an inhibitory effect, perhaps "afferent" in character, caused by switching on the stimulus. If this is so, it could be assumed that complete inhibition lasted 26 msec, after which it gradually became weaker, disappearing altogether after 150 msec.

Discussion

Single units of the auditory cortex of the cat were classified here on the basis of the stability of their responses to repeated auditory stimuli. Units whose latent period, spike counts, and response type are consistent functions of some stimulus parameters despite its repeated application constituted only 37% of the total number studied and were described as "stable" units. For these units, the relationships between the response characteristics and certain parameters of the stimulus are very similar to those found for the slow-wave primary response (PR) [1, 10, 26, and others].

For both spike and slow activity (PR) the increase in the response and the shortening of the latent period reached a maximum for stimulus intensity of up to 20 to 25 dB above threshold. It may thus be suggested that spatial summation reaches a saturation level at 20 to 25 dB. This range of intensities is also the limit for temporal summation in both fast and slow forms of activity. Furthermore, the degree of temporal summation (the change of threshold depending on stimulus duration) for the two types of activity is of the order of 9 dB, while the critical summation time (the time during which this shift takes place) is of the order of 10 to 12 msec for both types of activity.

Similarity between response characteristics of the initial discharge of "stable" units and PR is likewise observed in double-click experiments (Fig. 10). The amplitude of PR as well as the number of spikes produced by a single unit are enhanced when the stimulus is a pair of clicks. The optimal interval between two clicks which causes maximal facilitation was of the order of 4 msec for both forms of response. Finally, the coincidence in time of the arousal of these two different forms of activity seems significant. All these facts probably indicate that the PR and the initial discharges of "stable" units of the auditory cortex are in some way interconnected and mutually dependent.

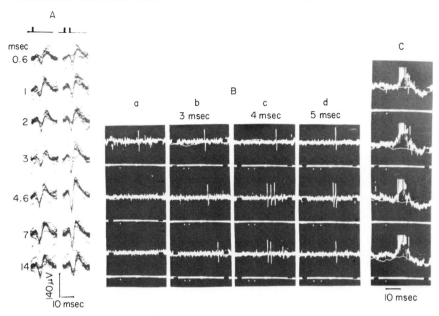

FIG. 10. Similarities between the characteristics of primary response (PR) and the early discharge of "stable" units in response to a pair of clicks. A: left column: PR to single click at an intensity of 15 dB above visual detection level; right column: PR to a pair of clicks at the same intensity with different intervals between clicks (numbers at left denote intervals between clicks in msec). Each record is a superposition of several traces. B: a - successive unit responses to a single click; b, c, and d - responses to a pair of clicks (numbers at the top denote intervals between clicks in msec for each column). All records at stimulus intensity at 65-dB attenuation. Upper trace: unit response; lower traces. B: a successive unit responses to a single click; b, c, and d—responses to a pair primary evoked response. Stimulus: single click at an intensity of 9-dB attenuation. Upper trace: responses; lower trace: time of stimulation.

However, the more important feature distinguishing the cortical units from the units of the lower levels of the auditory system is the dynamic change in their reactions to repetition of the stimulus. In one group of units (29%), this change was apparent and regular. It was expressed in some units by a gradual increase in magnitude of the response with preservation of the response pattern (14%); in others, by gradual extinction and disappearance of the response with repeated stimulation (15%). The dynamic change in another group of units (22%) was irregular and revealed no apparent trend. However, the proposed classification of cortical units is based on the pattern of dynamic changes of responses, which are evoked in anesthetized animals, and to stimuli that differ greatly from natural acoustic signals. It is of great importance to extend the studies to unanesthetized animals, with application of more adequate acoustic signals.

The characteristics of the "stable" cortical units are similar to the characteristics of units in the relay nuclei of the auditory system, and it may be that this group of units is responsible for the stability of the information received. The analysis of this information and an estimate of its significance for the organism is perhaps carried out by units that show dynamic changes in their reactions.

The units whose response is extinguished with repeated stimulation but which respond to the presentation of a new stimulus may belong to the group of "attention" units, first described by Hubel et al. [16] in the auditory cortex of an unanesthetized cat.

Evidently the extinction of the response with repeated application of the stimulus is not caused by adaptation. This is concluded because with a change in the characteristics of the stimulus, the response is immediately restored, and in some cases (for example, with frequency modulation of the stimulus), the extinguished response is not merely restored, but actually increases in magnitude, changing from a phasic-type to tonic-type response (Fig. 1). This phenomenon also indicates that cortical units can change their type of response abruptly depending on the conditions of stimulation.

Units which, with repetition of a stimulus, retain the information gained from that stimulus for some time are of special interest. With the presentation of another stimulus with different parameters, the newly obtained information does not obliterate the previous one, but joins it and is also stored for a long time. This phenomenon may be associated, in all probability, with a "short-term" or "operative" memory at the neuronal level.

The two opposed phenomena observed upon repetition of the stimulus i.e., a gradual increase of activity for some units and extinction of activity for others, may probably be understood if synaptic facilitation, analogous to post-tetanic potentiation, found in excitatory as well as inhibitory synapses [4, and others], is accepted as the mechanisms responsible for these phenomena.

It is common for cortical units to respond with sustained activity, which occasionally lasts for some seconds, even to stimuli a few milliseconds in duration. This prolonged activity of some cortical units is probably the result of reverberations [3, 10, 24, and others]. The possibility that other factors are responsible, e.g., dc potential changes [13, and others] cannot be excluded. It may be supposed that repeated application of the stimulus may cause potentiation of the discharges and their prolonged circulation in reverberating circuits, in which traces of the sensory stimulus are fixed ("short-term memory"). With further repetition, the stimulus is recognized from the stored trace and "habituation" to the signal occurs. According to Sokolov [25], habituation to repeated identical stimuli is the simplest form of acquisition of individual experience, of learning, i.e., of the conditioned reflex. However, the present results were obtained in anesthetized cats (chloralose), and not on waking animals and fluctuation of responses is more marked in waking animals than during sleep and anesthesia [5, 21, and others].

In these experiments, despite the presence of anesthesia, certain phenomena, observed for some of the neurons of the cortical projection zone of the auditory analyzer, must be regarded as true "learning" at the neuronal level. Consequently, one can speculate that a "waking" state of the analyzer is not essential, at least for some processes of "learning." The present study shows that under anesthesia the auditory analyzer is still capable of fixing information about an incoming signal and detecting and discriminating new sound signals. In all probability, the phenomena described can be associated with neurophysiological mechanisms for complex psychological manifestations which take place in the "subconscious" sphere of the brain and may be directly related to the "subsensory sensitivity" described by Gersuni [9].

Conclusions

If the stability of the response to repeated presentation of an auditory stimulus is used as a criterion, units of the auditory cortex of anesthetized cats may be divided into stable and a variable types.

"Stable" units are characterized by a response to each or most subsequent stimuli and by constancy of the temporal pattern of the response despite frequent repetitions of the stimulus. The possibility that the early discharges of stable units and the primary evoked potential in the auditory cortex may be interrelated and mutually dependent is discussed.

With frequent repetition of the stimulus, some "variable" units retain the information received about the stimulus for a long time, which is reflected in the pattern of the impulses corresponding to that particular stimulus. This phenomenon is regarded as a reflection of a "short-term" or "operative" memory at the neuronal level. The response of other "variable" units to repetition of the stimulus undergoes extinction when the stimulus is repeated.

Another group of "variable" units shows no apparent pattern in the variability of the response when stimuli are repeated.

It is common for some auditory cortical units to perform complex sensory functions, e.g., retention of the information received about a past sound signal, and detection and discrimination of new sound signals. Such "active" sensory functions which in respect to their integration level differ greatly from "passive-reflective" functions, are present even in the state of anesthesia.

It is postulated that a protracted storage of information about a signal for some units and extinction of the response for other neurons when the signal is repeated, may be due to "habituation" to the signal, or in other words, to "learning."

The possible significance of the phenomena described for the neurophysiological mechanisms underlying the "subconscious" or "subsensory sensitivity" is considered.

REFERENCES

1. Altman, J. A., and Maruseva, A. M. Evoked potentials of the auditory system. *J. Higher Nervous Activity (USSR)*, 15, 539-549 (1965) (in Russian).
2. Baru, A. V. Frequency differential limens as a function of tonal signal duration after ablation of the auditory cortex in animals (dogs). *In* "Problems of Physiological Acoustics" (G. V. Gersuni, ed.), Vol. 6: Mechanisms of Hearing, pp. 121-135. Nauka, Leningrad, 1967 (in Russian).
3. Burns, B. D. "The Mammalian Cerebral Cortex." Arnold, London, 1958.
4. Eccles, J. C. "The Physiology of Synapses." Springer, Berlin, 1964.
5. Erulkar, S. D., Rose, J. E., and Davies, P. W. Single Unit activity in the auditory cortex of the cat. *Johns Hopkins Hosp. Bull.* 99, 55-86 (1956).
6. Evans, E. F., and Whitfield, I. C. Classification of unit responses in the auditory cortex of the unanesthetized and unrestrained cat. *J. Physiol. (London)* 171, 476-493 (1964).
7. Evans, E. F., Ross, H. F., and Whitfield, I. C. The spatial distribution of unit characteristic frequency in the primary auditory cortex of the cat. *J. Physiol. (London)* 179, 238-247 (1964).
8. Galambos, R., and Bogdanski, D. F. Studies of the auditory system with implanted electrodes. *In* "Neural Mechanisms of the Auditory and Vestibular Systems" (G. L. Rasmussen and W. F. Windle, eds.), pp. 137-151. Thomas, Springfield, Illinois, 1960.
9. Gersuni, G. V. A study of subsensory reactions during the activity of the sense organs. *Sechenov Physiol. J. USSR*, 33, 393-412 (1947) (in Russian).
10. Gersuni, G. V. Organization of afferent inflow and the process of discrimination of signals of various duration. *J. Higher Nervous Activity (USSR)*, 15, 260-273 (1965) (in Russian).
11. Gersuni, G. V. On the mechanisms of hearing (in connection with studies of time and time-frequency characteristics of the auditory system. *In* "Problems of Physiological Acoustics" (G. V. Gersuni, ed.), Vol. 6: Mechanisms of Hearing, pp. 3-32. Nauka, Leningrad, 1967 (in Russian).
12. Gerstein, G. L., and Kiang, N.Y-S. Responses of single units in the auditory cortex. *Exp. Neurol.* 10, 1-18 (1964).
13. Gumnit, R. J. D. C. potential changes from auditory cortex of the cat. *J. Neurophysiol.* 23, 667-675 (1960).
14. Hind, J. E., Rose, J. E., Davies, P. W., Woolsey, C. N., Benjamin, R. M., Welker, W. I., and Thompson, R. F. Unit activity in the auditory cortex. *In* "Neural Mechanisms of the Auditory and Vestibular Systems" (G. L. Rasmussen and W. F. Windle, eds.), pp. 201-210. Thomas, Springfield, Illinois 1960.
15. Hubel, D. H. Single unit activity in striate cortex of unrestrained cats. *J. Physiol. (London)* 147, 226-240 (1959).
16. Hubel, D. H., Henson, C. O., Rupert, A., and Galambos, R. "Attention" units in the auditory cortex. *Science* 129, 1279-1280 (1959).
17. Katsuki, Y., Neural mechanisms of auditory sensation in cats. *In* "Sensory Communication" (W. A. Rosenblith, ed.), pp. 561-583. M.I.T. Press, Cambridge, Massachusetts, 1961.

18. Katsuki, Y., Watanabe, T., and Maruyama, N. Activity of auditory neurons in upper levels of brain of the cat. *J. Neurophysiol.* **22**, 343-359 (1959).
19. Lorente de Nó, R. Cerebral Cortex. *In* "Fulton's Physiology of the Nervous System" (J. F. Fulton, ed.), pp. 274-299. Oxford Univ. Press, London, 1943.
20. Maruseva, A. M. On the time characteristics of neurons of different types in the inferior colliculus of the rat. *In* "Problems of Physiological Acoustics" (G. V. Gersuni, ed.), Vol. 6: Mechanisms of Hearing, pp. 50-62. Nauka, Leningrad, 1967 (in Russian).
21. Murata, K., and Kameda, K. The activity of single cortical neurons of unrestrained cats during sleep and wakefullness. *Arch. Ital. Biol.* **101**, 306-331 (1963).
22. Oonishi, S., and Katsuki, Y. Functional organization and integrative mechanisms of the auditory cortex of the cat. *Jap. J. Physiol.* **15**, 342-365 (1965).
23. Radionova, E. A. On the significance of time characteristics of the response of the cochlear nucleus neurons. *In* "Problems of Physiological Acoustics" (G. V. Gersuni, ed.), Vol. 6: Mechanisms of Hearing, pp. 32-49. Nauka, Leningrad, 1967 (in Russian).
24. Shkolnik-Yarros, E. G. Neurons and Interneuronal Connections (The Visual Analyzer). "Meditzina," Leningrad, 1965 (in Russian).
25. Sokolov, E. N. Habituation as the simplest form of conditioned reflex. *J. Higher Nervous Activity (USSR)*, **15**, 249-259 (1965) (in Russian).
26. Vardapetian, G. A. Electrophysiological study of temporal summation in different levels of the auditory system of cats. *J. Higher Nervous Activity (USSR)*, **16**, 470-479 (1966) (in Russian).
27. Vardapetian, G. A. Dymanic classification of single unit responses in the auditory cortex of the cat. *J. Higher Nervous Activity (USSR)*, **17**, 95-106 (1967) (in Russian).
28. Vardapetian, G. A. Characteristics of single unit responses in the auditory cortex of the cat. *In* "Problems of Physiological Acoustics" (G. V. Gersuni, ed.), Vol. 6: Mechanisms of Hearing, pp. 74-90. Nauka, Leningrad, 1967 (in Russian).
29. Vartanian, I. A., and Ratnikova, G. I. Frequency localization and temporal summation in the auditory centers of the midbrain. *In* "Problems of Physiological Acoustics" (G. V. Gersuni, ed.), Vol. 6: Mechanisms of Hearing, pp. 62-74. Nauka, Leningrad, 1967 (in Russian).
30. Whitfield, I. C., and Evans, E. F. Responses of auditory cortical neurons to stimuli of changing frequency. *J. Neurophysiol.* **28**, 655-672 (1965).
31. Zaboeva, N. V. Temporal summation in the auditory cortex for stimuli of different frequencies and white noise. *In* "Problems of Physiological Acoustics" (G. V. Gersuni, ed.), Vol. 6: Mechanisms of Hearing, pp. 90-101. Nauka, Leningrad, 1967 (in Russian).

15

Absolute Thresholds and Frequency Difference Limens as a Function of Sound Duration in Dogs Deprived of the Auditory Cortex

A. V. Baru

The tonotopic organization of the auditory cortex, i.e., the spatial differentiation of neurons possessing selective sensitivity to various frequencies, which was established by determining thresholds for the evoked potentials, strychnine spikes, and discharges of single neurons [10, 20-23, 36, 37, 39, 41] suggested that the auditory cortex plays an essential role in the detection and discrimination of tonal pulses. However, a number of investigations [7, 8, 18, 30, 34, 35, 38] demonstrated that in cats and dogs the absolute thresholds for frequency discrimination of the long-lasting tonal pulses do not change after a bilateral ablation of areas AI, AII, Ep, IT, SII, and SS of the cerebral cortex.

This divergence between the results of the behavioral investigations and the data obtained from electrophysiological experiments concerning the primary evoked responses and single unit activity of the auditory cortex, is to some degree explained by recent investigations in which the function of the auditory cortex was studied by presenting sound signals of different duration. It was established that the information pertaining to the signal influences the primary evoked response for a critical time period of the order of 7 to 20 msec [16, 17]. It was found also that for signals of brief duration there was an increase in absolute thresholds for tonal and noise pulses in patients with local lesions of the auditory cortex [6, 15] and in animals with the auditory cortex removed, when the measurements were made on the ear contralateral to the side of the operation (1, 2, 3, 5).

The results of these studies led to an assumption that the earlier behavioral investigations failed to reveal the role of the auditory cortex in the detection and discrimination of the signal frequencies, because the thresholds were measured only for long-lasting tonal pulses (t=1 to 5 sec).

The purpose of the present work was to investigate in greater detail the role that the auditory cortex may have in discrimination of signals of different duration. For the work at hand we had to develop a method for monaural threshold measurements in animals; to establish the dependence of absolute thresholds and frequency difference limens on the duration of tonal pulses in intact controls; and to study the effect of auditory cortex ablation on the absolute threshold and frequency discrimination for tonal pulses with different duration.

Methods

SUBJECTS AND APPARATUS

The work was carried out on 20 dogs. We examined the audibility thresholds in 15 animals and the frequency difference limens for sound signals of 1- to 1000-msec duration in five dogs.

A Zg-2A generator of sound frequencies was used as a source of tonal signals; a G-2-12 generator produced a noise with a bandwidth of 20 to 20000 Hz. The duration of the pulses was controlled by a transistorized electronic switch with a low level of disturbances and smooth regulation of the phase [25]. Sound bursts were delivered through attenuators, calibrated in nepers, to a TD-6 electrodynamic earphone. The irregularity of the frequency characteristics of the earphone did not exceed ±4 dB in the range of 100 to 8000 Hz. The rise-fall time constant of the earphone was 0.6 msec for 1000 Hz. The segment of the sinusoid was switched on and off in zero phase. The experiments were conducted in a sound-deadened chamber. In order to avoid the difficulties inherent in maintaining an uniform free-field stimulation, we used a closed system with earphones mounted directly on the dog's head.

GENERAL PROCEDURE OF TRAINING

Avoidance technique was used to establish conditioned reflexes in the dogs. The advantage of this method was that when a conditioned reflex was established it was possible to obtain responses to 200 to 300 presentations of the signal during one experiment. The shock punishment in such an experiment was applied not more than 10 to 15 times, i.e., only when the animal did not lift its paw despite the application of a positive stimulus (a tone of

1000 Hz). A fixed position of the animal during the experiment made it possible to measure the monaural thresholds.

MEASUREMENT OF ABSOLUTE THRESHOLDS

When the animals began to respond—with a probability of 0.85 to 1.0—to signals with a duration of 1000 msec at an intensity of 60 to 70 dB above threshold for the motor avoidance reaction, we started to measure the absolute thresholds and frequency-difference limens. For the purpose of measuring the absolute thresholds, an extensive generalization of the response was developed, the dog was trained to respond to signals of different duration and intensity (from 1 to 1000 msec and from 80 dB above threshold to threshold value). The thresholds were measured by the method of limits. The intensity of the signals was reduced from an audible to an inaudible one initially in steps of 0.5 neper (4.33 dB) and then, with a gradual approach to the threshold, in steps of 0.1 Np (0.87 dB). The lowest intensity of the signal, at which the probability of detection was 0.5, has been taken as threshold. Measurements for the right and left ears were made alternately. The data obtained from measurements of the absolute thresholds were evaluated statistically. The values for threshold were averaged at each stimulus duration in individual animals, and in the whole series of experiments, and the dispersion of the data determined. When the distributions of the threshold values were estimated, the significance of the differences obtained in separate series of experiments, and the differences in the effect of the auditory cortex ablation were determined with Student's t-test.

MEASUREMENT OF FREQUENCY DISCRIMINATION

The difference limen for frequency (DL) was measured in two series of experiments which differed in the method of stimulus presentation (Fig. 1). In the first series [Fig. 1(a)] the animal was trained to lift its paw in response to a 1000-Hz signal of any duration, and not to lift it to signals of any other frequency, within the range of 500 to 990 Hz. In the second series* [Fig. 1(b)] the animal was trained to respond only to a change in the signal frequency. In the course of such experiments, a background signal—1000 Hz tonal pulses of definite durations which varied in different experiments—was presented with a frequency of 1.5 Hz. In response to a change in the frequency of the pulses the animal had to lift its paw; otherwise the paw was stimulated by a near-threshold current. In both series of experiments, the

---

* The methods for signal presentation and frequency-discrimination measurements in this series of experiments were the same as those described in previous investigations [7, 8, 34, 38].

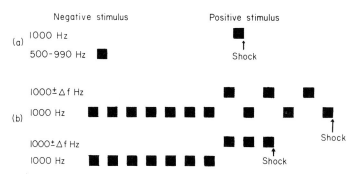

FIG. 1. Two methods (a) and (b) of stimulus presentation used in frequency-discrimination experiments. Lower squares in both successive rows represent standard (background) frequency; upper squares; comparison frequency.

frequency of the stimuli was changed so that it approached the frequency of the conditioned or background signal. In the second series of experiments this approach was gradual in steps of 20 Hz within the range of 800 to 900 Hz, and in steps of 10 Hz within the range of 900 to 1000 Hz. In the course of measuring the difference limen, tonal pulses of equal duration but of different frequencies were presented in a random order. In each experiment the measurements were performed only for signals of the same duration. The difference limens were measured for the following durations of tonal pulses: 1000, 220, 180, 100, 60, 40, 20, 10, 8, and 4 msec.

The measurements were done with signals of equal loudness. The loudness of signals of different duration was equalized to the loudness of a 1000 Hz tonal pulse with a duration of 1000 msec at an intensity of 60 to 65 dB above the threshold of the animal's hearing. This threshold was determined for tonal pulses of 1000-msec duration. In order to equalize the loudness of sound pulses of different duration, the intensity of the signals of 2- to 70 msec duration was, in accordance with Port [31], increased by 10 dB for a tenfold decrease of the duration of the pulses.*

The value of the differential threshold was calculated according to the χ^2 criterion. The significance of the difference between the distribution of responses to negative and positive stimuli was established at a confidence level of $p < 0.05$.

SURGERY AND HISTOLOGICAL PROCEDURES

After completion of preoperative testing, the auditory cortex was ablated under fully aseptic conditions. The operation was done under intratracheal

* The application to dog of the results obtained by Port [31] on human beings, does not apparently cause any substantial errors, since the dependence of the absolute thresholds on the duration of the sound signals is similar in man and dog.

anesthesia using a mixture of ether and oxygen which were introduced through an intubator. The brain tissue was removed by subpial aspiration with a small-gauge sucker. Bilateral ablations were done in two stages with an interval of 7 months, during which threshold measurements were carried out. In nine dogs extensive ablations of the auditory cortex were performed, including the cortex of the middle and superior parts of the anterior and posterior Sylvian gyri, as well as the cortex of the anterior, medial, and posterior ecto- and suprasylvian gyri. In some animals the ablation extended from above to the ectolateral gyrus, and from below to the posterior rhinal gyrus. In 11 dogs ablations were restricted to some parts of the auditory cortex, namely, to fields AI, AII, AIII, AIV, IT, SS, the entire ectosylvian or suprasylvian gyri. The testing started 10 to 14 days after the operation.

After completion of the experiments the dogs were sacrificed. The brains were removed, dehydrated in alcohol, embedded in celloidin and serially sectioned at 20 μ in a frontal plane. Every tenth section was stained with thionin or cresyl-violet. The sections were studied for retrograde degeneration of the cells in the posterior group of nuclei of the thalamus, the medial geniculate body and the inferior colliculus.

Results

THRESHOLD OF AUDIBILITY AS A FUNCTION OF SIGNAL DURATION BEFORE AND AFTER ABLATION OF THE AUDITORY CORTEX

The results of measuring the absolute thresholds for broadband noise pulses and tonal pulses of 1000 and 250 Hz, which vary in duration from 1000 to 1 msec, are presented in Fig. 2.

Figure 2(I) shows the thresholds for three normal dogs when sound signals were switched on and off at a random phase. Figure 2(II) shows the thresholds when the signals were switched on at a zero phase. When the duration of the signal exceeds 200 msec, the threshold for tonal pulses of 1000 Hz does not depend on the signal duration. At durations of less than 200 msec, the values for absolute threshold are an inverse function of the pulse duration. For signals of 1000 Hz this function may be approximated by two linear sections having a different slope. Within the duration range of 10 to 200 msec the slope of the curve is 10 dB per decade (i.e., for a tenfold increase in the duration of the pulse).

Probability functions for the animal's response to tonal pulse of 1000 Hz at different intensities are shown in Fig. 2(III). Each point on the curve represents an average of 100 to 1000 measurements in 11 dogs. A different duration of the pulses constitutes the parameter for the different curves. The data indicate that the deviations of the threshold values do not differ significantly from a logarithmic normal distribution.

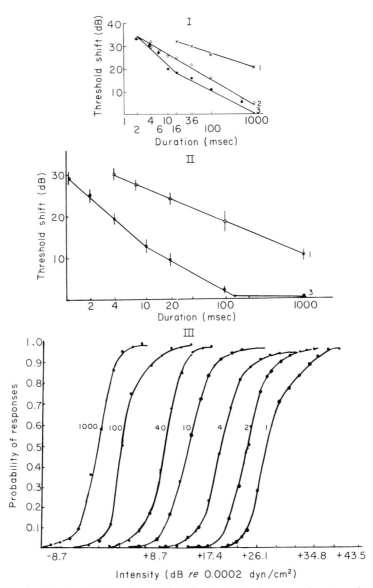

FIG. 2. (I) and (II) Mean threshold shifts in intact dogs as a function of stimulus duration. All measurements in reference to the threshold for 1000-Hz tone of 1000-msec duration. (I) Average values for three dogs for signals presented at random phase. Each point is a mean of 30 to 50 measurements. (II) Average values for 14 dogs for signals presented at zero phase. Each point is the mean of 400 to 1000 measurements. Curve 1 indicates the signal of 250 Hz; curve 2; white noise; curve 3; signal of 1000 Hz. (III) Graphs plotting the intensity of a 1000-Hz tonal signals of different duration against probability of the response. Each point is a mean of 100 to 1000 measurements. Data pertain to 11 dogs. Duration of the signal in msec is indicated for each curve.

The decrease in the absolute threshold, when the duration of the signal increases from 1 to 1000 msec, amounts to 29.5 ± 4.8 dB for pulses of 1000 Hz,* 33.1 ± 2.0 dB for pulses of 4000 Hz, and 28.0 ± 4.1 dB for broadband noise pulses; when the duration of the signals decreases from 1000 to 4 msec the threshold intensity of a pulse of 250 Hz increases by 18.75 ± 1.8 dB.

Prior to the operation the threshold values, measured by delivering the sound to the right or the left ear, did not differ by more than 2 dB in any animal.

The difference between threshold intensities for pulses of 1 and 1000 msec in duration, measured for six human subjects in the same experimental setup, was 24.5 dB for broadband noise and 27.0 dB for tonal pulses of 1000 Hz. These results are close to those of other authors [9, 42]. Thus, in intact dogs the dependence on their duration of the absolute thresholds for broadband noise pulses and tonal pulses of 250, 1000, and 4000 Hz does not essentially differ from that in human beings.

After a unilateral extensive ablation of the temporal cortex, including the superior parts of the anterior and posterior ecto- and suprasylvian gyri, the entire middle ecto- and suprasylvian gyri, as well as the superior portions of the anterior and posterior Sylvian gyri (areas AI, AII, Ep, SS), an increase in threshold was observed for signals with a duration of less than 16 msec, when measured for the ear contralateral to the side of the operation. When the sound signal was presented to the ear which was homolateral to the side of the operation, the thresholds did not change in comparison with the pre-operative values.

After removal of the auditory cortex of the other hemisphere in the same animals, similar changes in the threshold for brief signals were observed. However, even after bilateral ablations there was no change in thresholds for sound signals of long duration.

Figure 3 illustrates typical results of measuring threshold intensities for sound signals of different duration in the same animal before and after an extensive unilateral ablation of the auditory cortex. The thresholds for 1000-Hz tonal pulses of 1 to 2 msec in duration increased by 20 to 25 dB during the first 1 to 2 months. Eight to ten months after the operation this difference was 14 dB, while for white noise pulses of the same duration, it amounted only to 8.7 ± 0.4 dB. Further observations for 2 to 2.5 years after the operation did not reveal any further changes.

Similar results were in evidence after a removal of only the middle ecto-sylvian gyrus or of only the area AI. Figure 4 shows the results for two animals after ablation of a limited part of the auditory region. In dog No. 18,

---

* In our previous investigation [2] carried out on three dogs, we obtained a larger difference between the threshold intensities for 1000 Hz pulses of 1000 and 2 msec in duration (34.0 ± 4 dB). This is accounted for by the fact that the previous experiments we applied tonal signals presented at random phase [see Fig. 2(I)].

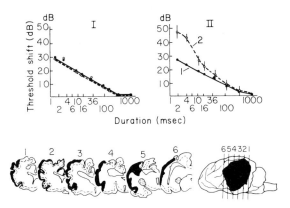

FIG. 3. Mean threshold shifts as a function of the duration of a 1000-Hz tone and extent of the cortical lesion in dog No. 4. Audibility thresholds before operation (I), and after a unilateral ablation of the auditory cortex (II). The solid line indicates measurements for the ear homolateral to the ablation area; dashed line, measurements for the ear contralateral to the side of operation. The lower right depicts the extent of cortical ablation. On the frontal sections (1 to 6) the areas of the ablated cortex are shown in black; the areas of the damaged and degenerated cortex and of the medial geniculate body are stippled.

area AI was fully removed. During the postoperative period of 1 to 1.5 months, the thresholds for short signals in both these animals increased by 20 to 22 dB, i.e., the increase was less by only 4 to 5 dB than for animals that had extensive ablations of the auditory region, including areas AI, AII, Ep, and SS. For these dogs the threshold increase is statistically significant only for durations of less than 10 msec. During the postoperative period of 2 to 4 months, the difference between the threshold intensities in these animals for brief signals (1 to 2 msec) before and after the removal of the auditory cortex amounted to 10 dB on the average [Fig. 4(I) and 4(III)], i.e., it did not essentially differ from the threshold increase in dogs with extensive ablations of the auditory cortex.

In animals with small ablations the maximal possible recovery of the thresholds was manifest 2 to 4 months after the operation; in animals with extensive ablations the maximal recovery did not occur before some 8 to 10 months postoperatively. Further recovery did not take place after both the small and the extensive ablations, even with the survival periods of 1 to 2 years.

After a partial removal of area AI, a small increase in absolute thresholds for brief signals was observed. But in contrast to the results with more extensive ablations, the defects in the perception of brief signals were fully compensated 2 to 4 months after the operation [Fig. 4(II)].

A unilateral isolated removal of Tunturi's third auditory area (AIII) did not result in any increase in thresholds. Similarly, an isolated removal of the

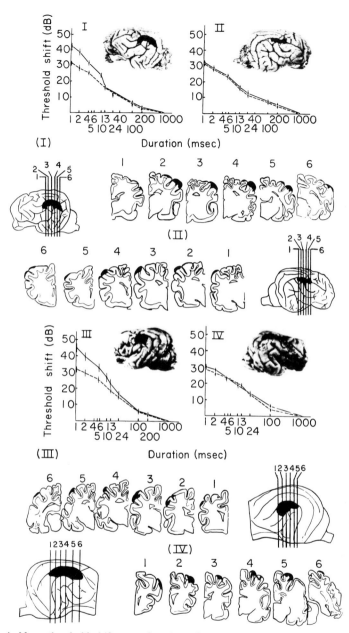

FIG. 4. Mean threshold shifts as a function of the duration of a 1000-Hz tone signal and extent of cortical lesions for two dogs. (I) Dog No. 18 after ablation of area AI in the left hemisphere. Measurements made in the 3 months after operation; (II) same dog after ablation of a part of area AI in the right hemisphere. Measurements 6 months after operation; (III) dog No. 19 after ablation of large part of the middle ectosylvian gyrus. Measurements made 4 months after operation; (IV) same dog after removal of the middle suprasylvian gyrus. Measurements made 5 months after operation. The solid line shows measurements for the ear contralateral to the side of ablation; dashed line, measurements for the ear homolateral to the side of ablation.

insulotemporal area (IT) or of the AIV area did not result in any threshold increase. However, a combined ablation of the IT and AIV areas led to a statistically significant increase in threshold intensity for sound signals of less than 10 msec in duration.

An ablation of the cortex of the middle syprasylvian gyrus, which was equal in its extent to an ablation of the cortex of the middle ectosylvian gyrus, but exceeded the extent of the brain substance removed during the ablation of the area AI, did not cause any permanent increase in thresholds for either the long-lasting or for brief signals [Fig. 4(IV)]. Only during the first postoperative month a small increase in the threshold for brief signals was observed. Apparently this was due to some traumatic effect on the adjoining parts of the middle ectosylvian gyrus possibly to a pressure exerted by a hematoma, or to a tissue edema.

A comparison of absolute thresholds after extensive and limited ablations of the auditory region indicates that during the early postoperative period an increase in thresholds after extensive ablations (for 1000-Hz pulses of 1 to 2 msec in duration) exceeds that observed after limited ablations by 4 to 5 dB; the maximal duration of the signal for which deficit occurs is 16 and 10 msec, respectively. The maximal recovery of function develops more slowly with extensive ablations. However, the noncompensated increase in thresholds is similar for both extensive and small (AI) ablations of the auditory region and amounts to 9 to 12 dB.

FREQUENCY DIFFERENCE LIMENS AS A FUNCTION OF DURATION OF TONAL PULSES IN DOGS BEFORE AND AFTER ABLATION OF THE AUDITORY REGION

Frequency difference limens were determined in five animals in two series of experiments that differed in the method of stimulus presentation (see "Methods," p. 266). The dependence between the value for DL (Δf) and the duration of the tonal pulse (Δt) obtained for all five dogs before the operation, is shown in Fig. 5 (curves 1 and 2 indicate the first series of experiments, and curve 3, the second series). The values for DL are averages from 20 to 40 experiments on individual animals (each point of the curve is a mean of 20 to 150 measurements). For animals No. 7 and No. 20 (curve 2), DL does not depend on the signal duration for $\Delta t > 100$ msec; for dog No. 8 (curve 1), the same is true for $\Delta t > 180$ msec. For shorter duration of the tonal pulses, the difference limen decreases as the duration of the pulses increases.

For two dogs (No. 7 and No. 20), in which the results of the measurements coincided, the limit of frequency discrimination for $\Delta t > 100$ msec was 20 Hz for a tone of 1000 Hz, i.e., 2% of the frequency value ($p < 0.001$). On different days during the whole experimental period of dog No. 8 could discriminate 1015 to 1020 Hz from 1000 Hz, the duration of the pulse being

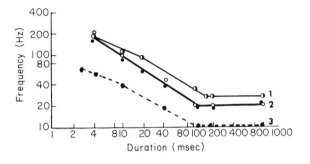

FIG. 5. Mean frequency difference limens in intact dogs as a function of the duration of 1000-Hz tone. Abscissa, signal duration in msec; ordinate, value of DL in Hz. Curve 1 demonstrates results of measurements in dog No. 8; curve 2, in dogs No. 7 and No. 20; curve 3, in dogs No. 27 and No. 29.

1000 msec. However, when the data for 20 experiments were averaged, the value of DL for this dog amounted to 30 Hz ($p < 0.002$). The values for frequency-difference limens in dog No. 8 were somewhat higher than in the two previous animals also in regard to other durations.

For dogs No. 27 and No. 29 (Fig. 5, curve 3), with a different method of stimulus presentation [see Fig. 1(b)], the limits for frequency discrimination were smaller than for the other animals for all durations of the signals. For the time range in which DL is independent of the signal duration ($t > 140$ msec), the DL value was 8 to 10 Hz or 0.8 to 1.0% of the frequency. For shorter signal duration ($t < 100$ to 180 msec) the curves, indicating the frequency difference limens as a function of the stimulus duration, can be approximated by two linear sections with different slopes (provided that the frequency and duration are plotted on a logarithmic scale). Irrespective of the absolute values of DL in the first and second series of experiments, the slope of the curves within the range from 100 to 180 msec to 10 to 20 msec does not manifest any substantial difference. For signal durations of less than 10 to 20 msec the slopes of the curves differ.

It should be noted that in the intact dogs, the DL for a given stimulus duration was the same regardless of whether the tone was delivered to the right or to the left ear.

Figure 5 indicates that the animals differed insignificantly from one another as regards DL values when a similar method of threshold measurement was used. Considerably greater differences between the animals were observed in tests characterizing the process of training.* Thus, in dogs No. 7 and No. 20, a conditioned reflex was established within a relatively short period of time

---

* The work of Rosenzweig [33] also revealed greater differences between the animals in tests involving learning (rate and stability of a habit, runs in a labyrinth) than in measuring the difference limen for signal intensity.

(during 30 experimental sessions) since within this time the animals reached the desired learning criterion (95-100% correct responses to presentations of signals of 1000 and 500 Hz). For dog No. 8, 60 sessions were required to reach the same criterion. Subsequently, when we passed from measuring the DL's for signals with a duration of 1000 to 100 msec to short signals with a duration of 20, 10, and 4 msec, dogs No. 7 and No. 20 had to be trained only in two or three sessions, while dog No. 8 required additional training in ten sessions.

The values of DL could be determined considerably faster in the second series of experiments when the responses of the animals to a change in the frequency of the signal were studied.

Difference limens obtained in the first series of experiments [method of stimulus presentation, see Fig. 1(a)] before and after an extensive ablation of the auditory cortex are presented in Fig. 6. This figure illustrates for three dogs the distributions of responses to tonal pulses which differed to a various degree from the frequency of the reinforced signal [preoperative Fig. 6(I); postoperative, Fig. 6(II)]. Despite individual variations among the animals, it is apparent that when the duration of the signal increases, the precision of the discrimination of the frequency (which is given by the slope of the curves) increases.

After a unilateral ablation of the auditory cortex no signs of postoperative amnesia were observed, since in the first postoperative session the animals properly responded to positive and negative stimuli during the presentation of long-lasting signals. The difference limen for a sound of 1000 msec in duration was somewhat larger than in the preoperative period (it amounted to 30 to 40 Hz); however, this DL increase did not substantially differ from that observed in intact animals after comparable time intervals between the experimental sessions. Moreover, during the second or third session, the DL values for tones 1000 msec in duration did not exceed 20 Hz, i.e., the limen value became the same as in the preoperative period.

Columns II and III in Fig. 6 present frequency-discrimination data for tones of different duration when the signal was delivered to the ear contralateral to the side of the auditory cortex ablation. The graphs in Fig. 6(III) illustrate the dependence of DL on the duration of the tonal pulse in the intact animal (solid line) and after the operation (dashed line). There is clearly an increase in the DL value for signals of 4 to 20 to 40 msec in duration. For all other durations the difference limen did not increase; in one of the dogs we even observed a statistically significant decline of the difference limen for signals of 1000 and 100 msec after the operation.

Ablation of the auditory cortex in the other hemisphere (the second operation) did not cause any substantial changes in the DL's, when the sound was delivered to the ear contralateral to the side of the first operation;

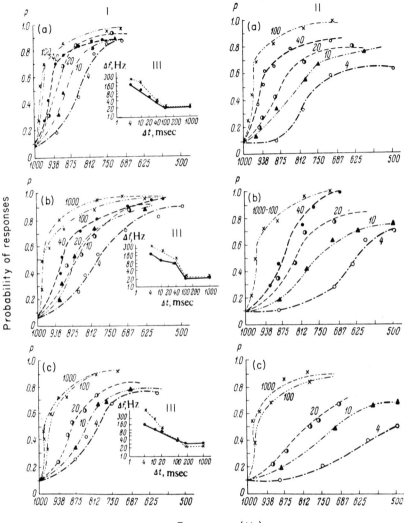

FIG. 6. Discrimination of frequencies by three dogs before (I) and after (II) unilateral ablation of the auditory cortex (the extent of the respective lesions for dogs No. 7 and No. 8 is shown in Fig. 8). Duration of the signal in msec is indicated for each curve. Abscissa, frequency in Hz; ordinate, probability of correct responses to nonreinforced stimuli. (a) Dog No. 20; (b) dog No. 7; (c) dog No. 8. (III) Difference limens for frequency (Δf) as a function of the duration of a 1000-Hz tone. Solid line: results before the operation; dashes: findings after the operation.

however, there was an increase in DL values for signals with a duration of less than 20 msec when the tones were delivered to the other ear.

Similar results were observed in the second series of experiments after an extensive ablation of the auditory cortex. Figures 7(I) and 7(II) show DL data after a bilateral ablation of the auditory cortex in dog No. 29. As was the case in the first experimental series, discrimination values for signal durations of 1000, 200, and 100 msec did not change after the operation in comparison with these values in the intact animal. By contrast, the discrimination for signals of 40, 20, 10, 6, and 4 msec in duration showed a considerable increase [Fig. 7(III)]. Dispersion of the DL values for signal of 2-msec duration was so large in different sessions that it was inpractical to plot these data. At this signal duration, the DL was 300 to 400 Hz in most sessions, although in some sessions it was as low as 200 Hz.

For signals that were 20 msec or shorter, all the animals, irrespective of the method of stimulus presentation, showed a considerable increase of the DL values (by 20 to 60 Hz, $p < 0.001$) after ablation of the auditory cortex. In dogs No. 7 and No. 29 such an increase was observed for a signal of 40-msec duration. The slope of the psychometric function was changed for all frequencies.

HISTOLOGY

Figures 3, 4, and 8 illustrate sections through the lesioned regions of the brain and indicate the extent of the ablations. The histological changes in brains of animals with extensive ablations of the auditory cortex are considered in some detail in dogs No. 7 and No. 8 [Figs. 8(a) and 8(b)].

In dog No. 8 the cortex of the superior parts of the anterior and posterior Sylvian gyri, as well as the whole cortex of the middle and posterior ectosylvian and suprasylvian gyri, have been removed in the left hemisphere. The cortex of the superior parts of the anterior ectosylvian and syprasylvian gyri was not directly affected by the operation, but the first and second layers were damaged as a result of scarring of tissue. The damage also partially affected a region in the occipital cortex. In the right hemisphere the following areas were removed: the superior parts of the anterior and posterior Sylvian gyri, the whole cortex of the middle ectosylvian and suprasylvian gyri, as well as the superior parts of the anterior and posterior ectosylvian gyri. The first and second cortical layers of the anterior suprasylvian gyrus were damaged due to scarring. In both hemispheres the cortex in the depth of the ectosylvian and suprasylvian fissures remained partially intact. In the regions adjoining the lesion, cellular edema, disintegration of the tigroid substance, and intense vacuolization of the cells were observed. Outside the limits of the lesion the cellular changes were of a reactive nature.

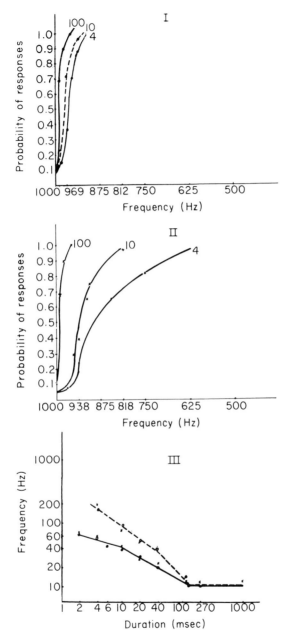

FIG. 7. Discrimination of frequencies for dog No. 29 (second experimental series) before (I) and after (II) bilateral ablation of the auditory region (areas AI, AII, Ep, SS). Duration of the signals in msec is indicated for each curve. Abscissa, frequency in Hz; ordinate, probability of correct response to a change in frequency. (III) Frequency-difference limens in Hz as a function of duration of a 1000-Hz tone. The solid line demonstrates results before the operation; dashed line, findings after the operation.

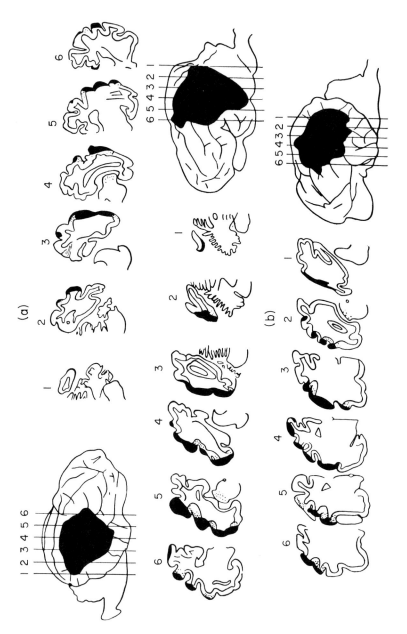

FIG. 8. Extent of cortical lesions in dog No. 7 (a) and dog No. 8 (b).

In dog No. 7 the ablation was less extensive; it included the cortex of the superior parts of the anterior and posterior Sylvian gyri, the whole cortex of the middle ectosylvian and suprasylvian gyri, and the superior parts of the anterior and posterior ectosylvian gyri. The cortex in the region of the anterior and posterior suprasylvian gyri was not primarily affected; however, the first and second layers were damaged due to scarring. The cortex in the depth of the ectosylvian and suprasylvian fissures remained intact. The nature of changes in the cells that adjoin the lesion is similar to that described for dog No. 8.

In both dogs degenerative changes occurred in the medial geniculate bodies, especially, in its small-celled part—a number of cells was destroyed, the amount of the tigroid substance in the preserved cells was decreased, and vacuolization and disintegration of cells were in evidence. Small-celled elements were almost totally absent in the anterior and middle thirds of the medial geniculate bodies. In the posterior third, the cell-changes were less pronounced. In dogs No. 7 and No. 8 the cells of the lateral geniculate bodies remained unchanged.

In dog No. 8 the more pronounced disturbances in the discrimination of brief sound signals corresponded to a somewhat more extensive ablation. This dog [Fig. 6(cII) and Fig. 6(cIII)] was unable to discriminate signals of 4-msec duration, even when the difference between the frequencies of the signals was 400 and 500 Hz.

For all animals with extensive ablations of the auditory region (particularly in dogs No. 7 and No. 8) degenerative changes were observed in some other thalamic nuclei. Some cells disappeared; in some others, the chromatophilic substance was dispersed; still other cells contained vacuoles in the cytoplasm and still others had irregular and rough outlines. Such changes were pronounced in the posterior nucleus and the pulvinar. A partial degeneration occurred also in the lateral nuclei (posterior, intermediate, and anterior), as well as in the posterior ventral nucleus of the thalamus. However, along with changed cells, a considerable number of intact cells remained in these nuclei.

In dog No. 7 the changes in the nuclei of the lateral thalamic group were less pronounced. Minimal degeneration of cells was observed in the posterior nucleus and in the pulvinar.

In dogs, in which only the primary auditory area (AI) was ablated, there were no degenerative changes in the lateral thalamic group; occasionally only single cells were encountered whose cytoplasm contained vacuoles.

Discussion

Our results suggest that there are two critical time periods when one measures the absolute thresholds, and the frequency difference limens as a function of duration of a tonal pulse in dogs before and after ablation of the auditory cortical region.

The first is that period of time of the signal duration within which one observes a dependence of the DL on the signal duration, i.e., when the auditory system performs a temporal integration of the signal. In dogs, this period is some 100 to 200 msec. Similar durations (about 200 msec) were established by us for man and this value agrees with the critical time during which the integration of a signal takes place in the human auditory system as determined by other [27, 42].

The second critical time period is 10 to 15 msec for absolute thresholds and 20 to 40 msec for the differential limen. This is that period of time of signal duration within which a deficit in frequency discrimination occurs after an extensive ablation of the auditory cortical region and within which an increase in absolute thresholds takes place after an extensive ablation of the temporal cortex, or after ablation of only area AI. It must be noted that the absolute threshold increases after a unilateral and bilateral ablation of the auditory cortex, do not depend on the spectral characteristics of the signals (tones of 1000, 4000 Hz, and a broadband noise).

As stated in the introduction, previous experimentation [7, 8, 34, 36] did not reveal any disturbances in the audibility thresholds, or frequency discrimination in the dog and cat after unilateral or bilateral ablation of the auditory cortex. The different results obtained in this study could conceivably be due to a different extent of the ablations, the method of investigation, different duration of the sound signals used. The deficit in frequency discrimination for brief signals cannot be explained by a greater extent of the ablation of the auditory region, since in our experiments such ablations were similar to, and in most cases even smaller than those described in the papers quoted. Moreover, an increase in absolute thresholds for signals of brief duration was also observed after an isolated ablation of only area AI. The methods of threshold measurement and of signal presentation are of great importance for disclosing deficits after ablation of the auditory cortex. Thompson [34], who with two different methods, investigated the discrimination of frequencies in cats after removal of the auditory cortex, showed that they could discriminate frequencies when the signals were long-lasting (t=1000 msec), when the method of training of Butler et al. [7, 8] was used, but when the method of Meyer and Woolsey [30] was applied the frequency discrimination by the same animals was deficient. In the present investigation an increase of frequency difference limens for signals with a duration of less than 20 to 40 msec was observed during the application of the two methods of stimulus presentation.

Consequently, the factor which disclosed the deficit in frequency discrimination in our experiments, a deficit which is demonstrable even after a unilateral and incomplete ablation of the auditory cortex was, we believe, the use of brief tonal pulses.

An increase in absolute thresholds for brief sound signals after an extensive ablation of the auditory region, or of area AI, is harmonious with previous work, in which an increase in absolute threshold for tonal and noise pulses of less than 7 to 10 msec in duration was observed in patients with lesions localized in the superior and medial divisions of the temporal lobe, or after ablation of these cortical regions [6, 14, 24].

A selective decline in thresholds for brief and long-lasting signals could be produced in normal subjects and in animals (before operation) by administering psychotropic substances with different mechanisms of action [caffein (Caf. natr. benz. 0.4) or amphetamine (0.015 to 0.02)]. After the administration of caffein we observed a statistically significant decrease in absolute thresholds (up to 5 dB) for sound signals of less than 16-msec duration ($p < 0.001$), while after the administration of amphetamine the absolute thresholds decreased for signals of all durations [4].

The data obtained suggest the existence in the auditory system of two spatially separate systems for analyzing signals with different time constants of integration: one with a short temporal integration of 20 to 40 msec; the second with a longer one of about 100 to 200 msec. Integration with a short time constant is possibly accomplished by short time constant neurons, which occur at all levels of the auditory system [12, 32, 39]. This system may be involved in transmission of information regarding spectral properties of the signal within very short time periods, in analysis of transients, in localization of the sound in space, and generally in operations that require precision timing [14]. It is possible that the role of the cortical projection zones in the discrimination of brief sounds is also connected with the capacity of some neurons in these zones to discharge for tens and hundreds of milliseconds after a sound signal (measured in milliseconds) has been delivered. This is probably due to reverberations in closed neuronal chains [11, 26, 28, 40]. Possibly, this mechanism is also responsible for the observation (made in a number of psychophysical experiments) that the perceived duration of a brief signal exceeds its physical duration [19]. In the intact animals, ablation of the auditory cortical region destroys some chains, in which reverberations may take place when a brief signal is presented and in this way may cause an increase in the absolute threshold and difference limens.

REFERENCES

1. Baru, A. V. Effects of lesions in the auditory cortex on detection of sound stimulus of different duration. *Abstr. 10th All-Union Conf. Physiologists, USSR, 1964,* Vol. 2, Pt. 1, pp. 79-80 (in Russian).
2. Baru, A. V. On the role of the temporal cortex in detection of sounds of different duration. *J. Higher Nervous Activity (USSR)* 16, 655-666 (1966) (in Russian).
3. Baru, A. V. Absolute and differential threshold for frequency as a function of signal duration after ablation of the auditory cortex in dog. *18th Int. Congr. Psychol. Symp. 15,* Publ. D-t, Moscow 1966. pp. 128-131.

4. Baru, A. V. Peculiarities in the detection of acoustic signals of different duration under the action of some drugs. *J. Higher Nervous Activity (USSR)* **17**, 107-115 (1967) (in Russian).

5. Baru, A. V. Frequency differential limens as a function of tonal signal duration after ablation of the auditory cortex in animals (dogs). *In* "Problems of Physiological Acoustics" (G. V. Gersuni, ed.), Vol. 6: Mechanisms of Hearing, pp. 121-135. Nauka, Leningrad, 1967 (in Russian).

6. Baru, A. V., Gersuni, G. V., Tonkonogii, I. M. Measurement of absolute auditory threshold of sound stimulus of different duration in temporal lobe lesions. *J. Neuropathol. Psychiat. (USSR)* **64**, 481-486 (1964) (in Russian).

7. Butler, R. A., Diamond, I. T., and Neff, W. D. Role of auditory cortex in discrimination of changes in frequency. *J. Neurophysiol.* **20**, 108-120 (1957).

8. Diamond, I. T., and Neff, W. D. Ablation of temporal cortex and discrimination of auditory patterns. *J. Neurophysiol.* **20**, 300-315 (1957).

9. Garner, W. R. The effect of frequency spectrum on temporal integration of energy in the ear. *J. Acoust. Soc. Amer.* **19**, 808-815 (1947).

10. Gerstein, G. L., and Kiang, N. Y-S. Responses of single cells in the auditory cortex. *Exp. Neurol.* **10**, 1-18 (1964).

11. Gersuni, G. V. Evoked potentials and discrimination of external signal. *J. Higher Nervous Activity (USSR)* **13**, 882-890 (1963) (in Russian).

12. Gersuni, G. V. Organization of afferent flow and the process of external signal discrimination. *Neuropsychologia* **3**, 95-109 (1965) (in Russian).

13. Gersuni, G. V. On the mechanisms of hearing in connection with studies of time and time-frequency characteristics of the auditory system. *In* "Problems of Physiological Acoustics" (G. V. Gersuni, ed.), Vol. 6: Mechanisms of Hearing, pp. 3-32. Nauka, Leningrad, 1967 (in Russian).

14. Gersuni, G. V., Baru, A. V., and Karaseva, T. A. On the role of the auditory cortical projection zone in discriminating acoustic signals. *J. Higher Nervous Activity (USSR)* **17**, 932-946 (1967) (in Russian).

15. Gersuni, G. V., Baru, A. V., Karaseva, T. A., and Tonkonogii, I. M. This volume, Chap. 16.

16. Gersuni, G. V., Gasanov, U. G., Zaboeva, N. V., and Lebedinsky, M. M. Evoked potentials of the auditory cortex and the time characteristics of the sound stimuli. *Biophysics (USSR)* **9**, 597-606 (1964) (in Russian).

17. Gersuni, G. V., Shevelev, I. A., and Likhnitsky, A. M. Dependence of the primary response of the auditory cortical area in alert cats on temporal parameters of the signal. *J. Higher Nervous Activity (USSR)* **14**, 489-497 (1964) (in Russian).

18. Goldberg, J. M., Diamond, I. T., and Neff, W. D. Frequency discrimination after ablation of cortical projection areas of the auditory system. *Fed. Proc. Fed. Amer. Soc. Exp. Biol.* **17**, 55 (1958).

19. Goldburt, S. N. Specifities of the human estimate of brief sound durations. *In* "Problems of Physiological Acoustics" (G. V. Gersuni, ed.), Vol. 6: Mechanisms of Hearing, pp. 150-158. Nauka, Leningrad, 1967 (in Russian).

20. Hind, J. E. An electrophysiological determination of tonotopic organization in auditory cortex of cat. *J. Neurophysiol.* **16**, 475-489 (1953).

21. Hind, J. E. Unit activity in the auditory cortex. *In* "Neural Mechanisms of the Auditory and Vestibular Systems" (G. L. Rasmussen and W. F. Windle, eds.), pp. 201-210. Thomas, Springfield, Illinois 1960.

22. Katchuro, I. I. Frequency localization within the auditory cortex of the cat. *Sechenov Physiol. J. USSR* **49**, 659-665 (1963) (in Russian).

23. Katchuro, I. I. Frequency localization in the acoustic cortex and the corpus geniculatum mediale. Dissertation, Leningrad, 1964 (in Russian).
24. Karaseva, T. A. Specifities of short sound signal estimate in cases of local injuries of the temporal lobe of the brain. *In* "Problems of Physiological Acoustics" (G. V. Gersuni, ed.), Vol. 6: Mechanisms of Hearing, pp. 135-146. Nauka, Leningrad, 1967 (in Russian).
25. Lebedev, A. P. Electronic gate with a low level of disturbances and the possibility of smooth phase control. *J. Higher Nervous Activity (USSR)* **16**, 742-746 (1966) (in Russian).
26. Livanov, M. N. The effect of inhibition on the neurons systems of cerebral cortex. *In* "The Reflexes of the Brain," pp. 64-72. IBRO, Nauka, Moscow, 1965 (in Russian).
27. Liang Chic-an and Chistovich, L. A. Frequency difference limens as a function of tonal duration. *Sov. Acoust. J.* **6**, 81-86 (1960).
28. Lorente de Nó, R. "Cerebral Cortex." *In* "Physiology of the Nervous System" (Fulton, J. F., ed.), pp. 274-300. Oxford Univ. Press, London, 1943.
29. Maruseva, A. M. On the temporal characteristics of the auditory neurons in the inferior colliculus of rat with different types of responses to sound stimuli. *In* "Problems of Physiological Acoustics" (G. V. Gersuni, ed.), Vol. 6: Mechanisms of Hearing, pp. 50-62. Nauka, Leningrad, 1967 (in Russian).
30. Meyer, D. R. and Woolsey, C. N. Effects of localized cortical destruction on auditory discriminative conditioning in the cat. *J. Neurophysiol.* **15**, 149-162 (1952).
31. Port, E. Über die Lautstärke einzelner kurzer Schallimpulse. *Acustica* **13**, 212-223, 1963.
32. Radionova, E. A. On the significance of time characteristics of the cochlear nucleus neurons. *In* "Problems of Physiological Acoustics" (G. V. Gersuni, ed.), Vol. 6: Mechanisms of Hearing, pp. 32-50. Nauka, Leningrad, 1967 (in Russian).
33. Rosenzweig, M. R. Discrimination of auditory intensities in the cat. *Amer. J. Physiol.* **59**, 127-136 (1946).
34. Thompson, R. F. The effect of training procedure upon auditory frequency discrimination in the cat. *J. Comp. Physiol. Psychol.* **52**, 186-190 (1959).
35. Thompson, R. F. Function of auditory cortex of the cat in frequency discrimination. *J. Neurophysiol.* **23**, 321-334 (1960).
36. Tunturi, A. R. Audio frequency localization in the acoustic cortex of the dog. *Amer. J. Physiol.* **141**, 397-403 (1944).
37. Tunturi, A. R. A difference in the representation of auditory signals for the left and right ears in the iso-frequency contours of the right middle ectosylvian auditory cortex in the dog. *Amer. J. Physiol.* **168**, 712-727 (1952).
38. Tunturi, A. R. Effects of lesions of the auditory and adjacent cortex on conditioned reflexes. *Amer. J. Physiol.* **181**, 225-229 (1955).
39. Tunturi, A. R. Anatomy and physiology of the auditory cortex. *In* "Neural Mechanisms of the Auditory and Vestibular Systems" (G. L. Rasmussen and W. F. Windle, eds.), pp. 181-200. Thomas, Springfield, Illinois, 1960.
40. Vardapetian, G. A. Characteristics of single unit responses in the auditory cortex of cat. *In* "Problems of Physiological Acoustics" (G. V. Gersuni, ed.), Vol. 6: Mechanisms of Hearing, pp. 74-90. Nauka, Leningrad, 1967 (in Russian).
41. Woolsey, C. N. Organisation of cortical auditory system: a review and a synthesis. *In* "Neural Mechanisms of the Auditory and Vestibular Systems" (G. L. Rasmussen and W. F. Windle, eds.), pp. 165-180. Thomas, Springfield, Illinois, 1960.
42. Zwislocki, J. Theory of temporal summation. *J. Acoust. Soc. Amer.* **32**, 1046-1060 (1960).

16
Effects of Temporal Lobe Lesions on Perception of Sounds of Short Duration

G. V. Gersuni, A. V. Baru, T. A. Karaseva, I. M. Tonkonogii

The purpose of the present work was to investigate the absolute thresholds for sound signals as a function of their duration in patients with temporal lobe lesions. The dependence of threshold intensity on the signal duration, which reflects the phenomenon of temporal integration (temporal summation), was repeatedly studied in psychophysical experiments [30].

The method of brief-tone audiometry is now widely used to establish the hearing capacity of patients with peripheral lesions of the auditory system [8, 15, 21, 26]. However, we do not know of any work that describes the application of this method for diagnosing central lesions of the auditory system, despite the fact that a number of electrophysiological, psychophysical, and behavioral investigations [11, 12, 13] suggest that detection and discrimination of brief sound signals are in fact significantly impaired when the lesion is localized in the auditory projection zone of the temporal lobe cortex.

In the patients examined, the local lesions in the temporal lobe were either of vascular origin, or were caused by extra- or intracerebral tumors or they were of traumatic or inflammatory origin. Some of the patients were examined before and after operative treatment. The control groups consisted of patients in whom the pathological focus was located outside the temporal lobe and of healthy untrained subjects.

Methods

In addition to the usual diagnostic methods practiced in the ear clinic, determinations of absolute thresholds for sound signals of varying duration were done in healthy, untrained adults and in pateints with focal brain lesions of various locations. We determined the threshold intensities for 1000-Hz tonal pulses and for broadband noise the durations of which ranged from 1.2 to 1200 msec. All thresholds were measured monaurally.

A sound generator of the Zg-24 type and a white-noise generator of the G-2-12 type served as sources of the sound signals. The required duration of the signals was obtained by means of an electronic switch with a low level of interferences and with a smooth regulation of the phase [22]. Rectangular signals with a minimal rise-fall time were generated. The segments of the sinusoid were switched on and off in the zero phase. The intensity of the pulses was regulated with attenuators calibrated in decibels. An electrodynamic TD-6 earphone with a time constant of 0.6 msec at a frequency of 1000 Hz was used as a sound emitter. The subject's verbal accounts were used for measuring the thresholds. In cases in which a verbal account was not practical, the subject was instructed to press a key. The thresholds were measured by the method of limits. The intensity of the signals was gradually reduced, at first by 5 dB, and subsequently near threshold by 1 dB. The lowest intensity of the signal, which the subject could detect with a probability of 0.5 was taken as the threshold value.

The sessions lasted 30 to 40 minutes. In order to exclude the influence of fatigue or training, the thresholds for the right and left ears were measured alternately.

The results of threshold measurements, for both individual subjects and for appropriate groups of subjects were successively averaged. The arithmetic and geometrical means, the median and the standard deviation, were the usual statistics determined. When the normal distribution of the threshold values was estimated, the significance of differences was determined by Student's *t*-test.

Two series of investigations were carried out. The first series consisted of patients with lesions of the cerebral cortex mainly of vascular origin who were hospitalized in the Bekhterev Psychoneurological Institute in Leningrad. The second series was composed of patients with brain lesions of varying etiology (brain tumors, consequences of cerebral traumas, inflammatory brain diseases) who were hospitalized in the Burdenko Neurosurgical Institute in Moscow.

Results

SERIES I

Thirteen patients* with focal brain lesions constituted this series. Twelve of these patients had softenings caused by disorders of cerebral circulation due to

---

* In addition, 23 patients with focal brain lesions of vascular origin have been recently investigated; in 13 of these patients, the pathological focus was localized in the temporal region [29].

atherosclerosis, hypertensive disease, or rheumatic vasculitis; in one patient an epidermoid cyst had been extirpated in the left temporoparietal region. In each case, the localization of the lesion was made on the basis of clinical, neuropsychological, and electroencephalographic data.

The patients were divided in two groups. The first group consisted of eight patients with lesions in the left temporal region—four with sensory-acoustic aphasia, three with sensory-amnestic aphasia and one with temporal conduction aphasia. The second group, which consisted of hospitalized control subjects, consisted of two patients with motor aphasia and right-sided hemiparesis, one patient with Gerstman's syndrome and apraxia, and of one with a softening focus in the brain stem. In one patient, not included in either of these groups, the softening focus was localized in the right temporoparietooccipital region. Three patients were 20 to 40 years old; 10 patients, 40 to 60 years old. The investigations were carried out 2 months to 2 years after the brain lesions had been diagnosed. Six healthy, adult, untrained subjects, aged 20 to 60 years, were investigated along with the hospitalized control subjects.

Audiometric determinations indicated that in all the subjects, including patients with temporal lesions, the thresholds for low and medium frequencies did not essentially differ from the normal levels. The observed rise in thresholds for high frequencies was within normal limits of such changes with age. Otoscopic examination did not reveal any abnormalities.

The results of measuring the threshold intensities for broadband noise pulses of different duration in normal subjects and in patients in the first and second groups are presented in Table 1.

In normal subjects, the threshold intensities for the right and left ear signals of the same duration were almost identical since the differences between them (up to 1 dB) are within limits of measuring errors and are statistically insignificant. The increase in threshold intensities caused by a shortening of the signals from 1000 to 1.2 msec is 24 to 25 dB. This value is in agreement with another work [9].

As was the case for the normal subjects, there was no asymmetry in thresholds for patients with lesions located outside the temporal lobe (Group II). The difference in threshold values between sounds of long and short duration amounted to 28 dB and was therefore somewhat higher than in the control group (24 to 25 dB).

In sharp contrast to these observations there are highly significant differences between the thresholds for the right and left ear signals of short durations (3.6 and 1.2 msec) in patients of the first group, in whom the pathological focus was located in the cortex of the temporal lobe. The threshold changes were due to an increase of the absolute thresholds for brief sounds delivered to the right ear, i.e., the ear contralateral to the temporal pathological focus. On the average, the threshold increase amounted to 9 dB, the individual values ranging from 6 to 23 dB. The difference in threshold values between the longest and shortest sounds for the right ear signal

TABLE 1

Dependence of Threshold Intensity for Broadband Noise Pulses (in dB) on Duration of the Signal.[a]

Group[c]		Sound duration in msec					
		1000	100	19	7.2	3.6	1.2
I	Right ear $\bar{X} \pm \sigma$	0	4.0 ± 1.3	9.0 ± 1.7	15.0 ± 1.9	26.0 ± 1.4	35.0 ± 0.7
	Left ear $\bar{X} \pm \sigma$	0	4.0 ± 1.8	9.0 ± 1.7	14.0 ± 1.8	18.0 ± 1.3	26.0 ± 1.2
	Difference in dB	0	0	0	1	8	9
	Significance	–	–	–	not sign.	$p < 0.001$	$p < 0.001$
II	Right ear $\bar{X} \pm \sigma$	0	3.0 ± 1.5	9.0 ± 2.1	17.0 ± 1.5	21.0 ± 1.6	28.0 ± 1.5
	Left ear $\bar{X} \pm \sigma$	0	4.0 ± 1.7	10.0 ± 1.8	18.0 ± 0.9	22.0 ± 1.1	28.0 ± 1.9
	Difference in dB	0	1	1	1	1	0
	Significance	–	–	–	not sign.	1	1
Normal	Right ear $\bar{X} \pm \sigma$	0	4.0 ± 1.5	12.0 ± 2.7	15.0 ± 2.7	19.0 ± 1.3	25.0 ± 2.2
	Left ear $\bar{X} \pm \sigma$	0	4.0 ± 2.2	12.0 ± 2.9	16.0 ± 3.1	18.0 ± 1.6	24.0 ± 2.4
	Difference in dB	0	0	0	1	1	1
	Significance	–	–	–	not sign.	1	1

[a] Threshold intensity of broadband noise pulses of 1000-msec duration was taken as a zero reference level.

[b] Symbol $\bar{X} \pm \sigma$ denotes the mean value of threshold intensity and the standard deviation of the mean.

[c] Group I; patients with lesions localized in the cortex of the temporal lobe; Group II; patients with lesions localized outside the temporal lobe; Normal healthy, untrained adults.

was 35 dB; for the left ear signal, i.e., on the side of the temporal pathological focus, this difference was 26 dB. The latter value closely approached that obtained for normal subjects.

Figure 1 illustrates typical findings for two patients with lesions in the left temporal lobe (II and III) and for one patient with a lesion in the left frontocentral region (IV). Data in Fig. 1 (II and III) indicate that in both patients with lesions localized in the left temporal lobe the thresholds for brief signals were higher for right ear signals, i.e., for signals delivered to the ear contralateral to the lesion, rather than for signals delivered to the left ear. No such difference is present for the patient with a lesion localized outside the temporal lobe or for the normal subjects (Fig. 1, I and IV).

The results lead to the following conclusion. The relation of threshold intensity to the duration of the sound reveals a selective deterioration in discrimination of brief sounds for certain brain lesions.* The thresholds for

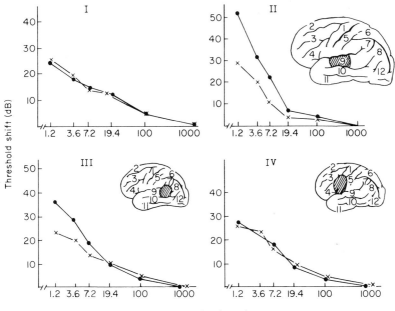

FIG. 1. Thresholds for audibility of broadband noise pulses of variable duration. I represents six normal subjects; II, a case of temporal conduction aphasia (patient G); III, a case of sensory-acoustic aphasia (patient Br); IV, a case of focal softening in the left frontal and anterior central region, with motor aphasia and right-side hemiparesis (patient Bo). Crosses indicate threshold values for the left ear signals; circles, threshold values for the right ear signals. Threshold for pulses of 1000 msec duration was taken as zero level.

* Similar results were obtained in 23 additional patients with local brain lesions of vascular origin [29].

brief sounds is increased for sounds presented to the ear contralateral to the lesion in those patients in whom the lesion occurs in the superior-posterior parts of the left temporal lobe, which is typical for sensory aphasia. However, we failed to established any peculiar features in threshold detection in patients with sensory-acoustic, sensory-amnestic and temporal conduction aphasias, i.e., when the lesion was localized in other parts of the left temporal lobe.

Since it is difficult to judge which particular temporal lobe structures may affect the thresholds in patients with vascular brain lesions, we studied the perception of sound signals of different duration in patients with focal brain lesions in a neurosurgical clinic, where more precise methods for localizing pathological foci are available, and where one can verify during surgical operation the affected brain area. Our aim was also to explore, in patients who were subjected to surgery, the relation between the increase in threshold intensity for sounds of short duration and the extent of the removal of the temporal lobe, as well as the relation of such thresholds to the duration of the pathological process.

SERIES II

This series consisted of 96 patients, ranging in age between 8 and 62 years and hospitalized in the Burdenko Institute of Neurosurgery in Moscow. The largest single group was formed by 68% of all patients who had brain tumors; 15% suffered from consequences of cerebral traumas, 14% from inflammatory brain diseases, and 3% from vascular diseases. Whereas the patients suffered from diverse diseases, a common clinical feature was the strongly pronounced character of the focal brain lesion against background of a satisfactory general state.

As regards the localization of the pathological focus, patients with lesions of the left or right temporal lobe constituted the largest group (52 patients). The control group consisted of 27 patients with lesions in the cerebral hemisphere where the focus was localized outside the temporal lobe, nine patients with lesions localized in the brain stem structures of the auditory system, eight patients with hypertensive-hydrocephalic syndrome, without any distinct localization of the pathological focus. The control group also included eight normal subjects whose age varied between 19 and 65 years.

Investigations took place in 47 patients before the operation, 32 after the operation, and 17 both before and after the surgical procedure.

The localization of the pathological focus was determined by extensive diagnostic procedures which included neurological, electrophysiological, and contrast roentgenological (angio- and pneumographic) methods. The status of higher cortical functions was evaluated by psychological procedures conducted according to the method of Luria [23]. Sixty-five diagnoses were verified during surgical operation and six during autopsy.

In no case did the tonal audiometry and tuning-fork examination reveal any changes which could be related to the localization of the pathological focus. Examination of eight normal, untrained subjects in this series showed that the difference between the threshold intensities for signals of 1200 and 1 msec duration was in either ear equal to 25 to 26 dB.

Threshold measurements, determined before and after the operation in 52 patients with lesions localized in different parts of the temporal lobe, demonstrated that an increase in threshold to sound bursts, the duration of which was less than 7 msec, was observed only when the pathological focus was localized in the superior part of the temporal lobe of 37 patients, irrespective of the nature of the lesion (tumors, vascular, traumatic, and inflammatory foci).

When the pathological process was localized in the basal or polar regions of the temporal lobe of 15 patients, no disturbances were observed in perception of brief sounds. There was no also increase in the absolute threshold for signals of short duration in 28 patients with lesions in the cerebral hemispheres when the pathological foci were localized outside the temporal lobe. Typical curves illustrating the relation of threshold intensities to the duration of the signal are shown in Fig. 2 (I, II, and III) for normal subjects and for patients with various localizations of the pathological focus.

The degree of threshold increase was a function of the extent of brain damage. Prior to the operation, the impairment in brief sound detection was, as a rule, most pronounced in patients with intracerebral tumors of the temporal lobe. This may be explained by damage to the auditory pathway passing in the depth of the temporal lobe as a compact bundle.

The defect in brief sound perception was most pronounced in those patients in whom the temporal lobe was either completely removed surgically (one observation) or in patients in whom a large resection of the superior temporal plane had been performed. In patients examined 2 to 12 weeks after excision of large portions of the superior and middle temporal gyri because of tumors, the findings for tonal pulses of 1000 Hz were as follows. The difference between the thresholds for pulses 1 msec long and those lasting 1200 msec was equal to 24 ± 3.35 dB if the sound was delivered to the ear homolateral to the lesion. This is 1.6 dB less than in the control group. By contrast, the difference in thresholds for such pulses delivered to the contralateral ear was equal to 40.3 ± 5.79 dB, i.e., 16.3 dB more than on the side homolateral to the lesion ($p < 0.02$), and 14.4 dB more than in the control group. For white-noise pulses, this difference amounted to 23.5 ± 1.2 dB on the side of the lesion, while on the opposite side it was 35.00 ± 1.93, i.e., 11.5 dB more ($p < 0.02$).

It should be noted that out of 37 patients with impairment of brief sound perception, the pathological focus was localized in the left hemisphere in 22 patients, in the right hemisphere in 15 patients. An increase in the contra-

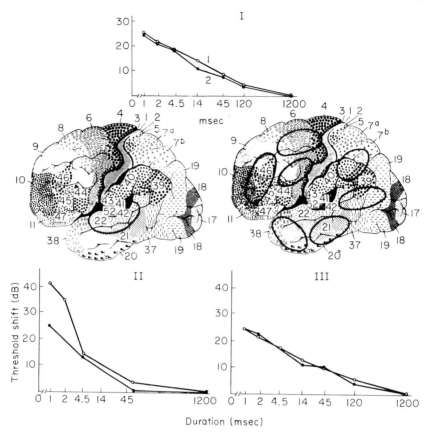

FIG. 2. Typical curves for audibility thresholds of 1000 Hz tone as a function of its duration. I represents normal subjects; II, patients with lesions localized in the superior part of the temporal lobe; III, patients with lesions localized in the basal and frontal regions of the temporal lobe and outside the temporal lobe. Open circles indicate threshold values for signals contralateral to the pathological focus; filled circles, threshold values for signals homolateral to the pathological focus. The affected areas are outlined on Brodmann's cytoarchitectonic chart of the human brain.

lateral threshold values for sounds of short duration was observed in all the patients regardless of whether the lesion was in the left or right hemisphere.

Figure 3(a) graphs threshold measurements for patient K, who had partial damage of the cortical auditory zone and its pathways in the right temporal lobe caused by an intracerebral tumor. Before the operation, the difference between threshold intensities for tonal pulses, the duration of which was 1200 and 1 msec, respectively, was 6 dB higher for the signal delivered to the ear contralateral to the focal lesion than for the homolateral signal. After the operation, during the course of which a considerable part of the right temporal lobe infiltrated by the tumor was resected, this difference increased to 17 dB.

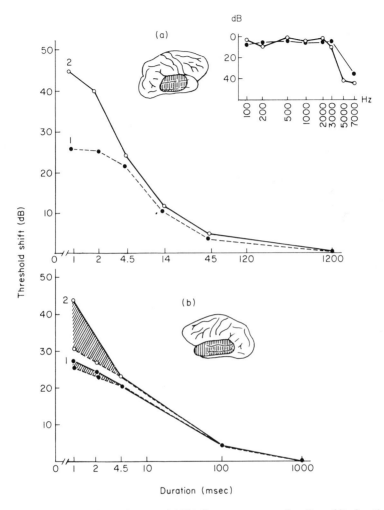

FIG. 3. Thresholds for audibility of 1000 Hz pure tone as a function of its duration in two patients with lesions of the superior part of the temporal lobe in the right and in the left hemisphere respectively. (a) Data for patient K. after resection of the superior and middle temporal gyri of the right hemisphere because of a tumor. Curve 1 indicates the curve for right ear, (signals homolateral to the cortical resection); curve 2 identifies the curve for left ear (signals contralateral to the cortical resection). (b) Data for patient S, shown before operation in curve 1, and after excision of the left temporal lobe infiltrated by a tumor, curve 2.

In patient S [Fig. 3(b)], who suffered from an intracerebral tumor in the left temporal lobe, the difference between the thresholds for the contralateral and ipsilateral signals was also 6 dB. After the removal of the left temporal lobe this difference was 16 dB.

These findings illustrate that the threshold intensities for brief signals increase for the signals delivered to the ear contralateral to the lesion regardless of whether the left (dominant) or the right (subdominant) hemisphere is damaged.

The increase in the threshold intensities for brief sound signals seems a permanent phenomenon. Thus, in three patients with intracerebral lesions caused by penetrating wounds in the left superior temporal area, who were examined 20 to 24 years after they had been wounded and 14 to 18 years after excision of the meningeal cicatrices, the threshold for brief sounds delivered to the ear contralateral to the lesion was increased by 6 to 9 dB.

In 20 patients, there was a temporal lobe lesion combined with a damage to the peripheral hearing apparatus. Of these, ten patients suffered from conductive-type deafness with a loss of hearing of more than 10 to 15 dB at all frequencies; ten others had perceptive-type deafness accompanied by a considerable loss of hearing for 4000 Hz and higher. The examination showed that lesions of the peripheral division of the auditory system do not prevent a manifestation of an increase of threshold intensities to brief signals contralateral to the temporal locus of the pathological process.

Measurements of the threshold intensities for sound signals of different duration were also carried out in nine patients who had lesions in the auditory brain stem structures at various levels (medulla oblongata near the bottom of the fourth ventricle, lateral lemniscus and posterior quadrigeminal bodies). These measurements did not reveal any clear disturbance in the perception of brief sound signals.

While most patients with lesions of the cortical auditory area did not exhibit any loss of hearing in the course of the usual audiometric examination, in which long-lasting sound signals were used, we observed an increase in thresholds for long-lasting signals up to 10 dB in patient R who had lesions localized in the quadrigeminal bodies. Moreover, in patient W who had lesions of the cochlear nuclei,* there was a considerable loss of hearing (20 to 35 dB). Therefore, the difference between the threshold intensities for signals with a duration of 1 and 1200 msec respectively was in all patients of this group smaller than in normal subjects. This can be explained by a predominant increase in the threshold values for long-lasting signals (Fig. 4).

A diminished capacity for temporal summation is, according to several authors [8, 15, 21, 26], characteristic also of patients with perceptive-type deafness.

Thus, only when the pathological process is localized in the cortex of the temporal lobe, there occurs an increase in threshold intensities for sound signals which are contralateral to the focus of the lesion and whose duration is less than 14 to 7 msec.

---

* These observations were verified during autopsy [19].

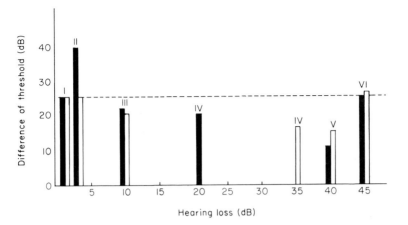

FIG. 4. Difference between threshold values for tonal pulses of 1000 Hz of 1200- and 1.2-msec duration in healthy, untrained subjects and in patients with lesions of the auditory system at different levels. I demonstrates normal subjects; II, patients with lesions of the auditory cortex; III, patient R with lesions in the inferior colliculus and lateral lemniscus; IV, patient W with lesions of the cochlear nuclei; V, patient M with perceptive-type deafness [21]; VI, patient P with conductive-type deafness [21]. White columns show difference in thresholds for signals delivered to the ear homolateral to the lesion; black columns, difference in thresholds for signals delivered to the ear contralateral to the lesion. Abscissa, hearing loss in decibels for a long-lasting 1000-Hz tone; ordinate, difference of threshold intensities in dB.

Morphological verification (six autopsies), performed by one of us [19], showed that in cases of defective detection of brief sounds, there was always in evidence a lesion involving the cortex of Heschl's gyrus as well as a lesion in the auditory tract, with subsequent retrograde degeneration of the cells in the medial geniculate body.

In two patients, in whom a tumor was localized in the temporal lobe, one could have expected some hearing deficits on the basis of clinical data. However, our examination revealed no defects of brief sound perception. This suggested that the auditory cortex was intact and this inference was confirmed by autopsy. Examination of serial histological sections of the brain revealed that the cortex of Heschl's gyrus, the central auditory tract and the medial geniculate body were intact.

Our data indicate that the destruction of the cortex of the superior temporal plane (projection of the auditory tract) resulting from a pathological process or its surgical removal, does not lead to any appreciable increase of the absolute thresholds for stationary sound signals. However, the removal or destruction of these regions both in the right (dominant) and left (subdominant) hemispheres results in an increase of the threshold intensities for sound signals if their duration is less than 10 msec and if these signals are delivered to the ear contralateral to the affected temporal lobe.

Thus, our data differ greatly from the results of previous investigations which failed to reveal any auditory disturbances characteristic of patients with cortical lesions. See references 6, 18, and 24.

The tests commonly used for diagnosing central auditory lesions present organized verbal or musical signals; they are applied under conditions where the excess of information is reduced by filters, temporal compression, periodical interruption, and introduction of interferences either by the announcer's text or by introduction of a background noise presented to the homolateral or contralateral ear.

This approach to the functional evaluation of the auditory cortex is based on utilization of its specifically human functions which cannot be revealed in experimentation on animals [7, 18, 20, 25, 27].

There is no doubt, however, that the human auditory cortex, which is the result of evolutionary development, must also possess some functions which are also present in animals. The functional deficits, which were established by us in patients with local lesions of the temporal lobe, are in full agreement with the results of experimental investigations carried out on animals. Thus, after an extensive removal of the temporal lobe cortex performed in dogs or after removal of area AI only, there is an increase in the absolute thresholds for sound signals of less than 10 to 16 msec in duration [2, 3]. If one performs an extensive ablation of the auditory cortex in the dog one observes an increase in the frequency difference limens and impaired discrimination of signals of short duration [4, 16]. This duration (10 to 16 msec) coincides with the time of temporal summation estimated by the threshold measurements of the primary evoked potentials and single units responses in the first auditory areas in animals [10, 28].

Moreover, we have demonstrated previously [1] that patients with lesions localized in the cortex of the temporal lobe do not discriminate tonal and noise pulses with different risetime constants. Similar data were obtained on dogs after a bilateral ablation of the temporal lobe [17].

The impairment in perception of sounds of short duration in patients with temporal lobe lesions may result from a defect in short-time memory. The hypothesis of the existence of a mechanism which makes possible the discrimination of brief sounds on the basis of "reproduction" (short-time memory), was advanced by Gersuni in 1963. As a consequence of relatively long reverberation of the excitatory process in neural circuits, this reproducing apparatus may put into operation a slowly reacting discriminating mechanism and prolong the effect of the brief signal action to the required extent.

REFERENCES

1. Avakian, R. V., Baru, A. V., Gersuni, G. V., and Tonkonogii, I. M. Threshold of audibility and discrimination of sound stimuli with different rise-time in patients with

temporal lobe lesions. *Rep. 20th Conf. Higher Nervous Activity, USSR, 1963*, p. 6 (in Russian).

2. Baru, A. V. Effects of lesions in the auditory cortex on detection of sound stimulus of different duration. *Abstr. 10th All-Union Conf. Physiologists, USSR, 1964*, Vol. II Pt. 1, pp. 79-80 (in Russian).

3. Baru, A. V. On the role of the temporal cortex in detection of sounds of different duration in the dog. *J. Higher Nervous Activity (USSR)* **16**, 655-666 (1966) (in Russian).

4. Baru, A. V. Frequency differential limens as a function of tonal signal duration after ablation of the auditory cortex in animals (dogs). *In* "Problems of Physiological Acoustics" (G. V. Gersuni, ed.), Vol. 6: Mechanisms of Hearing, pp. 121-135 Nauka, Leningrad, 1967 (in Russian).

5. Baru, A. V., Gersuni, G. V., and Tonkonogii, I. M. Measurement of absolute auditory threshold of sound stimulus of different duration in temporal lobe lesions. *J. Neuropathol. Psychiatry (USSR)* **64**, 481-486 (1964) (in Russian).

6. Bocca, E., and Calearo, C. Central hearing processes. *In* "Modern Developments in Audiology" (J. Jerger, ed.), pp. 337-370. Academic Press, New York, 1963.

7. Bocca, E., Calearo, C., and Cassinari, V. A new method for testing hearing in temporal lobe tumors. *Acta Oto-Laryngol.* **44**, 219-221 (1954).

8. Elliott, L. L. Tonal thresholds for short-duration stimuli as related to subject hearing level. *J. Acoust. Soc. Amer.* **35**, 578-580 (1963).

9. Garner, W. R. The effect of frequency spectrum on temporal integration of energy in the ear. *J. Acoust. Soc. Amer.* **19**, 808-815 (1947).

10. Gasanov, U. G. Threshold of evoked potentials of the auditory cortex in wakeful cats for signals of different duration. *In* "Problems of Physiological Acoustics" (G. V. Gersuni, ed.), Vol. 6: Mechanisms of Hearing, pp. 101-108. Nauka, Leningrad, 1967 (in Russian).

11. Gersuni, G. V. Evoked potentials and discrimination of external signal. *J. Higher Nervous Activity (USSR)* **13**, 882-890 (1963) (in Russian).

12. Gersuni, G. V. On the mechanisms of hearing in connection with studies of time and time-frequency characteristics of the auditory system. *In* "Problems of Physiological Acoustics" (G. V. Gersuni, ed.), Vol. 6: Mechanisms of Hearing, pp. 3-32. Nauka, Leningrad, 1967 (in Russian).

13. Gersuni, G. V., Gasanov, U. G., Zaboeva, N. V., and Lebedinsky, M. M. Evoked potentials of the auditory cortex and the time characteristics of the sound stimuli. *Biophysics (USSR)* **9**, 597-606 (1964).

14. Gersuni, G. V., Baru, A. V., and Karaseva, T. A. On the role of the auditory cortical projection zone in discriminating acoustic signals. *J. Higher Nervous Activity (USSR)* **17**, 932-946 (1967) (in Russian).

15. Harris, J. D., Haines, H. L., and Myers, C. K. Brief-tone audiometry (Temporal integration in the hypacusic). *A. M. A. Arch. Otolaryngol.* **67**, 699-713 (1968).

16. Hananashwili, M. M. The role of auditory cortex in sound discrimination in dogs. *Abstr. 10th All-Union Conf. Physiologists, USSR, 1964*, Vol. 2, Pt. 2, pp. 371-372 (in Russian).

17. Hananashwili, M. M. Discrimination of acoustic stimuli with different rise-time. *J. Higher Nervous Activity (USSR)* **15**, 788-795 (1965) (in Russian).

18. Jerger, J. Auditory tests for disorder of the central auditory mechanisms. *In* "Neurological Aspects of Auditory and Vestibular Disorders" (W. S. Fields, and B. R. Alford, eds.), pp.77-86. Thomas, Springfield, Illinois, 1964.

19. Karaseva, T. A. Testing of hearing in temporal lobe damage. Dissertation, the Burdenko Neurosurgical Institute, Moscow, 1967 (in Russian).

20. Kimura, D. Some effects of temporal lobe damage on auditory perception. *Can. J. Psychol.* **15**, 156-165 (1961).

21. Kishonas, A. P. Auditory thresholds as a function of sound duration in patients with hearing impairments. *In* "Problems of Physiological Acoustics" (G. V. Gersuni, ed.), Vol. 6: Mechanisms of Hearing, pp. 144-150. Nauka, Leningrad, 1967 (in Russian).

22. Lebedev, A. P. Electronic gate with a low level of disturbances and the possibility of smooth phase control. *J. Higher Nervous Activity (USSR)* **16**, 742-746 (1966) (in Russian).

23. Luria, A. R. Higher cortical functions in man and their disturbances in local brain lesions. Moscow Univ. Press, Moscow, 1962 (in Russian).

24. Matzker, J. Die zerebralen Hörstörungen und ihre Diagnostik. *In* "Studium Generale." Vol. 18, pp. 682-700. Springer, Berlin, 1965.

25. Milner, B. Laterality effects in audition. *In* "Interhemispheric Relations and Cerebral Dominance" (V. B. Mountcastle, ed.), pp. 177-195. Johns Hopkins Press, Baltimore, Maryland, 1962.

26. Miscolczy-Fodor, F. Monoaural loudness-balance-test and determination of recruitment-degree with short sound impulses. *Acta Oto-Laryngol.* **43**, 573-595 (1953).

27. Shankweiler, D. Effects of temporal lobe damage on perception of dichotically presented melodies. *J. Comp. Physiol. Psychol.* **62**, 115-119 (1966).

28. Vardapetian, G. A. Characteristics of single-unit responses in the auditory cortex of cat. *In* "Problems of Physiological Acoustics" (G. V. Gersuni, ed.), Vol. 6: Mechanisms of Hearing, pp. 74-90. Nauka, Leningrad, 1967 (in Russian).

29. Vasserman, L. J. Temporal integration in patients with temporal lobe lesions. *In* "Psychological Experiment in the Psychiatrical and Neurological Clinic" (I. M. Tonkonogii, ed.), pp. 17-34. Medicina, Leningrad, 1968 (in Russian).

30. Zwislocki, J. Theory of temporal summation. *J. Acoust. Soc. Amer.* **32**, 1046-1060 (1960).

17
Synaptic Transformation in the Auditory System of Insects

A. V. Popov

Many insects, especially Orthoptera, are characterized by complex acoustic behavior, including emission, perception, discrimination, and localization of specific sound signals used for communication between animals of the same species [2-5, 11, 12]. Moreover, many insects are highly sensitive to unspecific sounds such as noise or rustle, which provoke their escape reactions. Nonetheless, as evidenced by morphological and electrophysiological data, their auditory system, which is instrumental for all these reactions, consists of a very small number of neurons [6, 10, 13, 14, 23, 24, 31, 35]. It is therefore of great interest to know how such a simply organized system performs discrimination of the species-specific signals against a background of various noises in the environment.

Since the auditory system of insects evolved independently in different orders and even in families, it is natural to suppose that the mechanisms for sound signal analysis may be different in different groups of insects. In this chapter, we attempt to analyze the processes taking place in the receptors and the first synapses in the auditory system of four groups of insects (Acrididae, Tettigoniidae, Gryllidae, and Cicadidae). Some of the data were published earlier [20-27].

Material and Methods

The methods used for registration of electrical activity from tympanal organ receptors and single neurons of the thoracic ganglia, as well as the methods of recording and analyzing insect sounds were described in detail previously [20, 23, 26, 27]. The following insects were used in the experiments: Acrididae– *Locusta migratoria* L., *Calliptamus italicus* L., *Euthystira brachyptera* Ocsk., *Stenobotrus nigromaculatus* H.-Sch., *Celes variabilis* Pall., *Acrida bicolor* Thunb.; Tettigoniidae–*Decticus albifrons* Fabr.; Gryllidae–*Gryllus domesticus* L.; Cicadidae–*Cicada orni* L., *Tibicen plebeja* Scop., *Tibicina intermedia* Fieb., and *Cicadetta montana* Scop.

Results

ORGANIZATION OF THE AUDITORY SYSTEM IN LOCUSTS

Receptors

When a tungsten microelectrode in the form of a hook is introduced beneath the tympanal nerve through the wall of the air sack surrounding the organ, summated electrical potentials, (electrotympanogram - (ETG), produced by the excited tympanal organ receptors, are recorded during the sound delivery (Fig. 1). The ETG has a complex form and consists of three components: (1) initial discharge, consisting of some spikes of high amplitude (up to 2.5 mV) which appear only at the time of sharp rise of sound intensity; (2) asynchronous activity, the duration of which is a function of the sound duration; and (3) aftereffect, which consists either of asynchronous activity of small amplitude occurring after the termination of a sound of high intensity (80 to 90 dB),* or of inhibition of all activity after termination of sounds of intermediate and low intensity (Fig. 1). Detailed analysis of the dynamics of these ETG components during changes of various characteristics of the sound signal (duration, intensity, frequency, and transient and rhythmic pattern) before and after selective destructions of different groups of tympanal organ receptors, which are connected with different parts of the tympanal membrane, permit us to state the following conclusions about the functional organization of the locust tympanal organ.

Receptors connected with the elevated processes and the folded body and lying on the thick and soft part of the membrane, respond to sounds within the range of 500 Hz to 20 kHz. Optimum for their reaction is in the range of 4 to 9 kHz (best frequency, 6 kHz). These are the low-frequency (LF) receptors (Fig. 2). Moreover, Fig. 2 demonstrates a dynamic spectrogram of the warning song of the male and a summated spectrum of the normal song of a male and a warning song of a female of the same species (vertical stripes). It is clear that the

---

* Here and elsewhere intensity is measured in dB SPL *re* 0.0002 dyn/cm^2.

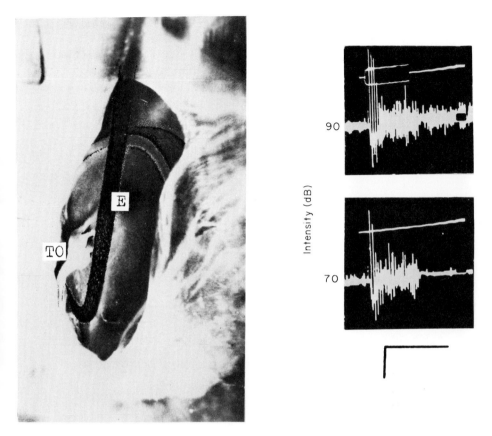

FIG. 1. Position of recording electrode during the registration of a summated electrical response of the tympanal nerve fibers and the response to sounds (6 kHz pure tone) at two intensities (*Locusta migratoria*). Duration of the signals is 60 msec; calibration, 100 msec and 0.5 mV. TO, tympanal organ; E, electrode.

LF receptors are most sensitive to those frequencies which are maximally present in the spectrum of communicative signals.

LF receptors in each group are distributed according to their thresholds. The mean threshold value for receptors, connected with the folded body, is 10 to 15 dB higher than the threshold for receptors, connected with the elevated processes.

The units connected with the elevated processes have a narrow range of latent periods, which makes the first impulses in their response appear nearly synchronously and form the initial component of the ETG. The amplitude,

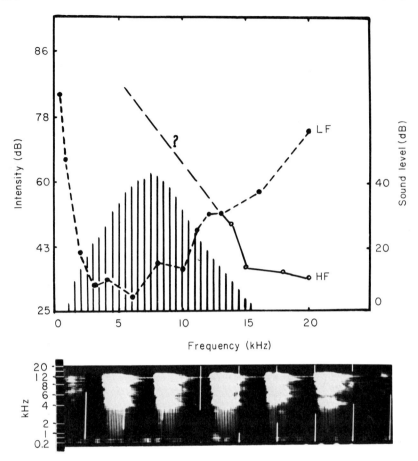

FIG. 2. Threshold-tuning curves for low-frequency (LF) and high-frequency (HF) receptors of the tympanal organ and the spectra of locust sounds (*L. migratoria*). The curves were obtained for sounds of about 120-msec duration. The LF segment of the HF curve is uncertain because it appeared to be impossible to destroy all the receptors except the HF ones. The interval between two vertical lines in the spectrogram is 100 msec. Ordinate on the right side of the graph: sound level of the songs in decibels relative to the 0 sensitivity of the spectrometer. For further explanations, refer to text.

number of spikes, and discharge pattern of this component reflect the depth and frequency of the amplitude modulation of a sound signal.

In addition to the LF receptors, the tympanal organ contains a small group (eight units) of high-frequency (HF) receptors that are connected with the more rigid and thinner part of the membrane. HF receptors are active in the range of frequencies from 4 to 5 kHz to 45 kHz.* The optimal range is about 15 to 20 kHz (Fig. 2, the HF curve).

* The upper limit of the frequency range of HF receptors is taken from the work of Katsuki and Suga [15, 16].

All the receptors of the tympanal organ are characterized by sustained discharges with a very slow adaptation rate. Phasic receptors are absent. In this respect, our data are in accord with those of Suga [32], who studied the response of single units. He also showed that the number of impulses produced by each receptor is proportional to the logarithm of stimulus intensity.

In all locusts studied, the organization of tympanal organs appeared to be similar.

Our findings were recently supported by Michelsen [19], who investigated the activity of single receptors using the microelectrode technique. In an unpublished communication, he stated that he had found a definite difference in the spectral sensitivity among the LF receptors. This is of interest because all the LF receptors are connected to the same locus of the tympanal membrane and hence there is no morphological basis for such diversity of receptors. In addition, Michelsen [19] describes a distinct group of receptors ("e" receptors) with rather long latent periods and a very slow increase of discharge frequency in their response to long sound stimuli. We have never seen any trace of such activity in the ETG. This may be explained by the small number of such units.

Ascending Neurons

Histological analysis, using degeneration technique and methylene blue staining, indicates that the axons of the tympanal organ receptors terminate in a well-defined region of the anterior neuropile of the metathoracic ganglion near the base of the anterior connectives. This region is the site of the first synapse of the auditory pathway in the locust. The impulses generated by the receptors are transferred here to four ascending neurons (two on each side), which send information about the sound to the brain, and to some segmental neurons. The properties of these neurons were described in detail elsewhere [13, 14, 21, 23, 24, 26, 27].

The axons of both ascending neurons on each side pass closely to each other through the whole thoracic nerve cord. This is the reason why their activity is often registered simultaneously by a microelectrode. However, identification of each axon is a simple matter because of great differences in the amplitude of their spikes (L, large and S, small fiber).

When a noise signal is used, and all the receptors are active, the ascending neurons produce sustained discharges in a definite range of intensities (Fig. 3). Since the threshold for the S fiber is 10 to 11 dB lower than the threshold for the L fiber, the activity of the former appears earlier during the step-by-step increase of sound intensity (Fig. 3, oscillograms on the left). The activity of the S fiber rises quickly, reaching the maximum value at a mean intensity of 8 to 9 dB above threshold, which is just about the intensity at which the L fiber becomes active. With further increase of stimulus strength, the activity of

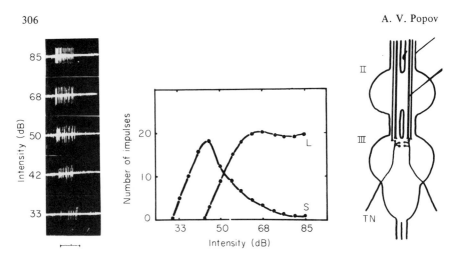

FIG. 3. Response of the L and S ascending fibers of *L. migratoria* to noises of different intensities. Duration, 120 msec; time calibration, 100 msec. Two recording methods used are shown in the scheme on the right. TN, tympanal nerve; II and III; meso- and metathoracic ganglion, respectively.

the S fiber declines slowly (nonmonotonic spike-count function; Fig. 3, S curve). This is accompanied by a transition from a tonic- to a phasic-type reaction. The same behavior is seen when high-frequency pure-tone signals are used (Fig. 4).

The number of impulses in the L fiber increases in proportion to the logarithm of stimulus intensity for 25 to 40 dB above threshold. With a further increase of stimulus strength, a saturation level is reached (monotonic spike-count function, Fig. 3, L curve). The discharges are thus sustained over the whole range of intensities (Fig. 3, oscillograms on the left).

Both neurons also behave in the way just described when high-frequency (above 12 kHz) pure-tone signals are used, and only HF receptors are active. The transition from a sustained to a phasic discharge pattern with an increase of intensity above a certain level (which is characteristic for the S fiber), is observed only in response to sounds longer than 15 to 20 msec. If the stimulus duration is shorter, the S fiber responds in a sustained manner with a long afterdischarge over the whole intensity range (Fig. 5, oscillograms on the left). As the signal duration becomes longer, inhibitory events appear at first only for a narrow range of high intensities and then progressively over a wide intensity range (Fig. 5, graph).

The sustained type of activity in the ascending fibers is characterized by (1) an independence of threshold from the risetime of the signal (transients); (2) a large dispersion of latent period values at thresholds; (3) a long-lasting and considerable summation capacity; and (4) a long afterdischarge in response to short sounds (shorter than 20 to 30 msec).

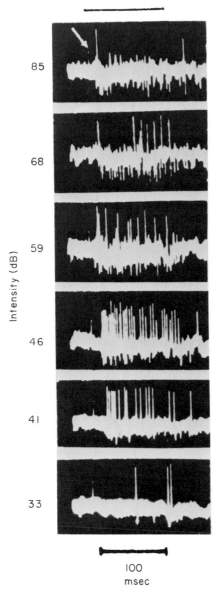

FIG. 4. Discharge patterns of the S fiber to a pure tone of high frequency (20 kHz) at different intensities of the tone. The transition from a sustained discharge pattern at low intensity (46 dB) to a phasic discharge pattern at high intensity (85 dB) is clearly seen. Signal duration, 120 msec. A deflection indicating the onset of the stimulus is marked by an arrow. The horizontal line above the oscillograms indicates the duration of the signal.

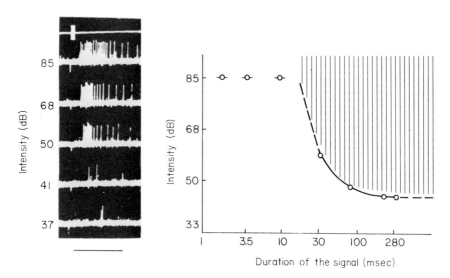

FIG. 5. Properties of the S fiber response to 20-kHz pure tones of different duration (*L. migratoria*). The signal duration for the records shown in the oscillograms is 9 msec. Time calibration, 100 msec. The relation between the threshold for inhibition for the S fiber response and signal duration is shown in the plot. The "inhibitory area" is striped.

Quite different results are obtained when low-frequency sounds are used and thus mainly the LF receptors are active (Fig. 6). Under these conditions, both ascending neurons give a typical phasic response, in which the impulses appear only at the moment of sharp increase in stimulus intensity. The response as such seems independent of sound intensity and thus differs sharply from the response of the tympanal organ receptors (Fig. 6, graphs).

The phasic-type activity of the ascending neurons is characterized, in contrast to the sustained type, by (1) a small dispersion of the latent periods at threshold; (2) a sharp increase in threshold and independence of the latency from the risetime of the stimulus (the shorter the risetime, the lower the threshold); (3) a short-lasting and limited summation capacity; and (4) an absence of a major afterdischarge in response to brief signals.

Thus, the sustained and phasic response types of ascending neurons can be distinguished not only on the basis of their discharge pattern, but also on the basis of other criteria.

The two types of the responses described are the same as those found in the central regions of the auditory system of mammals [7-9, 17, 18, 28-30]. The sustained type of activity of the locust neurons is identical with the "long-time constant regime" of cat neurons, described by Gersuni, and the phasic type of activity is similar to the "short-time constant regime." For both insects and mammals, the classification of the reaction type is based on a number of criteria (pattern of discharge, spike-count function, dependence of latency on intensity of the signal, summation characteristics, etc.).

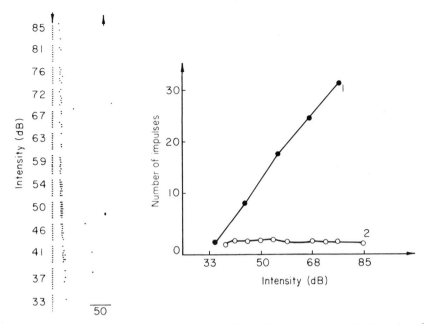

FIG. 6. Dependence of the response of the L fiber of *L. migratoria* on the intensity of a low-frequency signal. Discharge patterns of the neuron are shown at the left. The left-most string of dots in each block of data (identified by a downward-pointed arrow) indicates the beginning of the stimulus. Other dots indicate the time of spike occurrence. The upward-pointed arrow indicates the end of the stimulus. Stimulus, 5 kHz 120 msec in duration; time calibration, 50 msec. Graph at right plots the intensity of the stimulus against the number of spikes in the response. Curve 1 indicates the tympanal organ receptor calculated from the data of Suga [32]; curve 2 shows for the L fiber (mean values for three animals). Both curves pertain to 5-kHz signals 100 msec in duration.

Whereas the same auditory neuron changes its reaction type (polyfunctional neuron) in locusts, in mammals there are, as a rule, different and sharply separated groups of neurons with respective characteristics (short-time constant neurons with phasic or nonmonotonic discharges, and long-time constant neurons with sustained discharges). In addition, there are neurons which also change their activity from a short-time constant to a long-time constant regime with transition from a best frequency stimulus to a nonoptimal frequency, in a way similar to the ascending fibers of locust. The similarity observed may be due to the similarity of neural mechanisms for these two types of reactions in both locusts and mammals.

The phasic type of activity of the ascending fibers is well adapted for gathering information about the pattern of fast amplitude modulation of the sound, by means of which insects "recognize" the songs of their species [11, 12]. By contrast, the sustained type of activity seems poorly adapted for this task, but is well adapted for detection of small and slow changes of the absolute intensity levels, or for detection of slight shifts of the sound source in space. Such information is presumably useful for the insect to react in time to sounds of danger.

Segmental Neurons

Besides the two ascending neurons, at the level of the meso- and metathoracic ganglia, there are at least four segmental neurons on each side, whose fibers do not ascend higher than the mesothoracic ganglion.

One of these segmental neurons receives excitatory inputs from all the tympanal organ receptors of both sides, and hence responds with uniform sustained discharges to sounds of any frequency; this is perceived by the tympanal organ. Its spike-count function is monotonic in the range of 40 to 60 dB, just as is the case for the response of the receptors ("repeater neuron").

Another neuron differs from the first in that it does not react at all to pure tones and responds only to noise signals of sufficient duration (longer than 5 to 10 msec) when both LF and HF receptors of the tympanal organ are stimulated simultaneously ("noise-detector" neuron).

The third neuron responds to both tonal and noise signals but has only one optimum of sensitivity in the range of 4 to 6 kHz. This presumably means that it is connected to LF receptors of the tympanal organ ("low-frequency-detector" neuron). The neuron is characterized by a long afterdischarge (nearly 300 msec). The impulses occur at long intervals and the discharge train is independent of signal duration.

The response of the fourth neuron is similar to that of the L fiber but differs from the latter by a much lower discharge frequency and a higher threshold.

The responses of the segmental neurons were found both in the medial region ("repeater neuron") and dorsal region (other neurons) of the neuropile. Therefore, one can consider them to be either associative neurons or motoneurons participating in the formation of the segmental phonokinetic reactions [24, 26].

It can thus be concluded that at the level of the first synapses of the auditory pathway in the locust, information about the separate properties of the signal is selected from the entire afferent inflow, which is provided by the tympanal organ receptors. The information is then transferred in different channels to different parts of the central nervous system. Some of this information is conducted to the brain for subsequent processing (ascending neurons) and other data is utilized by the thoracic centers for the formation of segmental reactions, so that the output to the effectors is already provided at the level of the first synapse of the auditory pathway.

ORGANIZATION OF THE AUDITORY SYSTEM IN GRASSHOPPERS

Little is known about the auditory system of grasshoppers. Katsuki and

Suga [15, 16] found that the tympanal organ of these insects contains, as in locusts, two groups of receptors which differ in their spectral sensitivity. In Gampsocleis the LF receptors are sensitive to sounds in the frequency range from 0.6 to 30 kHz (with the best frequency of 6 to 7 kHz). The HF receptors are most sensitive to about 10 kHz, and they respond within the range from 3 to 60 kHz. The whole organ is thus capable of responding to frequencies from 0.6 to 60 kHz (optimum 6 to 10 kHz). Similar data concerning the frequency range for the tympanal organ were also obtained for other species of grasshoppers [33, 34].

In *Decticus albifrons*, studied in our laboratory, the tympanal organ appeared to be most sensitive to sounds of 18 to 21 kHz. The threshold for the leg nerve response to this optimal frequency is 25 to 26 dB. The threshold-frequency curve for this response has a small "hump" near 8 to 10 kHz and a well-defined optimum in the range of 18 to 20 kHz (Fig. 7, solid curve). It is possible that in this species as well the tympanal organ contains two types of receptors—one with a best frequency of about 8 to 10 kHz, and the other with a best frequency of about 18 to 20 kHz.

According to Katsuki and Suga (and our data confirm these observations) all the tympanal organ receptors of grasshoppers studied discharge in a sustained manner. The supposition of Autrum [1] that this organ contains receptors both phasic (producing only an initial discharge in the nerve) and tonic (producing an asynchronous activity) still lacks experimental support.

The axons of the tympanal organ receptors of one side connect with one gigantic fiber (T fiber) at the level of the first thoracic ganglion [33-35]. One branch of this fiber descends to the third thoracic ganglion and another ascends up to the brain. In addition to the connection with the T fiber on the same side, the sensory fibers connect with an interneuron, which inhibits the activity of the contralateral T fiber [36]. As a result, the discharge patterns of the two T fibers are different, depending on the location of the sound source.

In *Decticus albifrons* we also found only one ascending neuron on each side of the first thoracic ganglion. This neuron is most sensitive to frequencies of about 18 to 21 kHz (Fig. 7, broken line) which implies that the neuron is connected mainly to HF receptors of the tympanal organ (the findings are similar to those in other grasshoppers). It is characteristic for the response that a sustained discharge pattern of the ascending fiber is observed only for a narrow range of best frequencies. For lower frequencies the discharge train becomes shorter and impulses appear mainly at the onset of the signal for most stimulus intensities (Fig. 7). The interaction of the left and the right fibers in *Decticus albifrons* is similar to that in the Japanese species.

We conclude that the main transformations, taking place in the first auditory center of grasshoppers, are directed toward extraction of information concerning the location of the sound source.

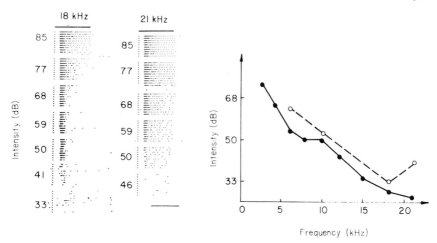

FIG. 7. Characteristics of the tympanal nerve response and of the ascending neuron response of *Decticus albifrons*. The signal duration of 120 msec is indicated by the length of a black line above each column of records. Time calibration, 100 msec. Threshold-tuning curves were obtained for signals 120 msec in duration.

ORGANIZATION OF THE AUDITORY SYSTEM IN CRICKETS

The tympanal organ of the cricket, *Gryllus domesticus*, contains at least two types of receptors. One of them is most sensitive to sounds of 4 to 5 kHz (the main energy content in calling songs of crickets is within the range of these frequencies). The second type is most sensitive in the range of 10 to 15 kHz (Fig. 8; see also Popov [26]). In the tympanal organ in crickets, similar data concerning the presence of receptors with different spectral sensitivity were obtained by Horridge [13]. As is the case for locusts and grasshoppers, the tympanal organ receptors of crickets are characterized by tonic responses and are able to synchronize the first impulses of the response with the time of sharp increase of stimulus intensity.

At the level of the first thoracic ganglion, the tympanal organ receptors connect with two ascending neurons on each side. One of them is connected with LF receptors; the second with HF receptors (Fig. 9). The LF neuron is spontaneously active. Its spontaneous impulses appear in bursts of two or three and are inhibited during the activity of the HF neuron. In analogy to the receptors, both ascending neurons are characterized by a sustained discharge pattern over the whole range of intensities. Response of the LF ascending neuron to a pure tone of 4 kHz is shown in Fig. 10. At a high-intensity level (85 dB) there is a marked afterdischarge. As the intensity is decreased, the afterdischarge is abolished, and inhibition of spontaneous activity occurs for some time after the stimulus ceases. Similar properties

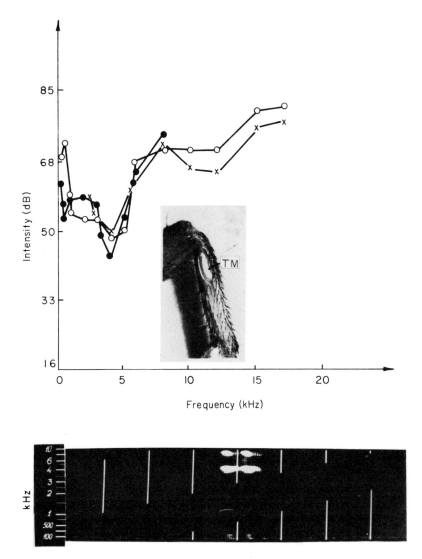

FIG. 8. Threshold-tuning curves for the tympanal nerve response and spectrum of the calling song of a male *Gryllus domesticus.* Curves for three animals are shown. Two humps on the curves can be seen. One corresponds to the optimal range of LF receptors; the second to the range of HF receptors. TM, tympanal membrane. The interval between two vertical lines in the spectrogram is 100 msec.

(afterdischarge or inhibition occurring with cessation of the stimulus) are characteristic for the tympanal organ receptors of locusts [20, 26]. The adaptation of the discharges in the ascending neurons is very slow.

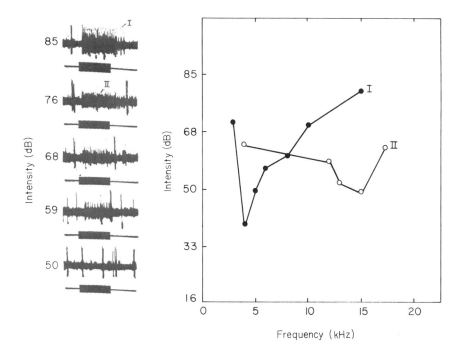

FIG. 9. Characteristics of the ascending auditory neurons of *Gryllus domesticus.* Recordings from the anterior part of the 1st thoracic ganglion by a microelectrode. Signal duration in the oscillograms, 120 msec; frequency, 15 kHz. Curves I and II indicate threshold-tuning curves for the LF and HF ascending neurons, respectively.

It appears that the ascending neurons of crickets repeat the pattern of the receptor response (sustained discharges in both cases), thus introducing no significant changes in the character of the information inflow. From this point of view, the auditory system of crickets is more primitive than that of locust.

THE AUDITORY SYSTEM OF CICADAS

The life of imago is very short in most singing cicadas (ordinarily a few days). During this time, the males and the females must find each other, and in this search the sound communication plays the main role. While it is very important for orthopterans, which live for a relatively long time, to perceive not only the sounds of their own species, but many other sounds in their

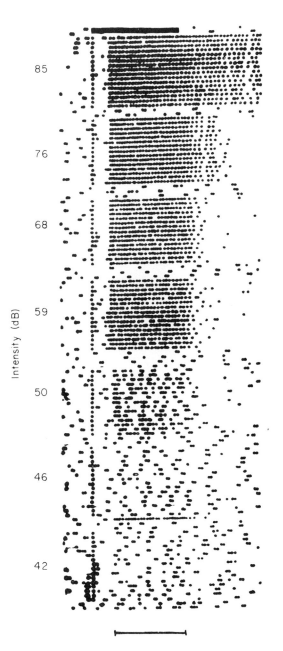

FIG. 10. Discharge patterns for the LF ascending neuron of *Gryllus domesticus.*
Microelectrode recordings from the 1st thoracic ganglion. Duration of the signal is
indicated by the length of a black line above the records. Time calibration, 100 msec.

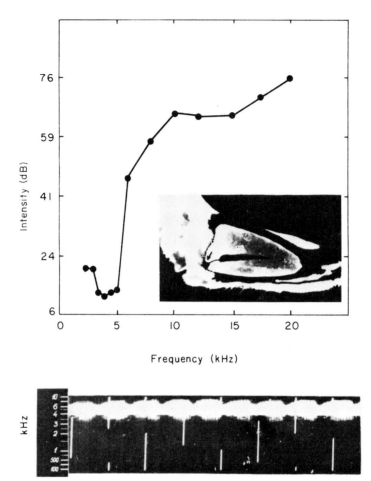

FIG. 11. Threshold-tuning curve for the tympanal nerve response of a female, and spectrum of the calling song of a male of *Tibicen plebeja*. Signal duration, 250 msec. Position of the tympanal organ receptors is marked by an arrow in the picture. The interval between two vertical lines in the spectrogram is 100 msec.

environment in order to secure their safety, the main task for cicadas is the perception of species-specific signals. The organization of the auditory system of the cicadas apparently reflects this demand since the main feature is a very sharp "tuning" of their tympanal organ receptors to frequencies, which are maximally present in the spectra of their calling songs (Fig. 11). All the tympanal organ receptors are tuned to the same range of frequencies, since they are connected with the same locus of the tympanal membrane. A large number of receptors (nearly 1500—see [37]) is evidently necessary in order to produce a powerful flow of the afferent impulses to activate the central ganglia. Similar to the receptors of orthopterans, the tympanal organ receptors of cicadas are able to synchronize the first impulses of their responses, as a result of which there appears a phasic component in the response. The amplitude of this component is proportional to the risetime of stimulus intensity. For rhythmic signals such as the songs of cicadas, the time pattern of these components follows the amplitude modulation pattern of the song.

The central transformations in the auditory system of cicadas are still unknown. One can suppose that there must be neurons in the central ganglia of females, which are selectively sensitive to the rhythmic structure of the calling song of the male.

Discussion

The data presented imply that the peripheral part of the auditory system of all Orthoptera in this study is constructed according to a similar plan. The tympanal organ possesses two groups of receptors differing in their spectral sensitivity and is thus sensitive to sounds in a wide range of frequencies. The spectrum of communicative sounds of these insects is much narrower than the range sensed by the tympanal organ, since only one group of receptors is tuned to frequencies that are maximally present in the song spectrum. Therefore, these insects can react not only to communicative sounds of their own species, but to various other sounds in their surroundings, particularly to sounds indicating danger. This capacity is absent in the auditory system of cicadas, whose imago life is short.

In the tympanal organ of all the insects studied those receptors which are tuned to communicative sounds are capable of synchronized activity and can thus transfer information about the amplitude modulation pattern of the song. Apparently this mechanism is used by insects in recognition of species-specific songs.

Although the principles of information coding by the tympanal organ receptors seem similar in different groups of insects, the principles for processing of this information in the first synapses of the auditory pathway are very different in the various groups. The organization of the first synapse in crickets seems most primitive since each of the two groups of receptors connects only with its own ascending neuron, which repeats the pattern of the receptor discharges. No inhibitory interactions are seen at this level [Fig. 12(a)]. In grasshoppers, there is only one ascending neuron on each side. It appears that the ascending neuron, connected with LF receptors, has been eliminated. Nonetheless, the first synapse is complex since two inhibitory interneurons are present. Each of them is excited by HF receptors of the ipsilateral side, and each inhibits the activity of the ascending neuron of the contralateral side. This interaction makes possible the extraction of information about the location of the sound source [Fig. 12(b)].

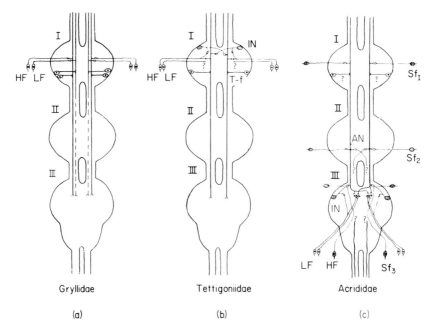

FIG. 12. Central connections at the first level of the auditory pathway in Gryllidae (a), Tettigoniidae (b), and Acrididae (c), as suggested by the electrophysiological experiments. LF and HF represent low- and high-frequency receptors of the tympanal organ; IN, inhibitory interneuron; T-f, T fiber; Sf_1, Sf_2, and Sf_3 are the sensory fibers of the different segmental mechanoreceptors, producing an inhibitory input for the auditory ascending neurons.

The most complex is the organization of the first synapse in locusts. A complex system of inhibitory interneurons appears to be present, and these interneurons can change activity patterns in the ascending neurons. In the scheme in Fig. 12(c), for the sake of clarity, the connections of only one ascending neuron (neuron S) are shown. The excitatory synapses are indicated by dots, the inhibitory ones by circles. Each ascending neuron is excited by tympanal organ receptors of both sides. Moreover, the LF receptors excite inhibitory interneurons, which in turn inhibit the ascending neuron by transforming its activity from a sustained to phasic type of discharge. The same neuron is further subjected to inhibitory influences caused by mechanoreceptors of the abdomen and the thorax at the level of the third, second, and evidently first thoracic ganglion, and thus its response to low frequencies is limited [38]. This inhibitory activity is produced not by the receptors themselves (as is shown in the scheme) but by interneurons that as yet have not been identified. At the level of the second thoracic ganglion, the S neuron receives inhibitory input from a unit (also unidentified as yet), which is selectively excited by HF tympanal organ receptors. The axon of this unit passes through contralateral meta- and mesothoracic connectives. Under the influence of this unit the activity of the S neuron changes from sustained to phasic, when high-frequency sounds of high intensity are presented. The scheme is constructed on the basis of data published elsewhere [24, 26].

Thus, it can be concluded that the auditory system of each of the investigated groups of insects is specialized in some way, and this specialization is expressed in the number of central units and in the organization of their connections in the thoracic center of the auditory system. The kind of this specialization depends upon the species and the acoustic environment, which is different for each group.

REFERENCES

1. Autrum, H. Phasische und tonische Antworten vom Tympanalorgan von *Tettigonia viridissima. Acustica* **10**, 339-348 (1960).
2. Busnel, R. G. On certain aspects of animal acoustic signals. *In* "Acoustic Behaviour of Animals" (R. G. Busnel, ed.), pp. 69-111. Elsevier, Amsterdam, 1963.
3. Dumortier, B. Morphology of sound emission apparatus in Arthropoda. *In* "Acoustic Behaviour of Animals" (R. G. Busnel, ed.), pp. 277-345. Elsevier, Amsterdam, 1963.
4. Dumortier, B. The physical characteristics of sound emissions in Arthropoda. *In* "Acoustic Behaviour of Animals" (R. G. Busnel, ed.), pp. 346-371. Elsevier, Amsterdam, 1963.
5. Dumortier, B. Ethological and physiological study of sound emissions in Arthropoda. *In* "Acoustic Behaviour of Animals" (R. G. Busnel, ed.), pp. 583-654. Elsevier, Amsterdam, 1963.
6. Eggers, F. Die stiftfürenden Sinnesorgane. *Zool. Bausteine.* **2**, 1-353 (1928).
7. Gersuni, G. V. On the mechanisms of hearing (in connection with studies of time and time-frequency characteristics of the auditory system). *In* "Problems of Physiological Acoustics" (G. V. Gersuni, ed.), Vol. 6: Mechanisms of Hearing, pp. 3-32. Nauka, Leningrad, 1967 (in Russian).
8. Gersuni, G. V. This volume, Chap. 6.
9. Gersuni, G. V., Altman, J. A., Maruseva, A. M., Radionova, E. A., Ratnikova, G. I., and Vartanian, I. A. This volume, Chap. 16.
10. Gray, E. D. The fine structure of the insect ear. *Phil. Trans. Roy. Soc. (London) Ser.* **B243**, 74-94 (1960).
11. Haskell, P. T. "Insect Sounds," p. 189. Witherby, Chicago, 1961.
12. Haskell, P. T. Sound production. *In* "The Physiology of Insecta" (M. Rockstein, ed.), Vol. I, pp. 563-608. Academic Press, New York, 1964.
13. Horridge, G. A. Pitch discrimination in Orthoptera (Insecta) demonstrated by responses of central auditory neurons. *Nature (London)* **185**, 623-624 (1960).
14. Horridge, G. A. Pitch discrimination in locusts. *Proc. Roy. Soc. (London) Ser.* **B155**, 218-231 (1961).
15. Katsuki, Y., and Suga, N. Electrophysiological studies on hearing in common insects in Japan. *Proc. Jap. Acad.* **34**, 633-638 (1958).
16. Katsuki, Y., and Suga, N. Neural mechanism of hearing in insects. *J. Exp. Biol.* **37**, 279-290 (1960).
17. Maruseva, A. M. On the time characteristics of neurons of different types in the inferior colliculus of the rat. *In* "Problems of Physiological Acoustics" (G. V.

Gersuni, ed.), Vol. 6: Mechanisms of Hearing, pp. 50-61. Nauka, Leningrad, 1967 (in Russian).

18. Maruseva, A. M. This volume, Chap. 11.
19. Michelsen, A. Pitch discrimination in the locust ear: observations on single sense cells. *J. Insect Physiol.* **12**, 1119-1131 (1966).
20. Popov, A. V. Electrophysiological studies of peripheral auditory neurons in the locust. *J. Evol. Biochem. Physiol.* **1**, 239-250 (1965) (in Russian).
21. Popov, A. V. The functional organization of the central part of the locust hearing system (Acrididae, Orthoptera). *Proc. 18th Int. Congr. Psychol. Moscow, Symp., 1966.* Vol. 15, pp. 177-187.
22. Popov, A. V. The structure and function of receptors in the auditory organ of insects. *In* "The Primary Processes in Receptor Elements of Sense Organs" (V. G. Samsonova, ed.), pp. 144-154. Nauka, Leningrad, 1966 (in Russian).
23. Popov, A. V. Synaptic transmission at the level of the first synapses of the auditory system in *Locusta migratoria. In* "Evolutionary Neurophysiology and Neurochemistry" (E. M. Kreps, ed.), pp. 54-67. Nauka, Leningrad, 1967 (in Russian).
24. Popov, A. V. Characteristics of activity of the central neurons in the auditory system of the locust. *In* "Problems of Physiological Acoustics" (G. V. Gersuni, ed.), Vol. 6: Mechanisms of Hearing, pp. 108-121. Nauka, Leningrad, 1967 (in Russian).
25. Popov, A. V. Principles of structural and functional organization of the first levels in the tympanal auditory system of different insects. *Proc. 6th Acoust. Conf., Moscow, 1968.* Sect. и. I-2, pp. 4-8 (in Russian).
26. Popov, A. V. Electrophysiological study of the functional properties of peripheral and central neurons in the auditory system of locust. pp. 1-231. Dissertation, Leningrad, 1967 (in Russian).
27. Popov, A. V. Comparative analysis of sound signals and some principles of auditory system organization in cicadas and Orthoptera. *In* "Modern Problems of Structure and Function of the Nervous System of Insects" (A. K. Voskresenskaja, ed.), pp. 182-221. Nauka, Leningrad, 1969 (in Russian).
28. Radionova, E. A. On the significance of time characteristics of the cochlear nucleus neurons. *In* "Problems of Physiological Acoustics" (G. V. Gersuni, ed.), Vol. 6: Mechanisms of Hearing, pp. 32-49. Nauka, Leningrad, 1967 (in Russian).
29. Radionova, E. A. This volume, Chap. 9.
30. Rose, J. E., Greenwood, D. D., Goldberg, J. M., and Hind, J. E. Some discharge characteristics of single neurons in the inferior colliculus of the cat. I. Tonotopical organization, relation of spike-counts to tone intensity, and firing patterns of single elements. *J. Neurophysiol.* **26**, 294-341 (1963).
31. Schwabe, J. Beiträge zur Morphologie und Histologie der Tympanalen Sinnesorgane der Orthopteren. *Zoologica (Stuttgart)* **50**, 1-154 (1906).
32. Suga, N. Peripheral mechanism of hearing in locust. *Jap. J. Physiol.* **10**, 533-546 (1960).
33. Suga, N. Central mechanism of hearing and sound localization in insects. *J. Insect Physiol.* **9**, 867-873 (1963).
34. Suga, N. Ultrasonic production and its reception in some neotropical tettigoniidae. *J. Insect Physiol.* **12**, 1039-1050 (1966).
35. Suga, N., and Katsuki, Y. Central mechanism of hearing in insects. *J. Exp. Biol.* **38**, 545-558 (1961).
36. Suga, N., and Katsuki, Y. Pharmacological studies on the auditory synapses in a grasshopper. *J. Exp. Biol.* **38**, 759-770 (1961).
37. Vogel, R. Über des Gehörorgan der Singzikaden. *Naturwissenschaften* **9**, 27-34 (1921).
38. Yanagisawa, K., Hashimoto, T., and Katsuki, Y. Frequency discrimination in the central nerve cords of locusts. *J. Insect Physiol.* **13**, 635-648 (1967).

AUTHOR INDEX

Numbers in parentheses are reference numbers and indicate that an author's work is referred to although his name is not cited in the text. Numbers in italics show the page on which the complete reference is listed.